Imaging and Intervention in Urinary Tract Infections and Urosepsis

Massimo Tonolini
Editor

Imaging and Intervention in Urinary Tract Infections and Urosepsis

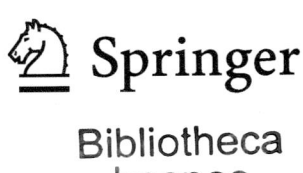

Springer

Bibliotheca
hospes

Editor
Massimo Tonolini
Department of Radiology
Luigi Sacco Hospital
Milan, Italy

ISBN 978-3-319-88574-2   ISBN 978-3-319-68276-1   (eBook)
https://doi.org/10.1007/978-3-319-68276-1

This Springer imprint is published by Springer Nature
The registered company is Springer International Publishing AG
The registered company address is: Gewerbestrasse 11, 6330 Cham, Switzerland

Contents

Part I

Clinicians' Current Perspectives on Urinary Tract Infections

Introduction

Massimo Tonolini

Arguably representing one of the most prevailing infectious illnesses worldwide, urinary tract infections (UTIs) are generally considered trivial by most physicians, since the majority of cases encountered in the general population are uncomplicated occurrences in otherwise healthy young women. However, UTIs account for hundreds of thousands of outpatient visits and emergency and hospital admissions yearly, resulting in a significant clinical and economic burden [1–3].

Indeed, UTIs encompass a heterogeneous spectrum of conditions ranging from asymptomatic bacteriuria to mild uncomplicated cystitis, potentially severe pyelonephritis and life-threatening sepsis. Clinical manifestations of UTIs may be limited or overlap with pre-existing complaints from chronic urinary tract dysfunction. According to the European Association of Urology (EAU) guidelines, severity of UTIs should be graded clinically as:

(a) Asymptomatic
(b) Causing local symptoms such as dysuria, urinary frequency, urgency, supra- or retropubic pain or bladder tenderness
(c) Causing general symptoms including fever, flank pain, nausea and vomiting

(d) Systemic inflammatory response syndrome with fever or hypothermia, hyperleucocytosis or leucopenia, tachycardia and tachypnoea
(e) Circulatory and organ failure [2]

Furthermore, UTIs represent the commonest (almost 40%) form of hospital-acquired infections, with bladder catheterisation as the key risk factor. The EAU guidelines define complicated UTIs (C-UTIs) as those associated with structural or functional abnormalities of the genitourinary tract, or with the presence of an underlying disease that interferes with host defence mechanisms, that result in an increased risk of acquiring infection or failing therapy. The commonest conditions predisposing patients to either acquiring infection or experiencing a more severe outcome are categorized with the mnemonic RENUC and summarized in Table 1.1 [2].

Traditionally, the vast majority of ascending UTIs were considered uncomplicated and did not routinely require imaging investigation, particularly in women of childbearing age. During my years as a resident in diagnostic imaging at the San Paolo Hospital in Milan (Italy) in the late 1990s, radiologists were only occasionally requested to investigate patients with suspected UTIs, in the vast majority of cases to exclude urinary obstruction with ultrasound and occasionally to study sequelae after acute pyelonephritis (APN) with intravenous pyelography. In fact, until a few years ago, the diagnosis of UTI was

M. Tonolini
Radiology Department, "Luigi Sacco" University Hospital, Via G.B. Grassi 74, Milan 20157, Italy
e-mail: mtonolini@sirm.org

© Springer International Publishing AG 2018
M. Tonolini (ed.), *Imaging and Intervention in Urinary Tract Infections and Urosepsis*,
https://doi.org/10.1007/978-3-319-68276-1_1

Table 1.1 Risk factors for acquiring urinary tract infection, developing complications and/or failing treatment (mnemonic RENUC) (Reproduced from Open Access Ref. no.[17], partially adapted from Ref.no. [2])

Type	Risk factors	Risk of more severe outcome
*R*ecurrent	Sexual behaviour	No
	Contraceptive devices	
	Postmenopausal hormonal deficiency	
	Controlled diabetes mellitus	
*E*xtra-urogenital	Pregnancy	Yes
	Male gender	
	Badly controlled diabetes	
	Immunosuppression including HIV, uraemia, transplant recipients, on corticosteroids, chemotherapy or immunosuppressants	
	Connective tissue disease	
*N*ephropathy	Impaired renal function	Yes
	Polycystic kidney	
*U*rological	Obstructive uropathy, e.g. congenital, lithiasis, stricture, tumour	Yes
	Short-term catheterisation	
	Neurogenic bladder	
	Urological surgery or instrumentation	
Permanent *c*atheter or non-resolvable urological risk factors	Long-term catheter	Yes
	Non-resolvable obstruction	
	Badly controlled neurogenic bladder	

primarily clinical and based upon a combination of clinical symptoms and signs plus consistent urinalysis and biochemical changes. At those days, imaging was reserved for:

(a) Patients with unusually severe symptoms, in which differentiation from renal colic or other acute abdominal disorders was required
(b) Patients with recurrent UTIs, to look for underlying treatable structural or functional abnormalities
(c) Patients with predisposing conditions to C-UTIs such as diabetes, immunosuppression, etc.
(d) Patients who failed to respond to conventional antibiotic therapy within 72 h [4–6]

Meanwhile, during the last decade, the scenario of UTI has changed, as discussed in the first section of this book which includes current clinical perspectives from prominent urologists, nephrologists and specialists in infectious diseases. In these chapters emphasis is placed on high-risk popula-

tions and on the increasingly concerning issue of bacterial resistance to antibiotics.

Furthermore, growing evidence has accumulated on the potential detrimental effect of UTI on renal function, which results from a combination of direct cellular injury and indirect effects of inflammatory mediators. In patients with preexisting normal renal anatomy and function, renal scarring has been reported to develop in up to 55% of patients after APN. Patients with chronic kidney disease or diabetes are particularly prone to progression of renal infection and deterioration of function, with the latter becoming permanent in the majority (77%) of cases [2, 7].

A highly prevalent disease, APN, reaches an annual incidence of 250,000 cases and yearly accounts for over 100,000 hospitalizations in the USA, with a non-negligible mean duration (11 days). However, there is no consensus on the definition of APN, which – until a few years ago – was almost invariably diagnosed clinically on the basis of fever, flank pain and tenderness, signs and symptoms of lower UTI, accompanied by leucocytosis, increased acute phase reactants, haematuria, bacteriuria and positive urine culture [2].

However, several recent studies-particularly those by G.B. Piccoli and C. Rollino-reported that APN presents with full-blown features in only a minority of patients. The correlation between clinical presentation, entity of abnormal biochemistry (C-reactive protein and leukocyte count) and extent of renal lesion in APN is often very limited: oligosymptomatic manifestations may correspond to multifocal lesion or abscesses, which require hospitalization and long-term therapy, and are associated with higher risk of developing renal scarring. Furthermore urine, blood cultures and both are positive only in 23.5–40%, 15.8–30% and 7.6% of cases, respectively, mostly because of previous empirical antibiotic therapies administered in the outpatient setting [8–10]. Conversely, a few other studies showed that some early available clinical predictors, namely, diabetes, hypotension, high leucocytosis and acute renal failure, may identify almost all patients with moderate (except for some cases of microabscesses) and severe APN [11].

Since choosing the most appropriate treatment relies on severity assessment, nowadays there is a growing need for "pathological" diagnosis of APN by radiological demonstration of parenchymal involvement; this is particularly true for abscessual forms, which require longer intensive in-hospital intravenous antibiotic therapy and are associated with higher risk of developing renal scars [2].

Meanwhile, state-of-the-art multidetector computed tomography (CT) and magnetic resonance imaging (MRI) reached extremely high accuracy in delineating the nature and extent of APN changes and consistently depict complications such as abscess and obstruction. Emergency physicians increasingly request early imaging of suspected APN, which is preferably carried out with MRI particularly in young patients and childbearing age women. Therefore, the following ample radiological section of this book reviews the role, techniques and imaging appearances of upper UTIs using ultrasound and contrast-enhanced ultrasound (CEUS), multidetector CT and MRI to assess severity and thus provide

a consistent basis for correct therapeutic choice. Emphasis is placed on the increasingly implemented diffusion-weighted (DW)-MRI sequences and apparent diffusion coefficient (ADC) maps to differentiate between spared parenchyma, nephritis and abscesses, particularly in children and patients with contraindication to intravenous contrast [12–16].

The third section of this volume reviews the imaging appearances of UTIs involving the prostate, seminal vesicles, urethra, perineum, penis and scrotum. Despite improved standards of care, "lower" UTIs are increasingly observed in patients with risk factors such as neurogenic dysfunction, bladder outlet obstruction, obstructive uropathy, urologic instrumentation or indwelling stent, urinary tract postsurgical modifications, chemotherapy or irradiation, renal dysfunction, diabetes and immunodeficiency [3]. With adequate technique and awareness of consistent findings, CT and MRI comprehensively assess the lower genitourinary structures and disorders and increasingly provide accurate detection of presence and extent of infectious changes, of possible complications, and assist in the differential diagnosis [17].

Furthermore, in our experience imaging signs of clinically unsuspected C-UTI may be incidentally detected in imaging studies performed to investigate other conditions such as urolithiasis, renal colic, gynaecologic pain or unspecific abdominal pain [17]. Cross-sectional imaging is paramount in the triage of sepsis, to confirm an underlying urological cause: albeit less severe compared to other sources, urosepsis remains associated with 20–40% mortality [2, 7].

Other dedicated chapters, respectively, review:

– The role of nuclear medicine (specifically with positron emission tomography) in the detection and follow-up of infections in polycystic kidneys
– The imaging of urogenital tuberculosis in the current CT era
– The imaging of UTI in patients with renal transplant
– The expanding role and possibilities of interventional radiology in the treatment of severe

urinary tract infections including drainage of infected urine and percutaneous treatment of abscesses collections

Finally, a specific chapter summarizes the current status of paediatric UTI imaging including anatomic, functional and reflux studies, borrowing from experience at hospitals especially devoted to children care.

As Editor, I hope that the effort made by all contributors will be effective in producing an up-to-date volume which will prove useful to practicing clinicians and radiologists who are daily confronted with potentially severe UTIs. Our aim is to increase familiarity with these disorders which frequently require in-hospital management, sometimes including intensive care admission, percutaneous interventions or even surgery, in order to decrease the associated morbidity.

References

1. Cardwell SM, Crandon JL, Nicolau DP et al (1995) Epidemiology and economics of adult patients hospitalized with urinary tract infections. Hosp Pract 44:33–40
2. Grabe M, Bartoletti R, Bjerklund-Johansen TE et al (2014) Guidelines on urological infections. European Association of Urology Available at: http://uroweb. org/wp-content/uploads/19-Urological-infections_ LR2.pdf
3. Roghmann F, Ghani KR, Kowalczyk KJ et al (2013) Incidence and treatment patterns in males presenting with lower urinary tract symptoms to the emergency department in the United States. J Urol 190:1798–1804
4. Browne RF, Zwirewich C, Torreggiani WC (2004) Imaging of urinary tract infection in the adult. Eur Radiol 14(Suppl 3):E168–E183
5. Stunell H, Buckley O, Feeney J et al (2007) Imaging of acute pyelonephritis in the adult. Eur Radiol 17:1820–1828
6. Craig WD, Wagner BJ, Travis MD (2008) Pyelonephritis: radiologic-pathologic review. Radiographics 28:255–277. quiz 327-258
7. Sorensen SM, Schonheyder HC, Nielsen H (2013) The role of imaging of the urinary tract in patients with urosepsis. Int J Infect Dis 17:e299–e303
8. Rollino C, Beltrame G, Ferro M et al (2012) Acute pyelonephritis in adults: a case series of 223 patients. Nephrol Dial Transplant 27:3488–3493
9. Abraham G, Reddy YN, George G (2012) Diagnosis of acute pyelonephritis with recent trends in management. Nephrol Dial Transplant 27:3391–3394
10. Piccoli GB, Consiglio V, Deagostini MC et al (2011) The clinical and imaging presentation of acute "non complicated" pyelonephritis: a new profile for an ancient disease. BMC Nephrol 12:68
11. Lim SK, Ng FC (2011) Acute pyelonephritis and renal abscesses in adults - correlating clinical parameters with radiological (computer tomography) severity. Ann Acad Med Singap 40:407–413
12. Martina MC, Campanino PP, Caraffo F et al (2010) Dynamic magnetic resonance imaging in acute pyelonephritis. Radiol Med 115:287–300
13. De Pascale A, Piccoli GB, Priola SM et al (2013) Diffusion-weighted magnetic resonance imaging: new perspectives in the diagnostic pathway of non-complicated acute pyelonephritis. Eur Radiol 23:3077–3086
14. Faletti R, Cassinis MC, Fonio P et al (2013) Diffusion-weighted imaging and apparent diffusion coefficient values versus contrast-enhanced MR imaging in the identification and characterisation of acute pyelonephritis. Eur Radiol 23:3501–3508
15. Vivier PH, Sallem A, Beurdeley M et al (2014) MRI and suspected acute pyelonephritis in children: comparison of diffusion-weighted imaging with gadolinium-enhanced T1-weighted imaging. Eur Radiol 24:19–25
16. Rathod SB, Kumbhar SS, Nanivadekar A et al (2015) Role of diffusion-weighted MRI in acute pyelonephritis: a prospective study. Acta Radiol 56:244–249
17. Tonolini M, Ippolito S (2016) Cross-sectional imaging of complicated urinary infections affecting the lower tract and male genital organs. Insights Imaging 7(5):689–711

Introduction to Urinary Tract Infections: An Overview on Epidemiology, Risk Factors, Microbiology and Treatment Options

Maria Diletta Pezzani and Spinello Antinori

2.1 Definitions

Urinary tract infections (UTIs) encompass a wide range of clinical conditions which can be asymptomatic or symptomatic. Based on the site of the infection, UTIs can be classified in:

- *Lower UTIs*: bacteriuria (urine), urethritis (urethra), cystitis (the urinary bladder).
- *Upper UTIs*: pyelonephritis (kidney).

According to the clinical presentation UTIs are divided in:

- *Uncomplicated*: whether they occur in a normal genitourinary tract with no prior instrumentation or comorbidities.
- *Complicated*: if they occur in presence of functional or structural abnormalities including instrumentation such as indwelling urethral catheters and significant medical or surgical comorbidities. This distinction has an important impact into clinical practice as complicated UTIs have major risk of worse outcome than expected from UTIs in people without identified risk factors.

Asymptomatic bacteriuria (ABU) is defined by a midstream sample of urine showing bacterial growth >10^5 colony forming units (CFU)/mL in two consecutive samples in women and in one single sample in men, in an individual without symptoms from the urinary tract. In a single catheterized sample, bacterial growth may be as low as 10^2 CFU/mL to be considered representing true bacteriuria in both men and women [1]. Guidelines of the Infectious Diseases Society of America (IDSA) defines catheter-associated bacteriuria as the presence of $\geq 10^5$ CFU/mL of ≥ 1 bacterial species in a single catheter urine specimen in a patient without symptoms compatible with UTIs. Catheter-associated UTIs (CA-UTIs) by contrastare defined by the presence of symptoms or signs compatible with UTIs with no other identified source of infection along with $\geq 10^3$ CFU/mL of ≥ 1 bacterial species in a single catheter urine specimen or in a midstream voided urine specimen from a patient whose urethral, suprapubic or condom catheter has been removed within the previous 48 h [2].

M.D. Pezzani (✉)
III Division of Infectious Diseases, Luigi Sacco Hospital, ASST Fatebenefratelli Sacco, Via GB Grassi 74, Milan, Italy
e-mail: diletta.pezzani@gmail.com

S. Antinori
Department of Biomedical and Clinical Sciences Luigi Sacco, University of Milano, III Division of Infectious Diseases, Luigi Sacco Hospital, ASST Fatebenefratelli Sacco, Via GB Grassi 74, Milan, Italy
e-mail: spinello.antinori@unimi.it

© Springer International Publishing AG 2018
M. Tonolini (ed.), *Imaging and Intervention in Urinary Tract Infections and Urosepsis*, https://doi.org/10.1007/978-3-319-68276-1_2

UTIs have a tendency to recur. A recurrence is defined as three symptomatic UTIs within 12 months or two symptomatic episodes half a year following clinical resolution of a previous UTI, and it implies a period of time without bacteriuria or signs of infection [3]. Clinically a recurrence occurring within 2 weeks from a previous episode is classified as a relapse otherwise is considered a reinfection. The majority of recurrences are thought to be reinfections [4]. Repeated ascending infection and chronic infection in the bladder seem to be the two mechanisms causing recurrences. This is supported by recent discoveries in the pathogenesis of UTIs leading to new insights about the persistence of bacteria and their ability to survive in the bladder [5].

2.2   Epidemiology

UTIs are one of the most common bacterial infections seen in both hospital and outpatient settings. In the United States in 2010, the emergency department (ED) visits with a primary diagnosis of UTI were more than 3 million: Of these 84.5% were women and among them approximately half of all UTIs presentations between 18 and 40 of age [6]. In 2012 UTIs accounted for 25.3% of all ID-related ED visits of elderly adults in the United States with a hospitalization rate of 17% [7]. It is difficult to estimate the real incidence of UTIs in the outpatient setting as studies differ for the case selection criteria, source of data and sample size. A Swiss study found an incidence rate of visits to a GP for lower UTIs at 1.6 per 100 inhabitants per year [8]. In Canada incidence rates of UTIs with positive cultures have been estimated at 17.5 per 1000 inhabitants per year [9]. In France the annual incidence rate of confirmed UTIs in general practice was estimated at 2400 per 100,000 women [10].

UTIs represent also an important burden among healthcare-associated infections (HAIs). A prevalence survey conducted in the United States estimated that there were 648,000 patients with 721,8000 HAIs in acute care hospitals in 2011. Among these, 93,3000 were UTIs and 35,600   CA-UTIs [11]. Another recent study

evaluating the impact of six healthcare-associated infections in Europe estimated an occurrence of 2,609,911 new cases of HAIs every year in the European Union and European Economic Area (EU/EEA). Hospital-acquired UTIs (HA-UTIs) represented almost 30% of the total burden, especially among hospitalized 65-year-old patients and above, with 777,639 cases yearly and an incidence of 152/100,000 population [12].

Except for infants and elderly, females are more likely to experience UTIs than males. In childhood, especially during the first year of life, the incidence of UTIs among uncircumcised boys is 20.3% against a 5% in girls [13, 14]. This trend is going to reverse in the prepubertal age when about 3% of girls are diagnosed with UTIs versus 1% of boys [13]. It is estimated that among young, healthy women around 50–60% of them will experience at least one UTI in their lifetime [15]. A surveillance study based on self-reported questionnaire found out an annual incidence of UTIs of 12%, and by the age of 32, half of all women report having had at least one UTI [16]. Women are also more susceptible to recurrences [17]. A study conducted among college women who had already experienced one UTI showed that 27% experienced a recurrence within 6 months after the first episode, and 2.7% had a second recurrence over the same time of period [3, 18]. Incidence of UTIs in men increases after the age of 60. This is essentially due to the physiologic changes that occur in the structure and function of urinary tract which impair normal voiding with benign prostatic hyperplasia as the most common cause of obstruction of urine flow [19]. The trend in the incidence of UTIs is similar among both genders in the eight decade of life [20].

Symptomatic UTI is the second most common infection in residents of long-term care facilities (LTCF) with an estimated incidence rate of 0.1–2.4 per 1000 resident-day [21]. Indwelling urinary catheters contribute to the burden of UTIs giving a daily risk of acquiring bacteriuria of 3–7% [22]. The extensive use of indwelling catheters, 17.5% in 66 European Hospitals and 23.6% among 183 US hospitals [11], is responsible of a four- to six-fold increase of having a symptomatic urinary tract infection with consequent excessive antimicrobial use and risk of adverse outcomes [23].

2.3 Risk Factors

Many classifications have been proposed to assess factors which expose the individual at risk for UTI. Genetic predisposition, behavioural factors, host factors and risk for UTIs results from a complex interaction between all of these elements [1, 24, 25].

The higher susceptibility of female sex is firstly due to anatomical characteristics with the proximity of the female urethra to the vaginal cavity and to the rectum. This increases the probability of colonization of the periurethral mucosa by potential uropathogens and thus facilitating the ascending route of infection to the bladder or the kidney. Specific behaviours have been associated to UTIs. Studies among college women have shown that sexual intercourse, use of spermicides and diaphragms and number of sexual partners increase risk of acquiring UTIs [26, 27].

A prior UTI is a well-known risk factor for further episodes. It is estimated that among young, healthy women, around 20–30% with a first UTI will experience two or more episodes, and around 5% will have recurrences. These high rates of recurrences were observed in studies conducted in different time, but they all confirmed these frequencies [3, 25]. In postmenopausal women, further predisposing factors are advancing age, comorbidities and urological abnormalities favouring incontinence; the role of oestrogens, which are believed to contribute to UTIs, is controversial [28].

Type 2 diabetes mellitus (DM2) has always been considered a predisposing factor for infections and most commonly UTIs [29]. Incidence of diabetes is increasing: in the United States, there were 1.7 million new diabetes cases among adults aged 20 years or older in 2012, and in the period 2009–2012, at least 37% of adults aged 20 years or older had prediabetes (altered fasting glucose or A1C levels) [30]. Previous epidemiological studies have shown a 1.2–2.2 increase in the relative risk of UTI in patients with diabetes compared with those without [31]. Moreover, a recent study examining the 1-year prevalence and healthcare costs implications of UTIs in a type 2 diabetes population in the United States observed an 8.2% risk of one or more UTIs diagnoses during a 1-year study period [32]. Prevalence of AB in women with DM is three to four times greater than in woman without DM as the frequency of symptomatic infection [33]. In particular, in a cohort of women with DM type 2, ABU was the most important risk factor for developing symptomatic UTI (34% in women with ABU vs. 19% in those without). Higher glucose urine concentration, decrease immune function, duration and severity of diabetes and possible autonomic neuropathy leading to urinary retention are all factors identified as possible responsible for increased susceptibility [31]. Surprisingly, HbA1c, which expresses the degree of glycaemia, does not seem to correlate with UTIs risk [31]. Despite bacterial aetiology is qualitatively the same, patients with type 2 diabetes are more likely to be infected with uropathogen-resistant strains and to be exposed to serious complications of UTIs such as emphysematous conditions of the bladder and the kidney, renal abscesses and papillary necrosis [29].

There is a growing evidence about the correlation between obesity and the risk of infection (*i.e.*, blood stream infection, ventilator-associated pneumonia, influenza infection, etc.), and in the last years, a few studies have specifically evaluated obesity as a possible additional risk factor for UTIs. It has come out that obese people have a fivefold increase of risk of developing pyelonephritis compared to those nonobese [34]. For males with a BMI of 50 kg/m^2 or more, there is an increased risk of 2.38 and for females 1.25 [35]. Recently, a study conducted in Israel among 122 premenopausal women have shown an overall prevalence of recurrent UTI (RUTI) of 23.4 and 49.5% of those were obese. The study took into account also age, the use of contraceptive, sexual intercourse, diabetes mellitus and metabolic syndrome, but there was no statistical difference between cases and controls except, interestingly, for maternal history of RUTI, use of probiotics and BMI [36]. It is presumable that, similar to diabetes even with different mechanisms, dysregulation of the immune system caused by altered levels of immunomodulatory adipokines (adiponectin) predisposes to infection.

Host genetics influence the susceptibility to infection. A case control study of 1,261 women revealed a positive correlation between recurrent cystitis/pyelonephritis and a urinary tract infection history in one or more female relative [37]. ABO blood group, secretory status and toll-like receptor polymorphisms have been associated to an increased susceptibility to UTI [38, 39]. Most likely, all of these factors interact and influence the immune response to the bacteria determining the severity of the disease.

2.4 Microbiology and the Emergence of MDR Bacteria

Gram-negative Enterobacteriaceae account for almost 80% of all UTI syndromes with *Escherichia coli* as the most frequent one followed by *Klebsiella pneumoniae*, *Proteus mirabilis* and *Pseudomonas aeruginosa*, while *Staphylococcus saprophyticus*, *Streptococcus agalactiae* and *Enterococcus* spp. are the major isolates among gram-positive bacteria [25, 40] (Table 2.1). However, many factors affect the aetiology of UTIs like age, gender, comorbidities and epidemiologic features [29, 41]. *E.* remains the predominant pathogen for both sexes regardless the age group, causing 74 and 65% of all syndromes in the outpatient and hospital setting,

Table 2.1 Most frequent uropathogens [40]

Uncomplicated UTIs microorganisms prevalence	Complicated UTIs microorganisms prevalence
Escherichia coli (75%)	*Escherichia coli* (65%)
Staphylococcus saprophyticus (6%)	*Enterococcus* spp. (11%)
Klebsiella pneumoniae (6%)	*Klebsiella pneumoniae* (8%)
Enterococcus spp. (5%)	*Candida* spp. (7%)
Group B *Streptococcus* (3%)	Group B *Streptococcus* (2%)
Proteus mirabilis (2%)	*Proteus mirabilis* (2%)
Pseudomonas aeruginosa (1%)	*Pseudomonas aeruginosa* (2%)

respectively [9]. It is more frequent in females than males (71% vs. 55%) [41] together with *Staphylococcus saprophyticus* (which is the main responsible for UTIs in young women after *E. coli*) [42, 43], whereas *P. aeruginosa* is more common in men (8.39% vs. 1.63%) [44]. The prevalence of UTIs caused by *K. pneumoniae*, *P. aeruginosa*, *Enterococcus* spp. and fungi is greater in the elderly (over the age of 60) [44]. This is because in this subpopulation underlying complicating factors (such as dementia, diabetes, bladder and bowel incontinence or urinary retention with need for catheterization, impaired immune function, residency in LTCF, exposure to broad spectrum antibiotics) favour complicated infections caused by resistant bacteria [40]. Less virulent organisms as *Proteus mirabilis*, *Candida* spp. and polymicrobial infections (20–30%) are also more frequent after the age of 60 [45, 46]. Noteworthy, *P. mirabilis* is of particular importance for patients with chronic indwelling catheters because of its ability to form biofilm [23].

The increase in antimicrobial resistance due to the spread of extended-spectrum beta-lactamases (ESBL)-producing organisms is of particular concern especially for the management of community-acquired infections [47] (Table 2.2). Approximately a decade ago, ESBL-producing Enterobacteriaceae began to appear in the community among patients with no documented contact with LTCFs, no recent antibiotic exposure and no other risk factors for ESBL carriage [48, 49]. A prevalence study conducted in Sweden between 2007 and 2011 showed an increase in the number of ESBL-producing *E. coli* from 3 to 4% with a peak among women aged 20–30 years associated to a decrease in the median age for acquiring ESBL. Authors stated that this increase was mainly due to urinary tract infections and partially related to the acquisition of ESBL *E. coli* during travels to countries of high endemicity [50]. In Japan, a 9-year period study on community-acquired ESBL Enterobacteriaceae infections revealed a gradual increase in the detection rate of ESBL producers (321 out of 5137 isolates) with ESBL *E. coli* prevalence raising from 1.2% in 2003 to 14.3% in 2011 [51]. Another prospective observational study conducted in five community hospitals in the United

Table 2.2 Characteristics of antimicrobial agents used for UTIs and mechanisms of resistance [47–49]

Antibiotic	Mechanism of action	Type of activity	Bacterial resistance mechanism
Beta-lactams	Inhibit bacteria cell wall biosynthesis	Bactericidal	Hydrolysis by β-lactamase Mutation of the target site (penicillin-binding protein)
Aminoglycosides	Inhibit protein synthesis by bacteria	Bactericidal	Inactivation through acetylation, nucleotidylation or phosphorylation Target site mutation (methylation of 16S rRNA)
Sulphonamides	Interfere with bacterial growth and multiplication	Bacteriostatic	Overproduction of dihydropteroic acid synthase (DHPS) or dihydrofolate reductase (DHFR) Altered DHPS—essential for folate synthesis in bacteria—leads to sulphonamide resistance and altered DHFR with loss of inhibition by trimethoprim
Quinolones	Interfere with bacteria DNA replication and transcription	Bactericidal	DNA gyrase mutations Protein binding of quinolone active
Polymyxin	Disrupt the structure of the bacterial cell membrane	Bactericidal	Mutation in lipopolysaccharide

States showed that among 291 patients infected or colonized with ESBL-producing *E. coli* as outpatients or within 48 h of hospitalization, 107 (36.8%) had community-associated infection of which 81.5% were urinary tract infection [49]. Recognized risk factors for community-onset ESBL infections are recurrent UTIs coupled with underlying renal pathology, recent exposure to fluoroquinolones, previous hospitalization, advanced age, diabetes mellitus and underlying liver disease. In the hospital setting, ESBL infections were significantly linked to intensive care unit stay, prolonged 'time at risk' (*i.e.*, time from admission to culture), presence of foreign medical devices (*i.e.*, central lines, nasogastric tube, urinary catheter and endotracheal tube), mechanical ventilation, recent prior invasive procedures and recent administration of antimicrobials (especially third-generation cephalosporins) [52].

2.5 Diagnosis

Diagnosis of UTI syndromes relies on clinical evaluation supported by laboratory findings. Symptoms like dysuria, frequency, urgency, suprapubic pain and haematuria are highly suggestive for lower UTI. However these manifestations do not occur necessarily all together or, by contrast, only dysuria can be present at the onset of the infection, so they need to be correlated with patient's clinical history (age, gender, presence of risk factors for UTIs). In women the differential diagnosis includes sexually transmitted diseases (STD) such as urethritis and vaginitis although they are usually accompanied by vaginal irritation or discharge [53]. A meta-analysis of studies of uncomplicated UTIs in women estimated that the probability of cystitis is greater than 50% in women with any symptoms of urinary tract infection and greater than 90% in women who have dysuria and frequency without vaginal discharge or irritation [54]. In men, bacterial prostatitis manifests with lower UTI symptoms plus fever and obstructive symptoms due to prostate inflammation such as hesitancy, nocturia, slow stream and dribbling [19]. Suspicion of pyelonephritis rises in the presence of systemic symptoms such as temperature >38 °C, chills, nausea or vomiting together with flank pain or costovertebral angle tenderness with or without cystitis symptoms. Complicated pyelonephritis may also present with sepsis or multiorgan system dysfunction [4]. The elderly might have an atypical presentation with nonspecific symptoms as fever or altered mental status [53].

Dipstick test and urine culture are the most supporting tests for the diagnosis of UTIs. The first one tests for leukocyte esterase, an enzyme present in host's urine polymorphonuclear leukocytes, and nitrites, which derives from the reduction of nitrate by the Enterobacteriaceae. Leukocyte esterase has a sensitivity of 62–98% and specificity of 55–96%. Urine nitrite is highly specific but has a poor sensitivity [6]. A positive dipstick test strongly supports the diagnosis of UTI in a patient with typical symptoms, but a negative one, if the clinical suspicion is high, does not rule it out. Urine microscopy reveals pyuria, which is present in the majority of patients with acute cystitis and pyelonephritis [4]. Noteworthy, in catheterised patients, pyuria is not diagnostic of catheter-associated bacteriuria or symptomatic UTI. Urine culture is the gold standard for the diagnosis. Traditionally a bacterial count $\geq 10^5$ CFU/mL has been considered the threshold predictive of bladder bacteriuria. However, because 30–50% of women with cystitis have between 10^2 and 10^4 CFU/mL in voided urine and the vast majority of patients with pyelonephritis have $\geq 10^4$ CFU/mL uropathogens in urine culture, a quantitative count $\geq 10^3$ is now suggested as a reasonable indicator of acute uncomplicated cystitis while count $\geq 10^4$ CFU/mL of pyelonephritis [1, 4, 53].

2.6   Treatment

Screening and treatment of asymptomatic bacteriuria are generally not recommended except for:

– Pregnant women, who are at major risk for symptomatic UTIs and pyelonephritis (between 15–45%) if not treated [55]
– Those subjecting to urological procedures, who are at risk for complicated infections [1]

The choice of the treatment should be guided by the antibiogram, and it should include same antibiotics recommended for uncomplicated or complicated UTIs considering host risk factors and comorbidities.

Guidelines [1, 2] recommend the following agents as first choice for the treatment of lower uncomplicated UTIs: nitrofurantoin macrocrys-

tal, fosfomycin trometamol and pivmecillinam. Trimethoprim–sulphamethoxazole remains highly effective only in areas where resistance rates of *E. coli* are known to be <20%; however, it should be avoided if used for UTI in the last 3 months. Aminopenicillins and oral cephalosporins, because of minor efficacy as short-course therapy and of resistance patterns, should be considered only when the other recommended drugs cannot be used. In the ARESC study, almost 20% of all the 2315 *E. coli* isolates exhibited low susceptibility to amoxicillin/clavulanate, cefuroxime and nalidixic acid, while resistance rates for ciprofloxacin exceeded 10%. In each country fosfomycin, mecillinam and nitrofurantoin were the most active drugs against *E. coli* [43]. These data are in line with those from the ECO SENS study which have registered higher resistance level in *E. coli* for amoxicillin/clavulanate, ciprofloxacin, ampicillin, TMP–SMX than mecillinam, fosfomycin trometamol and nitrofurantoin (<2%) with a rising trend from 1999 to 2008 [56]. For men, a longer antibiotic course has always been suggested (7–14 days) due to concerns of persistence of bacteria in the prostate favouring thus early recurrences [57]. Data on the best duration treatment are controversial. One observational study has shown no reduction in early or late UTI recurrences for treatment duration >7 days [58] contrasting with a clinical trial comparing 3 days vs. 14 days of ciprofloxacin which have underlined a clear benefit [59]. However, the first study was conducted among male veterans in an outpatient setting and the second one in spinal cord injury patients, a special subpopulation at risk so it is difficult to compare the results. Noteworthy, a long-duration therapy has to be balanced with the risk of *Clostridium difficile* infection [58]. In accordance to susceptibility testing and to local resistance patterns, TMP–SMX and quinolones, because of their better penetration in the prostatic tissue, should be preferred in men.

For acute uncomplicated pyelonephritis not requiring hospitalization, 7 days of a fluoroquinolone (in area with resistance <10%) or 14 days of TMP–SMX are the first-line choices. Quinolones have a broad spectrum of activity against many gram-negative bacteria so they have become a first-line choice for UTIs. However increasing resistance rates, from 1–4% to 6–15%, have been demonstrated, and even if in the community resistance remains <20%, MDR bacteria have displayed rates of resistance between 49 and 72% [60]. Surveillance data on TMP–SMX have estimated resistance rates ranging from 16% to 36% globally and between 60 and 77% among MDR [60]. For these reasons, these two agents should be considered carefully, and initiation with a parenteral antimicrobial such as ceftriaxone or an aminoglycoside may be warranted [2]. In case of pyelonephritis requiring hospitalization, suggested antimicrobials for intravenous therapy are aminoglycosides, extended-spectrum cephalosporins, beta-lactams in combination with beta-lactams inhibitors and carbapenems. The choice between these drugs has to take into account local resistance patterns and susceptibility testing [1, 2].

Treatment of CA-UTIs has to be considered only for those with appropriate signs and symptoms attributable to the urinary tract and after the exclusion of other sources of infection. In fact pyuria in patients with indwelling urinary catheters can be present with or without bacteriuria as a result of bladder inflammation, so it is not an indication whether to start antimicrobial therapy. If the catheter has been in place for more than 7 days, it should be removed before the initiation of an antibiotic. Duration of treatment can vary between 7 and 14 days according to the severity of the clinical presentation [1, 2].

Treatments for multidrug-resistant uropathogens rely on drugs which still retain antimicrobial activity and on a few new available options. A retrospective analysis on the use of oral fosfomycin for the treatment of MDR UTIs has shown a treatment success rate, defined by neither persistence nor recurrence by the same organism, of 55% [61]. A recent survey on 204 MDR urine isolates has found an overall resistance to fosfomycin of 21.6 and 19% among the ESBL producers with the lower rate in *E. coli* than that of *Klebsiella* spp. Noteworthy 83.3 and 63.7% of the isolates were resistant to fluoroquinolones and TMP–SMP, respectively [62]. Another retrospective cohort study performed to compare oral fosfomycin to intravenous ertapenem as step-down ther-

apy for the treatment of outpatient ESBL UTIs has shown noninferiority of fosfomycin with similar results between the two groups [63]. Nitrofurantoin exhibited a consistent antimicrobial activity against outpatient MDR *E. coli* isolated between 2001 and 2010 in the United States. Despite a decrease in the pan-susceptibility from 52.1% in 2001 to 42% in 2010, resistance to nitrofurantoin was found only in 2.1% in 2010 [64]. Another study evaluating the efficacy in vitro of five oral agents (including fosfomycin, nitrofurantoin, sulfamethoxazole–trimethoprim, ciprofloxacin and ampicillin) on 91 MDR uropathogens has found that fosfomycin and nitrofurantoin were the most active drugs with 96.7 and 76.7% of susceptibility against ESBLs producers, respectively [65]. The limit of fosfomycin and nitrofurantoin is their lack of tissue penetration so for UTIs due to MDR bacteria carbapenems and combination therapies with carbapenems, aminoglycosides and polymyxins are preferable [66]. The role of BLBLI is controversial. Piperacillin–tazobactam can be a carbapenem-sparing option against susceptible ESBL producers and for less serious infections [67]. However, new combinations have become available. Ceftolozane–tazobactam and ceftazidime–avibactam have been recently approved for the treatment of complicated UTIs. Ceftolozane is a novel cephalosporin with enhanced activity against gram-negative pathogens including *P. aeruginosa* and Enterobacteriaceae. The addition of tazobactam confers activity against class A and C ESBLs Enterobacteriaceae but not towards metallo-β-lactamases, *K. pneumonia* carbapenemases or others. The spectrum of activity of ceftolozane–tazobactam includes also streptococcal species and *Bacteroides fragilis*, but it has limited coverage against *Staphylococcus* spp. and other gram-negative anaerobes [68]. Avibactam is a novel β-lactamase inhibitor which restores the in vitro activity of ceftazidime against Ambler class A, class C and some class D β-lactamase producers; it is not active against metallo-β-lactamases (Table 2.3). Noninferiority of ceftazidime–avibactam vs. doripenem has been demonstrated in phase III clinical trials [69]. These new combinations are good carbapenem-sparing options but

Table 2.3 Types of beta-lactamase [66]

B-lactamase	Species	Effect
Class A: contain serine residues Example: TEM, SHV, CTX-M. KPC Carbapenemase	Enterobacteriaceae such as *Escherichia coli, Klebsiella* spp., *Proteus* spp. and *Pseudomonas* spp.	Cephalosporinase activity and resistance to third-generation cephalosporins Usually inhibited by clavulanate–tazobactam in vitro
Class B: contain metal ions Example: IMP, NDM, VIM carbapenemase	*Escherichia coli, Klebsiella* spp. and other Enterobacteriaceae, *Acinetobacter* spp.	Carbapenemase activity Not inhibited by clavulanate/tazobactam Aztreonam not hydrolysed by class B β-lactamases
Class C: contain serine residue (called also 'AmpC' enzymes) Example: CMY, DHA, ACT	*Enterobacter cloacae, E. aerogenes, Serratia marcescens, Citrobacter freundii, Pseudomonas aeruginosa, Providencia* spp. and *Morganella morganii* all contain inducible AmpC enzymes that are chromosomally encoded Plasmid-mediated AmpC (i.e. CMY) increasing in *E. coli*	Cephalosporinase activity including towards third-generation cephalosporins but cefepime stable Not inhibited effectively by clavulanate or tazobactam
Class D: contain serine residue Example: OXA-type carbapenemase	Enterobacteriaceae, *Pseudomonas* spp., *Acinetobacter baumannii*	Carbapenemase activity Weakly inhibited by clavulanate

ACT AmpC type, *CMY* cephamycins, *CTX-M* cefotaxime hydrolysing capabilities, *DHA* Dhahran Hospital, *IMP* imipenem, *KPC Klebsiella pneumoniae* carbapenemase, *NDM* New Delhi metallo-β-lactamase, *OXA* oxacillin hydrolysing capabilities, *SHV* sulphydryl variable, *TEM* Temoneira, *VIM* Verona integron-encoded metallo-β-lactamase.

have to be used wisely through the implementation of programmes of antimicrobial stewardship to limit the development of further resistance.

References

1. Grabe M, Bartoletti R, Bjerklund Johansen TE et al (2015) Guidelines on urological infections. European Association of Urology, The Netherlands. http://uroweb.org/guideline/urological-infections
2. Gupta K, Hooton TM, Naber KG et al (2011) International clinical practice guidelines for the treatment of acute uncomplicated cystitis and pyelonephritis in women: a 2010 update by the Infectious Diseases Society of America and the European Society for Microbiology and Infectious Diseases. Clin Infect Dis 52:e103–e120
3. Glover M, Moreira CG, Sperandio V, Zimmern P (2014) Recurrent urinary tract infections in healthy and nonpregnant women. Urol Sci 25:1–8
4. Hooton TM (2012) Uncomplicated urinary tract infection. N Engl J Med 366:1028–1037
5. Schwartz DJ, Chen SL, Hultgren SJ, Seed PC (2011) Population dynamics and niche distribution of uropathogenic *Escherichia coli* during acute and chronic urinary tract infection. Infect Immun 79:4250–4259
6. Takhar SS, Moran GJ (2014) Diagnosis and management of urinary tract infection in the emergency department and outpatient settings. Infect Dis Clin N Am 28:33–48
7. Goto T, Yoshida K, Tsugawa Y, Camargo CA, Hasegawa K (2016) Infectious diseases – related emergency department visits of elderly adults in the United States, 2011–2012. J Am Geriatr Soc 64:31–36
8. Kronenberg A, Koenig S, Droz S, Muhlemann K (2011) Active surveillance of antibiotic resistance prevalence in urinary tract and skin infections in the outpatient setting. Clin Microbiol Infect 17:1845–1851
9. Laupland KB, Ross T, Pitout JDD, Church DL, Gregson DB (2007) Community-onset urinary tract infections: a population-based assessment. Infection 35:150–153
10. Rossignol L, Vaux S, Maugat S et al (2016) Incidence of urinary tract infections and antibiotic resistance in the outpatient setting: a cross sectional study. Infection 45:33–40
11. Magill SS, Edwards JR, Bamberg W et al (2014) Multistate point-prevalence survey of health care-associated infections. N Engl J Med 370:1198–1208
12. Cassini A, Diamantis Plachouras P, Eck T et al (2016) Burden of six healthcare-associated infections on

European population health: estimating incidence- based disability-adjusted life years through a population prevalence-based modelling study. PLoS Med 13:e1002150

13. Stein R, Dogan HS, Hoebeke P et al (2015) Urinary tract infections in children: EAU/ESPU guidelines. Eur Urol 67:546–555

14. Wiswell TE, Enzenauer RW, Holton ME, Cornish D, Hankins CT (1987) Declining frequency of circumcision: implications for changes in the absolute incidence of male to female sex ratio of urinary tract infections in early infancy. Pediatrics 79:338–342

15. Foxman B, Barlow R, D'Arcy H, Gillespie B, Sobel JD (2000) Urinary tract infection: self-reported incidence and associated costs. Ann Epidemiol 10:509–515

16. Foxman B (2003) Epidemiology of urinary tract infections: incidence, morbidity, and economic costs. Dis Mon 49:53–70

17. Gupta K, Trautner BW (2013) Diagnosis and management of recurrent urinary tract infections in nonpregnant women. BMJ 346:f3140

18. Hooton TM (2001) Recurrent urinary tract infection in women. Int J Antimicrob Agents 17:259–268

19. Schaeffer AJ, Nicolle LE (2016) Urinary tract infections in older men. N Engl J Med 374:562–571

20. Caljouw MA, den Elzen WP, Cools HJ, Gussekloo J (2011) Predictive factors of urinary tract infections among the oldest old in the general population. A population-based prospective follow-up study. BMC Med 9:57

21. Nicolle LE (2009) Urinary tract infections in the elderly. Clin Ger Med 25:423–436

22. Hooton TM, Bradley SF, Cardenas DD et al (2010) Diagnosis, prevention, and treatment of catheter-associated urinary tract infection in adults: 2009 International Clinical Practice Guidelines from the Infectious Diseases Society of America. Clin Infect Dis 50:625–663

23. Nicolle LE (2014) Urinary tract infection in long-term care facilities. Healthcare Infect 19:4–12

24. Ronald A (2003) The etiology of urinary tract infection: traditional and emerging pathogens. Dis Mon 49:71–82

25. Foxman B (2014) Urinary tract infection syndromes: occurrence, recurrence, bacteriology, risk factors, and disease burden. Infect Dis Clin N Am 28:1–13

26. Foxman B, Chi JW (1990) Health behavior and urinary tract infection in college-aged women. J Clin Epidemiol 43:329–337

27. Vincent CR, Thomas TL, Reyes L et al (2013) Symptoms and risk factors associated with first urinary tract infection in college age women: a prospective cohort study. J Urol 189:904–910

28. Hu KK, Boyk EJ, Scholes D et al (2004) Risk factors for urinary tract infections in postmenopausal women. Arch Intern Med 164:989–993

29. Ronald A, Ludwig E (2001) Urinary tract infections in adults with diabetes. Int J Antimicrob Agents 17:287–292

30. Centers for Disease Control and Prevention (2014) National diabetes statistics report: estimates of diabetes and its burden in the United States, 2014. US Department of Health and Human Services, Atlanta

31. Chen SL, Jackson SL, Boyko EJ (2009) Diabetes mellitus and urinary tract infection: epidemiology, pathogenesis and proposed studies in animal models. J Urol 182:S51–S56

32. Yu S, Fu AZ, Qiu Y, Engel SS et al (2014) Disease burden of urinary tract infections among type 2 diabetes mellitus patients in the US. J Diabetes Complicat 28:621–626

33. Hoepelman AI, Meiland R, Geerlings SE (2003) Pathogenesis and management of bacterial urinary tract infections in adult patients with diabetes mellitus. Int J Antimicrob Agents 22:35–43

34. Semins MJ, Shore AD, Makary MA, Weiner J, Matlaga BR (2012) The impact of obesity on urinary tract infection risk. Urology 79:266–269

35. Saliba W, Barnett-Griness O, Rennert G (2013) The association between obesity and urinary tract infection. Eur J Intern Med 24:127–131

36. Nseir W, Farah R, Mahamid M et al (2015) Obesity and recurrent urinary tract infections in premenopausal women: a retrospective study. Int J Infect Dis 41:32–35

37. Scholes D, Hawn TR, Roberts PL et al (2010) Family history and risk of recurrent cystitis and pyelonephritis in women. J Urol 184:564–569

38. Sheinfeld J, Schaeffer AJ, Cordon-Cardo C, Rogatko A, Fair WR (1989) Association of the Lewis blood-group phenotype with recurrent urinary tract infections in women. N Engl J Med 320:773–777

39. Hawn TR, Scholes D, Li SS et al (2009) Toll-like receptor polymorphisms and susceptibility to urinary tract infections in adult women. PLoS One 4:e5990

40. Flores-Mireles AL, Walker JN, Caparon M, Hultgren SJ (2015) Urinary tract infections: epidemiology, mechanisms of infection and treatment options. Nat Rev Microbiol 13:269–284

41. Magliano E, Grazioli V, Deflorio L, Leuci AI, Mattina R, Romano P, Cocuzza CE (2012) Gender and age-dependent etiology of community-acquired urinary tract infections. Sci World J 2012:349597

42. Kahlmeter G (2003) An international survey of the antimicrobial susceptibility of pathogens from uncomplicated urinary tract infections: the ECO.SENS project. J Antimicrobl Chemother 51:69–76

43. Schito GC, Naber KG, Botto H et al (2009) The ARESC study: an international survey on the antimicrobial resistance of pathogens involved in uncomplicated urinary tract infections. Int J Antimicrob Agents 34:407–413

44. Đorđević Z, Folić M, Janković S (2016) Community-acquired urinary tract infections: causative agents and their resistance to antimicrobial drugs. Vojnosanit Pregl 73:218–218

45. Tandogdu Z, Wagenlehner FM (2016) Global epidemiology of urinary tract infections. Curr Opin Infect Dis 29:73–79

46. Genao L, Buhr GT (2012) Urinary tract infections in older adults residing in long-term care facilities. Ann Longterm Care 20:33

47. Pitout JD, Laupland KB (2008) Extended-spectrum β-lactamase-producing Enterobacteriaceae: an emerging public-health concern. Lancet Infect Dis 8:159–166

48. Ben-Ami R, Rodriguez-Bano J, Arslan H et al (2009) A multinational survey of risk factors for infection with extended-spectrum betalactamase-producing enterobacteriaceae in nonhospitalized patients. Clin Infect Dis 49:682–690

49. Doi Y, Park YS, Rivera JI et al (2013) Community-associated extended-spectrum beta-lactamase-producing Escherichia coli infection in the United States. Clin Infect Dis 56:641–648

50. Brolund A, Edquist PJ, Mäkitalo B et al (2014) Epidemiology of extended spectrum β-lactamase-producing Escherichia coli in Sweden 2007–2011. Clin Microbiol Infect 20:O344–O352

51. Chong Y, Shimoda S, Yakushiji H et al (2013) Community spread of extended-spectrum β-lactamase-producing Escherichia coli, Klebsiella pneumoniae and Proteus mirabilis: a long-term study in Japan. J Med Microbiol 62:1038–1043

52. Tal Jasper R, Coyle JR, Katz DE, Marchaim D (2015) The complex epidemiology of extended-spectrum beta-lactamase-producing Enterobacteriaceae. Future Microbiol 10:819–839

53. Pietrucha-Dilanchian P, Hooton TM (2016) Diagnosis, treatment, and prevention of urinary tract infection. Microbiol Spectr 4(6). https://doi.org/10.1128/microbiolspec.UTI-0021-2015

54. Bent S, Nallamothu BK, Simel DL, Fihn SD, Saint S (2002) Does this woman have an acute uncomplicated urinary tract infection? JAMA 287:22–29

55. Widmer M, Lopez I, Gülmezoglu AM, Mignini L, Roganti A (2015) Duration of treatment for asymptomatic bacteriuria during pregnancy. Cochrane Database Syst Rev 11(11):CD000491

56. Kahlmeter G, Poulsen HO (2012) Antimicrobial susceptibility of Escherichia Coli from community-acquired urinary tract infections in Europe: the ECO SENS study revisited. Int J Antimicrob Agents 39:45–51

57. Lipsky BA (1999) Prostatitis and urinary tract infection in men: what's new; what's true? Am J Med 106:327–334

58. Drekonja DM, Rector TS, Cutting A, Johnson JR (2013) Urinary tract infection in male veterans: treatment patterns and outcomes. JAMA Intern Med 173:62–68

59. Dow G, Rao P, Harding G et al (2004) A prospective, randomized trial of 3 or 14 days of ciprofloxacin treatment for acute urinary tract infection in patients with spinal cord injury. Clin Infect Dis 39:658–664

60. Walker E, Lyman A, Gupta K et al (2016) Clinical management of an increasing threat: outpatient urinary tract infections due to multidrug-resistant uropathogens. Clin Infect Dis 63:960–965

61. Seroy JT, Grim SA, Reid GE, Wellington T, Clark NM (2016) Treatment of MDR urinary tract infections with oral fosfomycin: a retrospective analysis. J Antimicrob Chemother 71:2563–2568

62. Linsenmeyer K, Strymish J, Weir S et al (2016) Activity of Fosfomycin against extended-spectrum-β-lactamase-producing uropathogens in patients in the community and hospitalized patients. Antimicrob Agents Chemother 60:1134–1136

63. Veve MP, Wagner JL, Kenney RM, Grunwald JL, Davis SL (2016) Comparison of fosfomycin to ertapenem for outpatient or step-down therapy of extended-spectrum β-lactamase urinary tract infections. Int J Antimicrob Agents 48:56–60

64. Sanchez GV, Baird AMG, Karlowsky JA, Master RN, Bordon JM (2014) Nitrofurantoin retains antimicrobial activity against multidrug-resistant urinary Escherichia coli from US outpatients. J Antimicrob Chemother 69:3259–3262

65. Hirsch EB, Zucchi PC, Chen A et al (2016) Susceptibility of multidrug-resistant Gram-negative urine isolates to oral antibiotics. Antimicrob Agents Chemother 60:3138–3140

66. Zowawi HM, Harris PN, Roberts MJ et al (2015) The emerging threat of multidrug-resistant Gram-negative bacteria in urology. Nat Rev Urol 12:570–584

67. Nguyen HM, Shier KL, Graber CJ (2014) Determining a clinical framework for use of cefepime and β-lactam/β-lactamase inhibitors in the treatment of infections caused by extended-spectrum-β-lactamase-producing Enterobacteriaceae. J Antimicrob Chemother 69:871–880

68. Giancola SE, Mahoney MV, Bias TE, Hirsch EB (2016) Critical evaluation of ceftolozane–tazobactam for complicated urinary tract and intra-abdominal infections. Ther Clin Risk Manag 12:787

69. Wagenlehner FM, Sobel JD, Newell P et al (2016) Ceftazidime-avibactam versus doripenem for the treatment of complicated urinary tract infections, including acute pyelonephritis: RECAPTURE, a phase 3 randomized trial program. Clin Infect Dis 63:754–762

Uncomplicated and Complicated Urinary Tract Infections in Adults: The Infectious Diseases's Specialist Perspective

3

Spinello Antinori and Maria Diletta Pezzani

Urinary tract infections (UTIs) are responsible in Western countries of thousands of outpatient visits as well as emergency and hospital admissions [1, 2]. The clinical syndromes associated with UTIs may range from asymptomatic bacteriuria to the more severe picture of pyelonephritis and urosepsis sometimes designated (including also prostatitis in men) as "febrile urinary tract infections" [3, 4].

However, the concept of uncomplicated and complicated urinary tract infection (c-UTI) still remains a matter of concern because severe infections or those with invasive tissue involvement are sometimes erroneously indicated as c-UTI [3, 5, 6]. The concept and the categorization of c-UTI were introduced by a panel of experts of the Infectious Diseases Society of America (IDSA) in order to make more easy the evaluation of antimicrobial treatment in different setting [7]. It should be acknowledged that the term "uncomplicated" refers to any infection observed in patients without known structural or functional risk factors that will render the individual more prone to develop UTI [8, 9].

Although the classification of any disease is generally far from to be perfect and acceptable by everyone involved in their management, we believe that the UTI classification developed by the European Association of Urology (EAU) and the European Section of Infection in Urology (ESIU) is currently the best working approach to be considered [10, 11].

This classification is organized in five main categories (clinical criteria, possible risk factors, pathogens, mode of acquisition of UTI and therapeutic options) (Table 3.1) [11, 12]. The clinical criteria are arranged by syndromes: urethritis (UR), cystitis (CY), pyelonephritis (PY), urosepsis (US) and male accessory gland infections (i.e., prostatitis, vesiculitis, epididymitis and orchitis). The latter, together with urethritis, is not considered here given the great variability of clinical presentation. It should be highlighted that asymptomatic bacteriuria is not considered an infection but rather a risk factor that needs to be treated only in selected circumstances such as pregnancy or surgery of the urinary tract. Considering the three clinical syndromes—CY, PY and US—a grading of severity was suggested with six items that include at the extremes the less severe form, cystitis (grade 1), and the more severe form, uroseptic shock (grade 6) (Table 3.2). As far as risk factors, the difficulty to weight all categories in a proper way due to the lack of solid

S. Antinori (✉)
III Division of Infectious Diseases, Luigi Sacco Hospital, ASST Fatebenefratelli Sacco, Department of Biomedical and Clinical Sciences Luigi Sacco, University of Milano, Via GB Grassi 74, Milan, Italy
e-mail: spinello.antinori@unimi.it;

M.D. Pezzani
Department of Biomedical and Clinical Sciences Luigi Sacco, University of Milano, Via GB Grassi 74, Milan, Italy
e-mail: diletta.pezzani@gmail.com

© Springer International Publishing AG 2018
M. Tonolini (ed.), *Imaging and Intervention in Urinary Tract Infections and Urosepsis*,
https://doi.org/10.1007/978-3-319-68276-1_3

Table 3.1 EAU/ESIU criteria for classification and patient assessment in urinary tract infection[a]

I. Clinical criteria	II. Possible risk factors	III. Pathogen/ aetiological agent	IV. Situation-circumstances under which UTI was acquired	V. Therapeutic options
1. Clinical presentation a. Urethritis (UR) b. Cystitis (CY) c. Pyelonephritis (PY) d. Urosepsis (US) e. Male adnexitis (MA)[a]	1. Patients characteristics a. Gender (male, female) b. Prematurity, newborn, young child, adolescent c. Premenopause d. Pregnancy e. Postmenopause f. Elderly (geriatric: physically or mentally handicapped)	1. Bacterial load 2. Pathogens (type, species) 3. Antimicrobial susceptibility/ resistance 4. Virulence	1. Community 2. Outpatient service a. Hospital setting b. Private practice 3. Inpatient service (hospital) 4. Long-term residential accommodation, nursing home 5. Healthcare associated	1. Pathogen(s) is (are) susceptible against commonly used antimicrobials a. Which are available b. Which are not easily available 2. Pathogen(s) has (have) limited susceptibility against commonly used antimicrobials a. But alternative antimicrobials are available b. But alternative antimicrobials are not easily available 3. Pathogen(s) is (are) multiresistant, and appropriate antimicrobials are not (or not easily) available

2. Specificity of symptoms
a. UTI specific
  i. Lower UTI (CY): dysuria, frequency, urgency, suprapubic pain
  ii. Upper UTI (PY): fever, flank pain CVA tenderness
b. UTI non-specific symptoms
  i. Catheter-associated UTI (bladder spasm, unexplained fever)
  ii. newborn and young children
  iii. Elderly patients (fever, confusion)
  iv. Patients with neurogenic disorders
	2. Relevant disease outside the urinary tract
	a. Immunosuppression
	  i. Innate
	  ii. Acquired (AIDS)
	b. Diabetes mellitus
	c. Other disorders			

3. Severity of symptoms a. Mild b. Moderate c. Severe d. Septic	3. Nephrological risk factors—status of the kidneys a. Impaired kidney function b. Kidney abscess c. Polycystic renal disease			

4. Pattern of infection
a. Isolated or sporadic
b. Recurrent
  i. Relapse
  ii. Reinfection
c. Unresolved or chronic
	4. Urological risk factors
	a. Functional disorders (reflux, neurogenic bladder disturbances)
	b. Obstruction without infectious nidus (tumour, noninfected stone)
	c. Obstruction with infectious nidus (stent, necrotizing tumour, infective stones)			

	5. External catheter a. Urethral b. Suprapubic c. Nephrostomy d. Others			
	6. Asymptomatic bacteriuria			

EAU European Association of Urology, *ESIU* European Society of Infectious Urology, *UTI* urinary tract infection, *CY* cystitis, *PY* pyelonephritis, *CVA* costovertebral angle
[a]Bjerklund Johansen TE, et al. Critical review of current definitions of urinary tract infections and proposal of an EAU/ESIU classification system. Int J Antimicrob Agents (2011); 385:64–70

Table 3.2 Clinical diagnosis of UTI and grading severity

Clinical diagnosis	Signs and symptoms	Laboratory alterations	Acronym	Grade of severity
Cystitis	Dysuria, urgency, frequency, suprapubic pain	WBC > 10,000/μL; urine dipstick: presence of nitritis Urine culture: positive 10^3 CFU/mL	CY-1	1
Mild and moderate pyelonephritis	Fever, chills, flank pain, costovertebral-angle tenderness	WBC > 10,000/μL; urine dipstick: presence of nitritis Urine culture: positive 10^4 CFU/mL	PN-2	2
Severe pyelonephritis	As PN-2 plus nausea and vomiting	WBC > 12,000/μL; urine dipstick: presence of nitritis Urine culture: positive 10^4 CFU/mL	PN-3	3
Urosepsis (simple)[a]	SIRS= Temperature > 38°C or <36°C Heart rate > 90 beats min Respiratory rate > 20 breaths/min PaCo2 < 32 mmHg With or without symptoms of cystitis or pyelonephritis	WBC > 12,000/μL or <4000/μL; Blood culture: positive for uropathogens	US-4	4
Severe urosepsis[b]	Hypotension (systolic pressure < 90 mmHg, hypoperfusion (i.e. lactic acidosis; oliguria; alteration of mental status)	WBC > 12,000/μL or <4000/μL; PLTs <80,000/μL or decrease >50% within 3 days; urine dipstick: presence of nitritis PaO_2 < 75 mmHg (at ambient air) Blood pH < 7.3; plasma lactate >1.5 fold of normal Blood culture: positive for uropathogens	US-5	5
Uroseptic shock	Hypotension unresponsive to adequate fluid resuscitation; hypoperfusion (i.e. lactic acidosis; oliguria; alteration of mental status)	Blood culture: positive for uropathogens Blood pH < 7.3; plasma lactate >1.5 fold of normal; ARDS ($PaO_2/FiO_2 \leq 200$)	US-6	6

WBC white blood cells, *ARDS* acute respiratory distress syndrome
[a]with SIRS
[b]As US-4 plus organ dysfunction or hypotension

data has led to the proposal to use a new system for phenotyping designated with the acronym ORENUC (Table 3.3).

In the era of widespread diffusion of multidrug-resistant bacteria in some cases with very limited or absent antimicrobial options, it is imperative to recognize and manage UTIs in the appropriate manner.

3.1 Asymptomatic Bacteriuria

Asymptomatic bacteriuria is defined as the absence of urinary symptoms and a positive urine culture (midstream sample of urine with at least 10^5 CFU/mL) with the same bacterial strain in two consecutive samples (for women) and in a single sample for men [13].

Table 3.3 Host risk factors categorized according to the ORENUC system[a]

Type	Risk factors	Risk of more severe outcome
O	No known risk factor (i.e., healthy premenopausal women)	No
Recurrent	Sexual behaviour Postmenopausal hormone deficiency Contraceptive devices Controlled diabetes mellitus	No
Extra-urogenital	Prematurity, newborn Male gender Pregnancy Uncontrolled diabetes mellitus Relevant immunosuppression	Yes
Nephropathy	Impaired renal function Polycystic kidney	Yes
Urological	Obstructive uropathy (i.e., stone, tumour) Short-term catheterization Urological surgery	Yes
Catheter	Long-term catheter Non-resolvable urinary obstruction Neurogenic bladder badly controlled	Yes

[a]Smelov V et al. Improved classification of urinary tract infection: future consideration. European Urology Supplements 2016;15:71–80

Screening and treatment for asymptomatic bacteriuria are not recommended unless in pregnant women and for individuals prior to perform transurethral resection of the prostate (TURP) or other instrumental procedures responsible for mucosal bleeding [13]. Asymptomatic bacteriuria is reported in 4–7% of pregnant women and should always be treated because of high risk of progression to UTI including pyelonephritis (20–30-fold compared with non-pregnant women) [14, 15]. A Cochrane meta-analysis regarding more than 2300 pregnant women shows that antibiotic treatment is effective in terms of eradication and prevention of pyelonephritis. The estimated number of individuals needed to treat to prevent one episode of pyelonephritis is seven [15]. Moreover, asymptomatic bacteriuria in pregnant women has been associated with preterm labour and low birthweight [16, 17].

3.2 Acute Uncomplicated Urinary Tract Infections

According to the EAU/ESIU classification, both sporadic or recurrent community-acquired acute cystitis and pyelonephritis in healthy individuals (O, R and partially E risk factors of the ORENUC classification) are enclosed in this category of UTI. Cystitis (or lower UTI) is the most common presentation characterized by dysuria, frequency, urgency, suprapubic pain and sometimes hematuria [8, 9]. It should be highlighted that dysuria can be present also in women with vaginitis and men with urethritis, and those sexually acquired infections should be ruled out [18, 19]. Absence of vaginal discharge in a woman with dysuria and urgency is indicative of UTI in more than 90% of cases [20].

In a study regarding women with no new vaginal discharge or change in discharge, the only variable predictive of STDs was more than one sex partner in the past year. However, it is worth noting that in women presenting to an emergency department with genitourinary symptoms, over-diagnosis of UTI is common (up to 52%), whereas sexually transmitted infection (STI) is underdiagnosed (37%) [21]. Women are most affected due to their anatomical conformation with a self-reported annual incidence of 12% and an estimated lifetime risk of UTI of 60% [22, 23].

Several risk factors for development of UTI among women have been recognized: sexual intercourse, the use of spermicidal products, a new sex partner and a previous history of cystitis [24, 25].

A possible genetic predisposition is suggested although unproved by the observed increased risk of recurrent cystitis and pyelonephritis among women reporting to have a first-degree relative with a history of UTI [26, 27].

3.2.1 Microbiology and Treatment of Acute Uncomplicated UTI

Escherichia coli is responsible for about 80% of all cases of uncomplicated community-acquired UTI followed by other Enterobacteriaceae (i.e., *Klebsiella* spp., *Proteus* spp., *Enterobacter* spp.) and to a lesser extent gram-positive microorganisms (*Staphylococcus saprophyticus*, enterococci) [28, 29].

A cause of concern is the increasing rate of resistance to several classes of antibiotics of *E. coli* isolates from individuals with uncomplicated UTI. Trimethoprim-sulfamethoxazole (TMP-SMX) is now considered an appropriate empirical antibiotic choice for uncomplicated UTI only if the surveillance studies show resistance rates under 20% [5, 8, 30, 31]. Unfortunately several surveillance studies conducted in North America (USA, Canada), in Europe and in Latin America (Brazil) reported resistance rates ranging from 16% (Canada) up to 30% in Europe and Brazil [32–35].

Therefore the use of TMP-SMX as an empirical therapy for uncomplicated UTI requires the knowledge by the treating physician of the rates of resistance in the local community and possible risk factors associated with *E. coli* non-susceptible to TMP-SMX. In a Greek study, patients treated with amoxicillin and/or TMP-SMX in the previous 3 months had a two-fold risk of having an infection with a TMP-SMX-resistant isolate [35]. Other studies showed that prior use of TMP-SMX and travel outside the United States in the previous 3–6 months was predictive of TMP-SMX resistance [36]. Nitrofurantoin, fosfomycin and pivmecillinam are recommended as empirical first-line therapy of acute uncomplicated cystitis by both the United States of America and European Infectious Diseases Society guidelines (IDSA and ESCMID) and by the European Association of Urology guidelines [12, 31]. Although the three previously mentioned drugs have inferior efficacy (especially fosfomycin or pivmecillinam) with respect of other antibiotics or are inactive against *Proteus* species and some *Enterobacter* and *Klebsiella* strains (nitrofurantoin) or are not approved in the United States and some other European countries (pivmecillinam), their low resistance rates together with minimal propensity to induce "collateral damage" are the reason for which they are recommended as first-line choices in the setting of acute uncomplicated cystitis (Table 3.4). Nitrofurantoin should not be used in patients with a creatinine clearance (CrCL) below 60 mL/min considering the potential risk of toxicity (especially pulmonary and neurologic toxicity), and it is considered a potentially inappropriate drug for patients older than 65 years of age [37, 38].

Both fosfomycin and nitrofurantoin should not be used if pyelonephritis is suspected [5]. The concept of "collateral damage" induced by some class of antibiotics (such as fluoroquinolones and cephalosporins), namely, selection of drug-resistant or multidrug-resistant organisms or increasing risk of *Clostridium difficile* infection, gained equal weight to drug efficacy in the treatment recommendations [39]. Fluoroquinolones are considered for the above-mentioned reasons a second choice for acute uncomplicated cystitis, but a recent study from the USA encompassing the period 2002–2011 shows that they are the most frequently prescribed antibiotics (49% overall) in the outpatient setting [40]. An even higher rate (62.7%) of prescribing a fluoroquinolone (i.e., ciprofloxacin) has been reported in a study regarding treatment of outpatient males with UTI [41]. Oral β-lactam antibiotics (i.e., amoxicillin, amoxicillin-clavulanate, cefaclor, cefpodoxime proxetil) are considered options when first-line agents cannot be used, but the increasing worldwide prevalence of extended-spectrum β-lactamase (ESBL)-producing *E. coli* is a matter of concern and can be associated with high rates of treatment failure [2, 42, 43].

As previously discussed an episode of pyelonephritis (or upper tract UTI) that occurs in a healthy premenopausal, non-pregnant women without other recognized risk factors (Table 3.1

Table 3.4 Acute uncomplicated cystitis and pyelonephritis treatment recommended by IDSA/ESCMID and EAU guidelines

Clinical syndrome	IDSA/ESCMID 2012	EAU 2015
Acute cystitis	**First-line therapy** Nitrofurantoin monohydrate/macrocrystal 100 mg bid for 5 days po[a] Or Trimethoprim/sulfamethoxazole (TMP-SMX) 160/800 mg bid for 3 days po Or Fosfomycin trometamol 3 g single dose po Or Pivmecillinam 400 mg bid for 5 days po	**First choice** Fosfomycin trometamol 3 g single dose po Or Nitrofurantoin monohydrate/macrocrystal 100 mg bid for 5 days po[a] Or Pivmecillinam 400 mg tid for 5 days po
	Second-line therapy Fluoroquinolones Ciprofloxacin 250 mg bid for 3 days po Levofloxacin 250 or 500 mg single dose for 3 days po **Beta-lactams** Amoxicillin-clavulanate Cefpodoxime-proxetil 100 mg bid for 5 days po	**Alternatives** Fluoroquinolones[b] Ciprofloxacin 250 mg bid for 3 days po Levofloxacin 250 mg single dose for 3 days po Ofloxacin 200 mg bid for 3 days **Cephalosporins** Cefadroxil 500 mg bid for 3 days po TMP-SMX 160/800 mg bid for 3 days po[b]
Acute pyelonephritis (mild and moderate)	**First-line therapy** Ciprofloxacin 500 mg bid for 7 days po with or without an initial dose of 400 mg intravenous ciprofloxacin[c] Ciprofloxacin 1000 mg (extended release)/day for 7 days po Levofloxacin 750 mg/day for 5 days po Plus 1 g ceftriaxone iv[d] or a consolidated 24-h dose of an aminoglycoside **Second-line therapy** TMP-SMX 160/800 mg bid for 14 days po Plus 1 g ceftriaxone iv[e] or a consolidated 24-h dose of an aminoglycoside	**First choice** Ciprofloxacin 500–750 mg bid for 7–10 days po Levofloxacin 500 mg/day for 7–10 days po Levofloxacin 500 mg/day for 5 days po **Alternatives**[f] Cefpodoxime proxetil 200 mg bid for 10 days po Ceftibuten 400 mg/day for 10 days po Trimethoprim-sulphamethoxazole 160/800 mg bid for 14 days po[g]

(continued)

Table 3.4 (continued)

Clinical syndrome	IDSA/ESCMID 2012	EAU 2015
Severe acute uncomplicated pyelonephritis	**Parenteral fluoroquinolone** Ciprofloxacin 400 mg bid iv Levofloxacin 500–750 mg/day iv **Aminoglycoside** Gentamicin 5–7 mg/day iv **Extended spectrum cephalosporin** Ceftazidime 1 g tid ± an aminoglycoside iv Ampicillin-sulbactam ± aminoglycoside (if gram-positive cocci are causative) iv	**First choice**[h] Ciprofloxacin 400 mg bid iv Levofloxacin 250–500 mg/day iv Levofloxacin 750 mg/day iv **Alternatives** Cefotaxime 2 g tid iv Ceftriaxone 1–2 g/day iv Ceftazidime 1–2 g tid iv Cefepime 1–2 g bid iv Co-amoxiclav 1,5 g tid iv[i] Piperacillin-tazobactam 2,5–4,5 g tid iv Amikacin 15 mg/kg/day[i] Gentamicin 5 mg/kg/day[i] Ertapenem 1 g/day iv Imipenem/cilastatin 0.5/0.5 g tid iv Meropenem 1 g tid iv Doripenem 0.5 g tid iv

IDSA/ESCMID Infectious Diseases Society of America/European Society of Clinical Microbiology and Infectious Diseases, *EAU* European Association of Urology

[a] Avoid in patients with glucose-6-phosphate dehydrogenase deficiency

[b] If local resistance pattern is known (*E. coli* resistance <20%)

[c] Where the prevalence of resistance of community uropathogens to fluoroquinolones is not known to exceed 10%

[d] If the prevalence of fluoroquinolone resistance is thought to exceed 10%

[e] When the susceptibility of TMP-SMX is not known

[f] Clinical but not microbiological equivalent efficacy compared with fluoroquinolones

[g] Not for initial empirical therapy

[h] After improvement, the patient can be switched to an oral regimen using one of the agents listed for oral antimicrobial therapy in mild and moderate acute uncomplicated pyelonephritis (if active against the infecting organism) to complete 1–2 week course of therapy. Therefore, only daily dose and no duration of therapy is indicated. *bid* twice daily, *tid* thrice daily, *iv* intravenous

[i] Not studied as monotherapy in acute uncomplicated pyelonephritis

and 3.3) is considered uncomplicated. A clinical diagnosis of pyelonephritis is suspected in the presence of fever (temperature > 38°C), chills, flank pain and costovertebral-angle tenderness; other systemic symptoms such as nausea and vomiting or mental confusion can be present [3, 4, 8, 10, 20]. Symptoms suggestive for cystitis are frequently absent.

Different from suspected acute uncomplicated cystitis where urinalysis and urine culture are not routinely needed, in case of pyelonephritis, it is recommended to always perform a urine culture before starting empirical antimicrobial treatment [31]. Especially in the emergency department, patients are frequently assessed for pyuria and bacteriuria with commercially available dipstick testing for leukocyte esterase and urinary nitrites [44]. Although blood cultures are not routinely recommended in acute uncomplicated pyelonephritis given the possibility of associated bacteremia, we believe that if feasible they should be done before antibiotic treatment. The recommendations about the use of radiological techniques such as ultrasound and computed tomography in the diagnosis of acute uncomplicated pyelonephritis are outside the scope of this review, and the readers are referred to the appropriate chapters in this book dealing with this issue.

Empiric antimicrobial therapy for acute uncomplicated pyelonephritis should be started quickly once the diagnosis is entertained; as a general rule, an antibiotic with broad-spectrum *in vitro* activity against the likely uropathogens should be used (Table 3.4). Additional factors to be considered in choosing an appropriate empiric drug are the local resistance data, history of exposure to the same class of antibiotics in the recent past (a factor that increase the probability of resistance), history of allergy and, if known, antimicrobial susceptibility of previous UTI strains. Oral regimens that can be used for the outpatient treatment of less severe acute uncomplicated pyelonephritis are reported in Table 3.4. Given the high direct and indirect costs associated with hospital treatment of acute uncomplicated pyelonephritis, there is suggestion to treat most episodes in the outpatient setting, but this probably is more frequently achieved in the USA than in Europe [45–47]. Clinical severe uncomplicated pyelonephritis as well as complicated pyelonephritis (risk factors and underlying disease) should be always managed with hospitalization of the patients. Criteria for severity of uncomplicated pyelonephritis requiring hospitalization include high fever (>40°C), dehydration, hypotension and high leukocyte count.

Both IDSA/ESCMID and EAU guidelines indicate fluoroquinolones as appropriate initial empiric antibiotic for uncomplicated pyelonephritis if the prevalence of fluoroquinolone resistance of community uropathogens is known to be less than 10% [12, 31]. Otherwise a long-acting intravenous antibiotic (i.e., ceftriaxone) should precede oral therapy, or a 24-h consolidated dose of an aminoglycoside is indicated. The use of TMP-SMX should be reserved only to episodes of uncomplicated pyelonephritis caused by susceptible microorganisms, and the duration of treatment was prolonged for 14 days. Oral β-lactam agents are associated with high failure rates and should be used only when susceptibility of causal microorganisms is known and for no more than 14 days [48]. However, a meta-analysis of randomized controlled trials shows that for pyelonephritis 7 days of treatment is equivalent to longer treatment in terms of clinical and microbiological failure, but trials that included β-lactamase were old and with small number of patients [49]. For this reason it is advisable to manage

patients with short-term treatment only when fluoroquinolones are used [50].

3.3 Acute Complicated Urinary Tract Infections

As previously indicated and acknowledged by the international guidelines, the concept of complicated UTI (c-UTI) refers to both structural and functional abnormalities of the genitourinary tract or to an underlying disease that poses an increased risk of complications or therapeutic failure or poor outcome [31, 51]. This definition does not account for severity or invasiveness of the infection thus giving reason for some ambiguity relative to classification, as recently suggested [6].

Male gender "per se" is considered, when a UTI is diagnosed, responsible for c-UTI; however, in young men without systemic symptoms and no medical history and/or physical examination indicative of a causative factor, it is suggested by some authors to consider UTI as uncomplicated [51, 52]. However, structural and functional abnormalities of the urinary tract associated with male's ageing increase either the risk or the complications of UTI [53]. Among men with febrile UTI, a study reported in more than 90% of cases a transient increase of serum prostate antigen and/or prostate volume [54]. It is always important to rule out unrecognized pathologies of the urinary tract that can require surgery (i.e., prostatic hypertrophy, urethral stricture, bladder and renal stones, bladder cancer) or prolonged antibiotic treatment (i.e., chronic prostatitis) [54].

3.3.1 Special Patient Groups

Diabetes mellitus is a well-known risk factor for recurrent UTIs, complications (persistent bacteriuria, bacteremia, bilateral renal involvement, urosepsis) and development of life-threatening peculiar picture of pyelonephritis such as emphysematous pyelonephritis [55–63]. Emphysematous pyelonephritis (EPN) is an acute necrotizing infection of the kidney characterized by the presence of gas within the renal parenchyma or perinephric tissues. Seventy-eighty percent of patients with a diagnosis of EPN had diabetes mellitus. Enteric gram-negative facultative anaerobes (i.e., *E. coli*, *Klebsiella* spp., *Proteus* spp.) able to ferment glucose and lactate to carbon dioxide are the more frequently responsible microorganisms [62, 63]. Based on the extent and distribution of gas observed on CT scan, a four-tier classification of EPN has been proposed with a prognostic intent [64]. However, a recent study failed to identify a mortality predictive role of such classification [63]. Percutaneous catheter drainage together with timely start of empiric antibiotic treatment (with ceftazidime or a carbapenem) seems to be able to lower mortality from 80% to 9–13% [63, 65]. Emergency nephrectomy can be necessary in patients with rapid deterioration of the clinical picture [66].

UTIs are the most common infectious complication after kidney transplantation with a reported incidence ranging from 26% to 76% [67–69]. A 38% pooled prevalence of UTI has been reported from a meta-analysis of 13 studies with more than 3,000 patients undergoing kidney transplantation [70]. A recent study shows that kidney transplant recipient had a 72-fold higher risk for first-time hospitalization for pyelonephritis compared to matched population controls [71]. Although in the same study, a declining incidence of pyelonephritis was reported during the 20 years of observation, the researchers found a 45% higher risk of graft loss and death among patients experiencing post-transplant pyelonephritis compared to those who do not have a diagnosis of pyelonephritis [71]. Female gender was a risk factor consistently associated with development of post-transplant UTIs with a pooled odds ratio of 3.11 (CI 95% 2.10–4.13) [70–73]. Other recognized risk factors for post-transplant UTIs are presence and duration of indwelling catheter, acute rejection episodes, cadaveric organ recipients, older age and recurrent UTIs before transplantation [70, 73–75]. UTIs are generally observed in the first 3 months after transplantation with 38% diagnosed during the first post-transplant month [76, 77].

Carbapenem-resistant *Klebsiella pneumoniae* (CRKP) and ESBL-producing *K. pneumoniae*, an emerging worldwide nosocomial problem, especially frequent in southern Europe (Greece, Italy, Romania) and with devastating consequence among frail patients, have been observed also in UTI following solid organ transplantation [77–79]. It should be noted that *Enterococcus* spp. are emerging microorganisms responsible for UTIs in the transplant setting with prevalence of 33–44% [77, 80]. Appropriate treatment of these infections poses several difficulties because of the profile of resistance especially for *E. faecium*.

Pregnant women are considered at increased risk of UTIs and those with asymptomatic bacteriuria also at increased risk of developing pyelonephritis compared to women without bacteriuria [13, 81]. Although most guidelines recommend screening for asymptomatic bacteriuria (ASB) as a routine pregnancy practice, a recent qualitative review failed to identify reliable evidence supporting screening for ASB in pregnancy probably as a consequence of the availability only of old studies and several methodological shortcomings [13, 82–84]. However, recent studies reported an incidence of acute antepartum pyelonephritis ranging from 0.5% to 1.3% which is less than historical reports [85–87]. Moreover, a randomized controlled trial aiming to assess the consequences of treated and untreated ASB in pregnant women did not show any difference using a composite end point (pyelonephritis and preterm birth) [88]. Although a significant association of ASB with pyelonephritis was evident (2.4% vs 0.6%, AOR 3.9), the absolute risk of pyelonephritis in untreated ASB is low [88]. As a rule, pregnant women with acute pyelonephritis should be hospitalized and treated with parenteral antibiotics is generally recommended [89].

Catheter-associated urinary tract infection (CA-UTI) represents the most common healthcare-associated infection worldwide with a four-fold increased risk of UTI compared to those without a urinary catheter [90, 91]. Placement of an indwelling urinary catheter is associated with the risk of development of bacteriuria of 3–10% per day, and by day 30 bacteriuria is considered universal [92–94]. The definition of CA-UTI is an infection occurring in an individual that is currently catheterized or has been catheterized within the past 48 h along with >10^3 CFU/mL of >1 bacterial species cultured from a single catheter urine specimen [90]. However, because signs and symptoms compatible with CA-UTI are nonspecific (i.e., new onset or worsening fever, malaise, altered mental status, lethargy), other possible infectious causes should be excluded before attributing them to catheter-associated bacteriuria. The actual definition of CA-UTI was introduced in 2009 excluding catheter-associated asymptomatic bacteriuria, a condition not requiring antimicrobial treatment [95]. Bacteremia is another complication of CA-UTI with an associated mortality of 9% [96]. *E. coli* is the single organism more frequently isolated in patients with bacteriuria after short-term catheterization, whereas infections among patients with long-term catheterization are generally polymicrobial and frequently with a reduced spectrum of susceptibility to most class of antibiotics [90, 97, 98]. The spectrum of microorganisms includes *Klebsiella* spp., *Enterobacter* spp., *Pseudomonas aeruginosa*, coagulase-negative staphylococci, *Enterococcus* spp., *Providencia* spp., *Proteus* spp., *Morganella* spp. and *Candida* species [99, 100]. The best way to avoid CA-UTI is to place a urinary catheter only when strictly indispensable as indicated by international guidelines as well as an early removal of it [90, 101]. Antibiotic prophylaxis is generally not recommended on the basis of weak evidences suggesting a protective role only in some settings [102–104]. Moreover, the worldwide increase in the rate of antibiotic resistance and the limited options of effective drugs in nosocomial-acquired infections are other reasons for not using prophylaxis for catheterized patients.

3.3.2 Management of Complicated UTI

Before starting an antibiotic treatment, c-UTI patients should undergo a urine culture as well as a blood culture when it is appropriate. Recommendations regarding empirical treatment of c-UTI that can be applied to every circumstance and every patient are obviously unfeasible, and therefore it is not surprising that there are no published consensus guidelines. The appropriate antibiotic choice should consider the characteristic of the patient (i.e., age, drug allergies, comorbidity), the severity of the infection, the spectrum of possible uropathogens implicated and the knowledge of surveillance national and local data regarding patterns of susceptibility of the different microorganisms [105, 106]. Moreover, the pharmacokinetic/pharmacodynamic characteristics of the drugs and their possible interactions should be considered in the appropriate choice. In general, fluoroquinolones are useless for urologic patients, when they were previously used for the same patient and in areas with more than 10% fluoroquinolone resistance. Carbapenem antibiotics have long been considered the drugs of choice for infections caused by ESBL-producing microorganisms [107]. However, the increasing isolation of carbapenem-resistant Enterobacteriaceae (CRE) clearly suggests the use of carbapenem-sparing regimens when appropriate. Cefepime and piperacillin-tazobactam may be reasonably alternative against ESBL-producing *E. coli* and *Klebsiella* spp. when the minimum inhibitory concentrations (MICs) are <2 μg/mL for the former drug and <16 μg/mL for the latter drug [108–110]. Ceftolozane-tazobactam, a recently approved combination of a cephalosporin with a β-lactamase inhibitor, provides better efficacy than levofloxacin in adults with c-UTI, including pyelonephritis [111, 112]. This is a drug of niche for c-UTI and should be reserved only for carbapenem-sparing regimens when other alternatives are not suitable and for multidrug-resistant (MDR) *Pseudomonas aeruginosa*. Another carbapenem-sparing drug regimen that can be used for c-UTI caused by MDR microorganisms is the combination of ceftazidime with avibactam, a non-β-lactam β-lactamase inhibitor which is able to restore the in vitro activity of ceftazidime against ESBL and *K. pneumoniae* carbapenemase and Ambler Class C (i.e., AmpC) and some class D β-lactamase-producing bacteria. It is not active against metallo-β-lactamase. In a randomized controlled trial, ceftazidime-avibactam demonstrates superiority versus doripenem for the treatment of c-UTI including acute pyelonephritis [113]. However, to preserve its efficacy as a salvage therapy for CRE, the use of ceftazidime-avibactam should be reserved for severe c-UTI caused by MDR microorganisms [114].

3.4   Urosepsis

Urosepsis is generally defined as a sepsis in which the source of the infection is the urinary tract and/or the prostate (in males) [115]. Urosepsis represents about 25% of all cases of adult sepsis and 5% of cases evolving to severe sepsis and septic shock [116, 117].

Obstructive uropathy is responsible for about 78% of cases of urosepsis with urolithiasis being the most frequent cause [118, 119]. A recent systematic review that aimed to identify risk factors for urosepsis and urosepsis-related mortality in older adults concluded for the lack of quality evidence regarding risk factors [120]. It should be recognized that a new sepsis definition published in 2016 has been adopted, but several concerns have raised, and its applicability in the field of urosepsis is presently unknown [121–123]. The administration of an initially adequate intravenous antibiotic is essential for optimal outcome, but inadequate coverage in urosepsis may be a problem due to the lack of solid microbiological data [124]. In a German study regarding sepsis, the bacterial spectrum of urosepsis consisted of *E. coli* in 61% of cases, followed by other enterobacteria in 16%, *S. aureus* in 8% and enterococci in 6% of cases [125]. A recent point prevalence study conducted in 70 countries from 2003 to 2013 shows that the overall prevalence of *E. coli* as a cause of urosepsis was 43% followed by *Enterococcus* spp. (11%) and *Klebsiella* spp. (10%) and *Pseudomonas aeruginosa* (10%) [126]. Patients with a diagnosis of urosepsis had the highest resistance rates to all class of antibiotics compared with patients with other healthcare-associated urinary tract infections (HAUTI) [126]. Overall resistance to fluoroquinolone in Europe was reported to be 59%, 42% for ceftazidime and 34% for piperacillin-tazobactam, but as highlighted knowledge of local resistance

rates is essential. More recent data from EARS-Net, the largest European surveillance system on antimicrobial resistance, shows that for *E. coli* isolates from invasive infections, the population-weighted mean percentage for fluoroquinolone resistance is 22.8% in 2015 [78]. However, eight countries (Greece, Romania, Spain, Bulgaria, Malta, Slovakia, Italy and Cyprus) had resistance prevalence higher than 30%. Among the *E. coli* isolates that are resistant to third-generation cephalosporins (mean percentage 13.1%), 88.6% were ESBL-positive. The resistance to carbapenems of *E. coli* in Europe remained rare with only two countries (Greece and Romania) with reported resistance rates above 1%. Combined resistance to third-generation cephalosporins, fluoroquinolones and aminoglycosides ranged from 0% (Iceland) to 17.1% (Slovakia) [78]. Antibiotic resistance against *K. pneumoniae* is a cause of concern in Europe with more than one third of isolates reported in 2015 that were resistant to at least one antimicrobial under surveillance (i.e., fluoroquinolones, aminoglycosides, third-generation cephalosporins and carbapenems) and 4.7% of all *K. pneumoniae* isolates resistant to all groups of antibiotics. An increasing rise of carbapenem-resistant strains was observed with three countries (Greece, Italy and Romania) with reported resistance percentages higher than any other country (61.9%, 33.5% and 24.7%, respectively) [78]. Moreover, the high percentages of ESBL-positive *K. pneumoniae* resistant to third-generation cephalosporins (85.3%) may lead to an increased use of carbapenems with an obvious increase of carbapenemase-producing Enterobacteriaceae. As far as *Pseudomonas aeruginosa* is concerned, MDR was observed cumulative for 5.5% of the isolates with also a confirmed increasing trend of resistance to piperacillin-tazobactam (from 16.7% in 2012 to 18.1% in 2015) [78]. Carbapenems resistance of *P. aeruginosa* is also high (>25% of isolates) in eight countries (Bulgaria, Lithuania, Hungary, Poland, Croatia, Greece, Slovakia and Romania). High-level gentamicin resistance of *Enterococcus faecalis* was reported in 31.3% of isolates in 2015 with seven countries (Spain, Bulgaria, Lithuania, Hungary, Poland, Italy, Slovakia) having percentages higher than 40%. A significant increase of vancomycin-resistant *E. faecium* was observed in 12 countries, although the increase at European level from 2012 to 2015 (8.1% and 8.3%) was not statistically significant. Since enterococci have intrinsic resistance to several classes of antibiotics and display the ability to acquire additional resistance, the epidemiologic situation regarding these bacteria is harmful owing to their role in HAUTI.

When urosepsis is suspected, blood cultures are mandatory before starting empiric antimicrobial therapy, whereas urine cultures have a low sensitivity and specificity in the presence of obstructive pyelonephritis [118]. Procalcitonin (PCT) is the best and more rapid biomarker of systemic inflammation and if available should be used for patients with suspected urosepsis. In a prospective observational study, a single determination using a cut-off of PCT > 0.25 µg/L had the best diagnostic performance (sensitivity 95%, specificity 50%) in predicting bacteremia among patients with urosepsis [127]. Despite the fact that the investigators of the above-cited trial suggested that adopting a PCT threshold of <0.25 µg/L can be associated with a 40% of blood culture utilization, we believe that the appropriate use of PCT in this setting is not as a blood culture sparing biomarker but as a guide to stop antibiotics [128].

3.5 Recurrent UTI

Recurrent UTI is frequently observed among young healthy women without any urological alteration, and it is defined as three or more urinary tract infections in the past 12 months or two episodes in the past 6 months (with at least one confirmed by a positive culture) [27]. Although several risk factors have been identified or suspected (use of spermicides; sexual intercourse; new sexual partner; tampon use; a relative with history of UTI), counselling and behavioural modifications as preventive measures are generally of little efficacy. Non-antimicrobial prophylaxis with immunoactive products (i.e., OM-89) and probiotics (i.e., intravaginal products containing *Lactobacillus* spp.), drinking cranberry (*Vaccinium macrocarpon*) juice and the use of

adhesion blockers (i.e., d-mannose) are sometimes useful [8, 12, 129]. Antimicrobial prophylaxis with long-term low dose antibiotics or post-coital antibiotic prophylaxis is the alternative strategy. It is generally employed with nitrofurantoin (100 mg per day), cephalexin (250 mg daily), fosfomycin (3 g every 10 days) or trimethoprim-sulfamethoxazole (40/200 mg daily) with an important reduction of the risk of recurrences [27, 130]. It should be highlighted that after stopping prophylaxis, women experience pretreatment rates of infection. Moreover, the increasing antimicrobial resistance needs to be considered because many antibiotics commonly employed to treat UTI are now ineffective [131]. Finally, the so-called patient-initiated treatment strategy should be considered for motivated women. This means that women learn to recognize signs and symptoms of cystitis and undergo a self-treatment with a 3-day course of an antimicrobial [27, 129].

Conclusions

Urinary tract infections are among the most frequent infectious complications with a high impact in terms of suffering for the patients and cost for the healthcare systems. The increasing worldwide antimicrobial resistance of Enterobacteriaceae with ESBL and carbapenemase-producing microorganisms poses a high risk of treatment failure especially among hospitalized frail patients. Antimicrobial stewardship programme should be urgently implemented, and physicians need to be aware of "collateral damage" induced by several antibiotics and educated to use them accordingly with the appropriate guidelines.

References

1. Schappert SM, Rechtsteiner EA (2011) Ambulatory medical care utilization estimates for 2007. Vital Health Stat 169:1–38
2. Rossignol L, Vaux S, Maugat S, Blake A, Barlier R, Heym B et al (2017) Incidence of urinary tract infections and antibiotic resistance in the outpatient setting: a cross-sectional study. Infection 45:33–40

3. Schneeberger C, Holleman F, Geerlings SE (2016) Febrile urinary tract infections: pyelonephritis and urosepsis. Curr Opin Infect Dis 29:80–85

4. Stalenhoef JE, van Dissel JT, van Nieuwkoop C (2015) Febrile urinary tract infection in the emergency room. Curr Opin Infect Dis 28:106–111

5. Walker E, Lyman A, Gupta K, Mahoney MV, Snyder GM, Hirsch EB (2016) Clinical management of an increasing threat: outpatient urinary tract infections due to multidrug-resistant uropathogens. Clin Infect Dis 63:960–965

6. Johnson JR (2017) Definition of complicated urinary tract infection. Clin Infect Dis 64(4):529

7. Rubin USE, Andriole VT, Davis RJ, Stamm WE (1992) Evaluation of new anti-infective drugs for the treatment of UTI. Clin Infect Dis 15:216

8. Hooton TM (2012) Uncomplicated urinary tract infection. N Engl J Med 366:1028–1037

9. Pietrucha-Dilanchian P, Hooton TM (2016) Diagnosis, treatment and prevention of urinary tract infection. Microbiol Spectr 4(6). doi:101128/microbiolspec.UIT-0021-2015

10. Bjerklund Johansen TE, Botto H, Cek M, Grabe M, Tenke P, Wagenlehner FME, Naber KG (2011) Critical review of current definitions of urinary tract infections and proposal of an EAU/ESIU classification system. Int J Antimicrob Agents 38(Suppl):64–70

11. Smelov V, Naber K, Bjerklund Johansen TE (2016) Improved classification of urinary tract infection: future considerations. Eur Urol Suppl 15:71–80

12. Grabe M, Bartoletti R, Bjerklund Johansen TE, Cai T, Cek M, Koves B et al (2015) Guidelines on urological infections. European Association of Urology, The Netherlands

13. Nicolle LE, Bradley S, Colgan R, Rice JC, Schaeffer A, Hooton TM (2005) Infectious disease Society of America Guidelines for the diagnosis and treatment of asymptomatic bacteriuria in adults. Clin Infect Dis 40:643–654

14. Patterson TF, Andriole VT (1997) Detection, significance, and therapy of bacteriuria in pregnancy. Update in the managed health care era. Infect Dis Clin N Am 11:593–608

15. Smaill F, Vazquez JC (2007) Antibiotics for asymptomatic bacteriuria in pregnancy. Cochrane Database Syst Rev 8:CD000490

16. Mittendorf R, Williams MA, Kass EH (1992) Prevention of preterm delivery and low birth weight associated with asymptomatic bacteriuria. Clin Infect Dis 14:927–932

17. Romero R, Oyarzun E, Mazor M, Sirtori M, Hobbins JC, Bracken M (1989) Meta-analysis of the relationship between asymptomatic bacteriuria and preterm delivery/low birth weight. Obstet Gynecol 73:576–582

18. Shapiro T, Dalton M, Hammock J, Lavery R, Matiucha J, Salo DF (2005) The prevalence of urinary tract infections and sexually transmitted disease in women with symptoms of simple urinary tract infection stratified by low colony count criteria. Acad Emerg Med 12:38–44

19. Armed Forces Health Surveillance Center (2014) Relationships between diagnoses of sexually transmitted infections and urinary tract infections among male service members diagnosed with urethritis, active component, US Armed Forces, 2000–2013. MSMR 21:14–17

20. Bent S, Nallamothu BK, Simel DL, Finh SD, Saint S (2002) Does this woman have an acute uncomplicated urinary tract infection? JAMA 287:2701–2710

21. Tomas ME, German D, Donskey CJ, Hecker MT (2015) Overdiagnosis of urinary tract infection and underdiagnosis of sexually transmitted infection in adult women presenting to an emergency department. J Clin Microbiol 53:2686–2692

22. Foxman B, Brown P (2003) Epidemiology of urinary tract infection transmission and risk factors, incidence, and costs. Infect Dis Clin N Am 17:227–241

23. Foxman B, Barlow R, D'Arcy H, Gillespie B, Sobel JD (2000) Urinary tract infection: self-reported incidence and associated costs. Ann Epidemiol 160:509–515

24. Hooton TM, Scholes D, Hughes JP, Winter C, Roberts PL, Stapleton AE et al (1996) A prospective study of risk factors for symptomatic urinary tract infection in young women. N Engl J Med 335:468–474

25. Scholes D, Hooton TM, Roberts PL, Stapleton AE, Gupta K, Stamm WE (2000) Risk factors for recurrent UTI in young women. J Infect Dis 182:1177–1182

26. Scholes D, Hawn TR, Roberts PL, Li SS, Stapleton AE, Zhao LP et al (2010) Family history and risk of recurrent cystitis and pyelonephritis in women. J Urol 184:564–569

27. Hooton TM (2001) Recurrent urinary tract infection in women. Int J Antimicrob Agents 17:259–268

28. Dielubanza EJ, Schaeffer AJ (2011) Urinary tract infections in women. Med Clin North Am 95:27–41

29. Ronald A (2002) The etiology of urinary tract infection: traditional and emerging pathogens. Am J Med 113(Suppl.1A):9S–14S

30. Barber A, Norton JP, Spivak AM, Mulvey MA (2013) Urinary tract infections: current and emerging management strategies. Clin Infect Dis 57:719–724

31. Gupta K, Hooton TM, Naber KG, Wullt B, Colgan R, Miller LG et al (2011) Executive summary: international clinical practice guidelines for the treatment of acute uncomplicated cystitis and pyelonephritis in women: a 2010 update by the Infectious Diseases Society of America and the European Society for Microbiology and Infectious Diseases. Clin Infect Dis 52:561–564

32. Sanchez GV, Master RN, Bordon J (2011) Trimethoprim-sulfamethoxazole may no longer be acceptable for the treatment of acute uncomplicated cystitis in the United States. Clin Infect Dis 53:316–317

33. Zhanel GG, Hisanaga TL, Laing NM, DeCorby MR, Nichol KA, Weshnoweski B et al (2006) Antibiotic resistance in *Escherichia coli* outpatient urinary isolates: final results from the North American Urinary Tract Infection Collaborative Alliance (NAUTICA). Int J Antimicrob Agents 27:468–475

34. Schito GC, Naber KG, Botto H, Palou J, Mazzei T, Gualco L et al (2009) The ARESC study: an international survey on the antimicrobial resistance of pathogens involved in uncomplicated urinary tract infections. Int J Antimicrob Agents 34:407–413

35. Katsarolis I, Poulakou G, Athanasia S, Kourea-Kremastinou J, Lambri N, Karaiskos E et al (2010) Acute uncomplicated cystitis: from surveillance data to a rationale for empirical treatment. Int J Antimicrob Agents 35:62–67

36. Colgan R, Johnson JR, Kuskowski M, Gupta K (2008) Risk factors for trimethoprim-sulfamethoxazole resistance in patients with acute uncomplicated cystitis. Antimicrob Agents Chemother 52:846–851

37. Oplinger M, Andrew CO (2013) Nitrofurantoin contraindication in patients with a creatinine clearance below 60 ml/min: looking for the evidence. Ann Pharmacother 47:106–111

38. Campanelli CM (2012) American Geriatrics Society 2012 beers criteria update expert panel. America geriatrics society updated beers criteria for potentially inappropriate medication use in older adults. J Am Geriatr Soc 60:616–631

39. Paterson DL (2004) "Collateral damage" from cephalosporin or quinolone antibiotic therapy. Clin Infect Dis 38(Suppl 4):S341–S345

40. Kobayashi M, Shapiro DJ, Hersh AL, Sanchez GV, Hicks LA (2016) Outpatient antibiotic prescribing practices for uncomplicated urinary tract infection in women in the United States, 2002–2011. Open Forum Infect Dis 3:ofw159

41. Drekonja DM, Rector TS, Cutting A, Johnson JR (2013) Urinary tract infection in male veterans: treatment patterns and outcomes. JAMA Intern Med 173:62–68

42. Meier S, Weber R, Zhinden R, Ruef C, Hasse B (2011) Extended-spectrum beta-lactamase-producing gram-negative pathogens in community-acquired urinary tract infections. An increasing challenge for antimicrobial therapy. Infection 39:333–340

43. Lob SH, Nicolle LE, Hoban DJ, Kazmierczak K, Badal RE, Sahm DF (2016) Susceptibility patterns and ESBL rates of *Escherichia coli* from urinary tract infections in Canada and the United States, SMART 2010–2014. Diagn Microbiol Infect Dis 85:459–465

44. Takhar SS, Moran GJ (2014) Diagnosis and management of urinary tract infection in the emergency department and outpatient settings. Infect Dis Clin N Am 28:33–48

45. Brown P, Ki M, Foxman B (2005) Acute pyelonephritis among adults: cost of illness and considerations for the economic evaluation of therapy. PharmacoEconomics 23:1123–1142

46. Czaja CA, Scholes D, Hooton TM, Stamm WE (2007) Population-based epidemiologic analysis of acute pyelonephritis. Clin Infect Dis 45:273–280

47. Nicolle LE (2008) Uncomplicated urinary tract infection in adults including uncomplicated pyelonephritis. Urol Clin North Am 35:1–12

48. Hooton TM, Roberts PL, Stapleton AE (2012) Cefpodoxime vs ciprofloxacin for short-course treatment of acute uncomplicated cystitis: a randomized trial. JAMA 307:583–589

49. Eliakim-Raz N, Yahav D, Paul M, Leibovici L (2013) Duration of antibiotic treatment for acute pyelonephritis and septic urinary tract infection-7 days or less versus longer treatment: systematic review and meta-analysis of randomized controlled trials. J Antimicrob Chemother 68:2183–2191

50. Sandberg T, Skoog G, Hermansson AB, Kahlmeter G, Kuylenstierna N, Lannergard A et al (2012) Ciprofloxacin for 7 days versus 14 days in women with acute pyelonephritis: a randomised, open-label and double-blind, placebo-controlled, non-inferiority trial. Lancet 380:484–490

51. Geerlings SE (2016) Clinical presentations and epidemiology of urinary tract infections. Microbiol Spectrum 4(5). UTI-0002-2012). https://doi.org/10.1128/microbiobiolspec.UTI-0002-2012

52. Krieger JN, Ross SO, Simonsen JM (1993) Urinary tract infections in healthy university men. J Urol 149:1046–1048

53. Schaeffer AJ, Nicolle LE (2016) Urinary tract infections in older men. N Engl J Med 374:562–571

54. Ulleryd P, Zackrisson B, Aus G, Bergdahl S, Hugosson J, Sandberg T (1999) Prostatic involvement in men with febrile urinary tract infection as measured by serum prostate-specific antigen and transrectal ultrasonography. BJU Int 84:470–474

55. Boyko EJ, Fihn SD, Scholes D, Chen CL, Normand EH, Yarbro P (2002) Diabetes and the risk of acute urinary tract infection among post-menopausal women. Diabetes Care 25:1778–1783

56. Shah BR, Hux JE (2003) Quantifying the risk of infectious disease for people with diabetes. Diabetes Care 26:510–513

57. Carton JA, Maradona JA, Nuno FJ, Fernandez-Alvarez R, Perez-Gonzalez F, Asensi V (1992) Diabetes mellitus and bacteraemia: a comparative study between diabetic and non-diabetic patients. Eur J Med 1:281–287

58. Horcajada JP, Moreno I, Velasco M, Martinez JA, Moreno-Martinez A, Barranco M et al (2003) Community-acquired febrile urinary tract infection in diabetics could deserve a different management: a case-control study. J Intern Med 254:280–286

59. Kofteridis DP, Papademitraki E, Mantadakis E, Maraki S, Papadakis JA, Tzifa G et al (2009) Effect of diabetes mellitus and the clinical and microbiological features of hospitalized elderly patients with acute pyelonephritis. J Am Geriatr Soc 57:2125–2128

60. Bjurlin MA, Hurley SD, Kim DY, Cohn MR, Jordan MD, Kim R et al (2012) Clinical outcomes of nonoperative management in emphysematous urinary tract infections. Urology 79:1281–1285

61. Thomas AA, Lane BR, Thomas AZ, Remer EM, Campbell SC, Shoskes DA (2007) Emphysematous cystitis: a review of 135 cases. BJU Int 100:17–20

62. Y-C L, Chiang B-J, Pong Y-U, Chen C-H, Y-S P, Hsueh P-R et al (2014) Emphysematous pyelonephritis: clinical characteristics and prognostic factors. Int J Urol 21:277–282

63. Y-C L, Hong J-H, Chiang B-J, Pong Y-U, Hsueh P-R, Huang C-Y et al (2016) Recommended initial antimicrobial therapy for emphysematous pyelonephritis. 51 Cases and 14-year-experience of a tertiary referral center. Medicine 95:e3573

64. Huang JJ, Tseng CC (2000) Emphysematous pyelonephritis: clinicoradiological classification, management, prognosis, and pathogenesis. Arch Intern Med 160:797–805

65. Somani BK, Nabi G, Thorpe P, Hussey J, Cook J, N'Dow J (2008) ABACUS research group. Is percutaneous drainage the new gold standard in the management of emphysematous pyelonephritis? Evidence from a systematic review. J Urol 179:1844–1849

66. Moutzouris DA, Michalakis K, Manetas S (2006) Severe emphysematous pyelonephritis in diabetic patient. Lancet Infect Dis 6:614

67. Takai K, Tollemar J, Wilczek HE, Groth CG (1998) Urinary tract infections following renal transplantation. Clin Transpl 12:19–23

68. Pellé G, Vimont S, Levy PP, Hertig A, Ouali N, Chassin C et al (2007) Acute pyelonephritis represents a risk factor impairing long-term kidney graft function. Am J Transpl 7:899–907

69. Karakayali R, Emiroglu R, Arslan G, Bilgin N, Haberal M (2001) Major infectious complications after kidney transplantation. Transplant Proc 33:1816–1817

70. Wu X, Dong Y, Liu Y, Li X, Sun Y, Wang J et al (2016) The prevalence and predictive factors of urinary tract infection in patients undergoing renal transplantation. A meta-analysis. Am J Infect Control 44:1261–1268

71. Graversen ME, Dalgaard LS, Jensen-Fangel S, Jespersen B, Ostergaard L, Sogaard OS (2016) Risk and outcome of pyelonephritis among renal transplant recipients. BMC Infect Dis 16:264

72. Lee JR, Bang H, Dadhania D, Hartono C, Aull MJ, Satlin M et al (2013) Independent risk factors for urinary tract infection and for subsequent bacteremia or acute cellular rejection. A single-center report of 1166 kidney allograft recipients. Transplantation 96:732–738

73. Parasuraman R, Julian K (2013) The AST infectious diseases community of practice. Urinary tract infections in solid organ transplantation. Am J Transplant 13:327–336

74. Nicolle LE (2014) Urinary tract infections in special populations. diabetes, renal transplant, HIV infection, and spinal cord injury. Infect Dis Clin N Am 28:91–104

75. Singh R, Geerlings SE, Peters-Sengers H, Idu MM, Hodiamont CJ, ten Berge IJM et al (2016) Incidence, risk factors, and the impact of allograft pyelonephritis on renal allograft function. Transpl Infect Dis 18:647–660

76. Valera B, Gentil MA, Cabello V, Fijo J, Cordero E, Cisneros JM (2006) Epidemiology of urinary infections in renal transplant recipients. Transplant Proc 38:2414–2415

77. Golebiewska JE, Debska-Slizien A, Rutkowski B (2014) Urinary tract infections during the first year after renal transplantation:one center's experience and a review of the literature. Clin Transpl 28:1263–1270

78. European Centre for Disease Prevention and Control. Antimicrobial resistance surveillance in Europe (2017) 2015 Annual report of the European Antimicrobial Resistance Surveillance Network (EARS-Net). ECD, Stockholm

79. Brizendine KD, Richter SS, Cober ED, van Duin D (2015) Carbapenem-resistant *Klebsiella pneumoniae* urinary tract infection following solid organ transplantation. Antimicrob Agents Chemother 59:553–557

80. Bonkat G, Rieken M, Siegel FP, Frei R, Steiger J, Groschl L et al (2012) Microbial ureteral stent colonization in renal transplant recipients: frequency and influence on the short-time functional outcome. Transpl Infect Dis 14:57–63

81. Gilstrap LC III, Ramin SM (2001) Urinary tract infections during pregnancy. Obstet Gynecol Clin N Am 28:581–591

82. US Preventive Services Task Force (2008) Screening for asymptomatic bacteriuria in adults: US preventive services task force reaffirmation recommendation statement. Ann Intern Med 149:43–47

83. National Collaborating Centre for Women's and Children's Health (2008) Antenatal care: routine care for the healthy pregnant women. RCOG Press, London

84. Angelescu K, Nussbaumer-Streit B, Sieben W, Schibler F, Gartlehner G (2016) Benefits and harms of screening for and treatment of asymptomatic bacteriuria in pregnancy: a systematic review. BMC Pregnancy Childbirth 16:336

85. Sharma P, Thapa L (2007) Acute pyelonephritis in pregnancy: a retrospective study. Aust N Z Obstet Gynaecol 47:313–315

86. Wing DA, Fassett MJ, Getahun D (2014) Acute pyelonephritis in pregnancy: an 18-year retrospective analysis. Am J Obstet Gynecol 210:219.e1–219.e6

87. Bacak SJ, Callaghan WM, Diets PM, Crouse C (2005) Pregnancy-associated hospitalizations in the United States, 1999–2000. Am J Obstet Gynecol 192:592–597

88. Kazemier BM, Koningstein FN, Schneeberger C, Ott A, Bossuyt PM, de Miranda E et al (2015) Maternal and neonatal consequences of treated and untreated asymptomatic bacteriuria in pregnancy: a prospective cohort study with an embedded randomised controlled trial. Lancet Infect Dis 15:1324–1333

89. Wing DA (2001) Pyelonephritis in pregnancy: treatment options for optimal outcomes. Drugs 61:2087–2096

90. Hooton TM, Bradley SF, Cardenas DD, Colgan R, Geerlings SE, Rice JC et al (2010) Diagnosis, prevention, and treatment of catheter-associated urinary tract infection in adults: 2009 International Clinical practice Guidelines from the Infectious Diseases Society of America. Clin Infect Dis 50:625–663

91. Foxman B (2014) Urinary tract infection syndromes: occurrence, recurrence, bacteriology, risk factors, and disease burden. Infect Dis Clin N Am 28:1–13

92. Chenoweth CE, Saint S (2011) Urinary tract infections. Infect Dis Clin N Am 25:103–115

93. Saint S, Lipsky BA, Goold SD (2001) Indwelling urinary catheters: a one-point restraint? Ann Intern Med 137:125–127

94. Warren JW, Tenney JH, Hoopes JM, Muncie HL, Anthony WC (1982) A prospective microbiologic study of bacteriuria in patients with chronic indwelling urethral catheters. J Infect Dis 146:719–723

95. Press MJ, Metlay JP (2013) Catheter-associated urinary tract infection:does changing the definition change quality? Infect Control Hosp Epidemiol 34:313–315

96. Ortega M, Marco F, Soriano A, Almela M, Martinez JA, Pitart C et al (2013) Epidemiology and prognostic determinants of bacteraemic catheter-acquired urinary tract infection in a single institution from 1991 to 2010. J Infect 67:282–287

97. Warren JW (1997) Catheter-associated urinary tract infections. Infect Dis Clin N Am 11:609–622

98. Jacobsen SM, Stickler DJ, Mobley HL, Shirtliff ME (2008) Complicated catheter-associated urinary tract infections due to *Escherichia coli* and *Proteus mirabilis*. Clin Microbiol Infect 21:26–59

99. Nicolle LE (2005) Catheter-related urinary tract infection. Drugs Aging 22:627–639

100. Tenke P, Koves B, Johansen TEB (2014) An update on prevention and treatment of catheter-associated urinary tract infections. Curr Opin Infect Dis 27:102–107

101. Wald HL, Ma A, Bratzler DW, Kramer AM (2008) Indwelling urinary catheter use in the postoperative period: analysis of the national surgical infection prevention project data. Arch Surg 143:551–557

102. Lusardi G, Lipp A, Shaw C (2013) Antibiotic prophylaxis for short-term catheter bladder drainage in adults. Cochrane Database Syst Rev 7:CD005428

103. Marschall J, Carpenter CR, Fowler S, Trautner BW, Prevention Epicenters Program CDC (2013) Antibiotic prophylaxis for urinary tract infections after removal of urinary catheter: meta-analysis. BMJ 346:f3147

104. Niel-Weise BS, van den Broek PJ, da Silva EM, Silva LA (2012) Urinary catheter policies for long-term bladder drainage. Cochrane Database Syst Rev 8:CD004201

105. Koningstein M, van der Bij AK, de Kraker MEA, Monen JC, Muilwijk J, de Greeff SC et al (2014) Recommendations for the empirical treatment of complicated urinary tract infections using surveillance data on antimicrobial resistance in the Netherlands. PLoS One 9:e86634

106. Pallett A, Hand K (2010) Complicated urinary tract infections: practical solutions for the treatment of multiresistant gram-negative bacteria. J Antimicrob Chemother 65(Suppl.3):iii25–iii33

107. Toussaint KA, Gallagher JC (2015) Beta-lactam/beta-lactamase inhibitor combinations: from there to now. Ann Pharmacother 49:86–98

108. Nguyen HM, Shier KL, Grabber CJ (2014) Determining clinical framework for use of cefepime and beta-lactam/beta-lactamase inhibitors in the treatment of infections caused by extended-spectrum-beta-lactamase-producing Enterobacteriaceae. J Antimicrob Chemother 69:871–880

109. Pak SH, Choi SM, Chang YK, Lee DG, Cho SY, Lee HJ et al (2014) The efficacy of non-carbapenem antibiotics for the treatment of community-onset acute pyelonephritis due to extended-spectrum beta-lactamase-producing *Escherichia coli*. J Antimicrob Chemother 69:2848–2856

110. Rodriguez-Bano J, Navarro MD, Retamar P, Picon E, Pascual A (2012) Beta-lactam/beta-lactam inhibitor combinations for the treatment of bacteremia due to extended-spectrum beta-lactamase producing *Escherichia coli*: a post hoc analysis of prospective cohorts. Clin Infect Dis 54:167–174

111. Wagenlethner FM, Umeh O, Steenbergen J, Yuan G, Darouiche RO (2015) Ceftolozane-tazobactam compared with levofloxacin in the treatment of complicated urinary-tract infections, including pyelonephritis: a randomised, double-blind, phase 3 trial (ASPECT-cUTI). Lancet 385:1949–1956

112. Scott LJ (2016) Ceftolozane-tazobactam: a review in complicated intra-abdominal and urinary tract infections. Drugs 76:231–242

113. Wagenlehner FM, Sobel JD, Newell P, Armstrong J, Huang X, Stone GG et al (2016) Ceftazidime-avibactam versus doripenem for the treatment of complicated urinary tract infections, including acute pyelonephritis: RECAPTURE, a phase 3 randomized trial program. Clin Infect Dis 63:754–762

114. Temkin E, Torre-Cisneros J, Beovic B, Benito N, Giannella M, Gilarranz R et al (2017) Ceftazidime-avibactam as salvage therapy for infections caused by carbapenem-resistant organisms. Antimicrob Agents Chemother 61:e01964–e01916

115. Wagenlehner FME, Pilatz A, Weidners W (2011) Urosepsis-from the view of the urologist. Int J Antimicrob Agents 385:51–57

116. Hotchkiss RS, Karl IE (2003) The pathophysiology and treatment of sepsis. N Engl J Med 348:138–150

117. Bouza E, San Juan R, Munoz P, Voss A, Kluytmans J (2001) A European perspective on nosocomial urinary tract infections. I. Report on the microbiology workload, etiology and antimicrobial susceptibility (ESGNI-003 study). European Study Group on Nosocomial Infections. Clin Microbiol Infect 7:523–531

118. Dreger MN, Degener S, Ahmad-Nejad P, Wobker G, Roth S (2015) Urosepsis-etiology, diagnosis and treatment. Dtsch Arztebl Int 112:837–848

119. Serniak PS, Denisov VK, Guba GB, Zakharov VV, Chernobritsev PA, Berko EM et al (1990) The diagnosis of urosepsis. Urol Nefrol (Mosk) 4:9–13

120. Peach BC, Garvan GJ, Garvan CS, Cimiotti JP (2016) Risk factors for urosepsis in older adults: a systematic review. Gerontol Geriatr Med 2:1–7

121. Singer M, Deutschman CS, Seymour CW, Shankar-Hari M, Annane D, Bauer M et al (2016) The third international consensus definitions for sepsis and septic shock (Sepsis-3). JAMA 315:801–810

122. Simpson SQ (2016) New sepsis criteria: a change we should not make. Chest 149:1117–1118

123. Wagenlenher FME, Tandogdu Z, Bierklund Johansen TE (2017) An update on classification and management of urosepsis. Curr Opin Urol 27: 133–137

124. Flaherty SK, Weberr RL, Chase M, Dugas AF, Graver AM, Salciccioli ED et al (2014) Septic shock and adequacy of early empiric antibiotics in the emergency department. J Emerg Med 47: 601–607

125. Rosenthal EJ (2002) Epidemiology of septicaemia pathogens. Dtsch Med Wochenschr 127:2435–2440

126. Tandogdu Z, Bartoletti R, Cai T, Cek M, Grabe M, Kulchavenya E et al (2016) Antimicrobial resistance in urosepsis: outcomes from the multinational, multicenter global prevalence of infections in urology (GPIU) study 2003–2013. World J Urol 34:1193–1200

127. van Nieuwkoop C, Bonten TN, van't Wout JW, Kuijper EJ, Groeneveld GH, Becker MJ et al (2010) Procalcitonin reflects bacteremia and bacterial load in urosepsis syndrome: a prospective observational study. Crit Care 14:R206

128. Heyland DK, Johnson AP, Reynolds SC, Muscedere J (2011) Procalcitonin for reduced antibiotic exposure in the critical care setting: a systematic review and an economic evaluation. Crit Care Med 39:1792–1799

129. Nickel JC (2005) Practical management of recurrent urinary tract infections in premenopausal women. Rev Urol 7:11–17

130. Foster RT Sr (2008) Uncomplicated urinary tract infections in women. Obstet Gynecol Clin N Am 35:235–248

131. Nakamura T, Komatsu M, Yamasaki K, Fukuda S, Higuchi T, Ono T et al (2014) Susceptibility of various oral antibacterial agents against extended spectrum β-lactamase producing *Escherichia coli* and *Klebsiella pneumoniae*. J Infect Chemother 20:48–51

Perspective from the Urologist

4

Ai Ling Loredana Romanò
and Antonio M. Granata

4.1 Introduction

Traditionally, urinary tract infections (UTIs) are classified based on symptoms, laboratory data and microbiological findings. Practically, they can be divided into uncomplicated and complicated UTIs and sepsis.

Most episodes of cystitis and pyelonephritis in otherwise healthy individuals are generally considered uncomplicated. If associated with an underlying condition that increases the risk of infection or of failing therapy, they become complicated. Such conditions include poorly controlled diabetes mellitus; pregnancy; hospital-acquired infection; acute kidney injury or chronic kidney disease; suspected or known urinary tract obstruction; presence of indwelling urethral catheter, stent, nephrostomy tube or urinary diversion; functional or anatomic abnormality of urinary tract; renal transplantation; other immunocompromising condition (e.g. chronic high-dose corticosteroid use, use of immunosuppressive agents, neutropenia, advanced HIV infection, B or T leukocyte deficiency); and infection with a uropathogen with broad-spectrum antimicrobial resistance.

The European Association of Urology (EAU) proposed a classification based on anatomical level of infection and grade of severity of infection. The authors agree with this last classification.

4.2 Cystitis

Acute cystitis refers to infection of the bladder. It is a very common UTI among women. Almost half of sexually active young women experienced at least one episode of UTI during their lifetime [1]. Risk factors include sexual intercourse, use of spermicides, vaginal postmenopausal hormonal status, history of urinary tract infection (during childhood or mother), urinary incontinence and cystocoele [2]. Only few men suffer from acute uncomplicated cystitis [3].

4.2.1 Clinical Manifestations

The diagnosis can be easily made on focused history. Typically, symptoms described are dysuria, frequency, urgency and pain during micturition. In case of complicated cystitis patients can present suprapubic pain and hematuria.

4.2.2 Diagnostic Evaluation

Laboratory diagnostic tools consist of urinalysis. Urine dipstick testing is a reasonable alternative

A.L.L. Romanò (✉) • A.M. Granata
Department of Urology, "Luigi Sacco" Hospital,
Via G.B. Grassi 74, Milan 20157, Italy
e-mail: ailing.romano@asst-fbf-sacco.it;
antonio.granata@asst-fbf-sacco.it

© Springer International Publishing AG 2018
M. Tonolini (ed.), *Imaging and Intervention in Urinary Tract Infections and Urosepsis*,
https://doi.org/10.1007/978-3-319-68276-1_4

to culture. A colony count of $\geq 10^3$ CFU/mL of uropathogen is diagnostic [4]. *Escherichia coli* is the main microorganism involved in the pathogenesis.

Radiographic imaging is not necessary to diagnose cystitis. Ultrasound (US) can point out mucosal oedema associated with a diffuse thickening of the bladder wall. In clinical practice, it is required in case of recurrent episodes. Generally it is more useful to rule out some complications, such as bladder stones or other bladder diseases (tumours). Other radiological examinations don't add any important information.

4.2.3 Disease Management

Antibiotic therapy is recommended in symptomatic patients. The first choice in many European countries are fosfomycin 3 g single dose, pivmecillinam 400 mg tid for 3 days and nitrofurantoin 100 mg bid for 5 days [5–7].

Alternative antibiotics include trimethoprim combined with sulphonamide and fluoroquinolone class (ciprofloxacin, levofloxacin) in 3-day regimens.

In case of complicated cystitis or suspected concomitant pyelonephritis, oral therapy with fluoroquinolones becomes the first choice.

4.3 Pyelonephritis

Acute pyelonephritis is less common than acute cystitis; the annual incidence is about 0.12 per person-year [8]. Upper UTIs occur more frequently in patients with diabetes mellitus [9].

E. coli is the causative pathogen in 70–95% of cases. Occasionally, other *Enterobacteriaceae*, such as *Proteus mirabilis* and *Klebsiella pneumoniae*, are isolated [10].

4.3.1 Pathogenesis

Pyelonephritis develops when pathogens ascend to the kidneys via the ureters but can also be caused by seeding of the kidneys from bacteremia or from bacteria in the lymphatics. Host and microbial factors that underlie progression from bladder to kidney infection require further investigation.

4.3.2 Clinical Manifestations

Acute pyelonephritis is suggested by flank pain, nausea and vomiting, fever (>38 °C), chills and costovertebral angle tenderness. Symptoms of cystitis may or may not be present [11]. Patients with acute complicated pyelonephritis may present with sepsis. In some cases they may be associated with a period of insidious, non-specific, signs and symptoms such as malaise, fatigue or abdominal pain. In diabetic patients acute pyelonephritis may also develop progression of renal parenchymal infection sometimes caused by gas-forming organisms (emphysematous pyelonephritis), with a high mortality [12].

The risk of chronic renal disease and renal insufficiency caused by pyelonephritis is low.

It is important to differentiate very early between an acute uncomplicated and complicated obstructive form of pyelonephritis, because the latter can very quickly lead to urosepsis.

4.3.3 Diagnostic Evaluation

The diagnosis begins with accurate clinical history. Physical examination should include abdominal and pelvic examination, to exclude the presence of vaginitis or urethritis. Pregnancy testing is also appropriate in women of childbearing age. Urinalysis (either by microscopy or by dipstick), including the assessment of white and red blood cells and nitrites, is recommended [13].

Pyuria is present in almost all patients with complicated UTI. Colony counts $\geq 10^4$ CFU/mL of pathogen are considered indicative of relevant bacteriuria. However, pyuria and bacteriuria may be absent if the infection does not communicate with the collecting system or if it is obstructed.

Urine cultures should be obtained prior to therapy to evaluate for antimicrobial resistance.

Patients with persistent clinical symptoms after 48–72 h of appropriate antibiotic therapy should undergo radiologic evaluation of the upper urinary tract, initially with US. In addition, radiologic evaluation is warranted for patients with pyelonephritis who also present symptoms of renal colic or have history of renal stones, diabetes, history of prior urologic surgery, immunosuppression, repeated episodes of pyelonephritis or urosepsis [13].

Evaluation of the upper urinary tract with US should be performed to rule out urinary obstruction or renal stone disease. Computed tomography (CT) scan should be considered if the patient still presents fever after 72 h of treatment. CT without contrast has become the standard radiographic study for demonstrating gas-forming infections, haemorrhage, obstruction and abscesses. Contrast is needed to demonstrate localized hypodense lesions due to ischaemia. Magnetic resonance imaging (MRI) is preferred in pregnant women to avoid radiation risk to the foetus.

In clinical practice CT remains the most used exam because it is widely available, can be remotely reported and is the one that offers more information at one time, especially with regard to complications. MRI would be preferable but not always, and not in all hospitals, there is a real chance to perform such an examination in emergency conditions.

4.3.4 Disease Management

Empiric antimicrobial therapy should be initiated promptly. In mild and moderate cases of acute uncomplicated pyelonephritis, oral therapy for 10–14 days is usually sufficient. The first-line therapy is represented by fluoroquinolone (Table 4.1), contraindicated in pregnancy. A third-generation oral cephalosporin could be an alternative in case of resistance. In communities with high rates of fluoroquinolone-resistant and ESBL-producing *E. coli*, initial empirical therapy with an aminoglycoside or carbapenem has to be considered.

In patients with severe pyelonephritis, parenteral antibiotics have to be used. After

Table 4.1 Recommended initial empirical antimicrobial therapy

	Antibiotics	Daily dose	Duration of therapy	Note
Mild and moderate acute uncomplicated pyelonephritis	Ciprofloxacin	500 mg bid	7–10 days	
Oral therapy	Levofloxacin	500 mg qd	7–10 days	
	Cefotaxime	400 mg qd	10 days	Alternative, not microbiological equivalent efficacy to fluoroquinolones
	Trimethoprim-sulphamethoxazole	160/800 mg bid	14 days	Only if the pathogen is known to be susceptible
	Co-amoxiclav	0.5/0.125 g tid	14 days	
Severe acute uncomplicated pyelonephritis	Ciprofloxacin	400 mg bid		
	Levofloxacin	500 mg qd		
	Cefotaxime	2 g tid		
Parenteral therapy	Piperacillin/tazobactam	2.5–4.5 g tid		
	Amikacin	15 mg/Kg qd		
	Ertapenem	1 g qd		

improvement, the patient can be switched to an oral therapy for 1–2 weeks. Positioning urinary catheter is important in order to drain the urinary tract.

4.4 Urosepsis

Sepsis is a complex systemic inflammatory host response to bacterial infection (Table 4.2). In urosepsis the focus of infection is localized to the urogenital tract. Patients with urosepsis should be identified at an early stage and promptly treated to prevent development of organ failure and other complications. Mortality rates are high. The severity depends mostly upon the host response.

4.4.1 Pathogenesis

Complicated UTI is the commonest precursor of urosepsis. It is important to note that a patient can move from an almost harmless state to severe sepsis in a very short time. Structural and functional abnormalities such as obstruction (congenital or acquired), instrumentation, impaired voiding, metabolic abnormalities and immunodeficiencies can be associated to urosepsis.

Microorganisms reach the urinary tract byway of the ascending, haematogenous or lymphatic routes. For urosepsis to be established, the pathogens have to reach the bloodstream. Gram-negative bacilli account for majority of the cases of urosepsis. These include *E. coli* (50%), *Proteus* spp. (15%), *Enterobacter* and *Klebsiella* spp. (15%) and *Pseudomonas aeruginosa* (5%), while Gram-positive organisms are involved less frequently (15%) [14].

4.4.2 Clinical Manifestations

The clinical presentation may be varied. Signs and symptoms of systemic inflammatory response syndrome which were initially considered to be 'mandatory' for the diagnosis of sepsis [15] are now considered to be alerting

Table 4.2 Diagnostic criteria for sepsis

• *General signs*
– Fever >38.3 °C
– Hypothermia <36 °C
– Tachycardia >90/min or >2 SD above age-specific normal value
– Tachypnea >30/min
– Impaired neurologic status
– Oedema or positive fluid balance (>20 mL/kg/d)
– Hyperglycemia (blood sugar >120 mg/dL or 7.7 mmoL/L) in the absence of previously diagnosed diabetes mellitus
• *Signs of inflammation*
– Leukocytosis >12/nL
– Leukopenia <4/nL
– Normal leukocyte count with >10% immature forms
– C-reactive protein >2 SD above normal
– Procalcitonin >2 SD above normal
• *Hemodynamic signs*
– Hypotension (SBP <90 mmHg, MAP <70 mmHg or SBP drop by >40 mmHg or to <2 SD below the age-specific normal value)
– Cardiac index (CI) >3–5 L/min/m^2
• *Organ dysfunction*
– Arterial hypoxemia ($p_aO_2/F_iO_2 < 300$)
– Acute oliguria <0.5 mL/kg/h or 45 mmoL/L for (≥ 2 h)
– Creatinine rise by (≥ 0.5 mg/dL)
– Coagulopathy (INR >1.5 or aPTT >60 s)
– Thrombocytopenia <100/nL
– Hyperbilirubinemia (total bilirubin >4 mg/dL or >70 mmoL/L)
– Ileus
• *Tissue perfusion variables*
– Lactate >2 mmol/L
– Decreased capillary refill or mottling

symptoms [16]. Fever, tachycardia, tachypnea and respiratory alkalosis are the typical manifestation. Only one-third of the patients classically present with fever and chills along with hypotension.

4.4.3 Diagnostic Evaluation

History is crucial in the evaluation of any UTI, including any previous history of infections, antibiotic use and a timeline of symptoms. A patient can be considered to have sepsis if he or she has evidence of bacteremia or clinical suspicion of sepsis accompanied by greater than or equal to two criteria of systemic inflammatory response syndrome as mentioned in Table 4.2.

The diagnosis of UTI, from simple cystitis to complicated pyelonephritis with sepsis, can be established with absolute certainty only by quantitative urine cultures.

Blood cultures should be done before antibiotic treatment is started. Ideally, several aerobic and anaerobic blood cultures are taken when fever is rising.

In a critically ill patient with urosepsis, CT and MRI are very useful investigations. These are the most precise methods for identifying bacterial interstitial nephritis and micro-abscesses within the kidney, perinephric abscesses, emphysematous pyelonephritis and renal papillary necrosis and can determine therapeutic choices and intervention times. Urinary unblocking, with either ureteral stenting or percutaneous nephrostomy, is mandatory.

4.4.4 Disease Management

The treatment of urosepsis needs the collaboration of a team (urologists, intensive care and intensive diseases specialists), to coordinate an adequate life-supporting care, appropriate and prompt antibiotic therapy.

Levels of therapy are divided into causal therapy (antimicrobial treatment and source control), supportive therapy (haemodynamic stabilization and airways, respiration support) and adjunctive therapy (glucocorticosteroids and intensified insulin therapy).

The drainage of any obstruction in the urinary tract is essential as first-line treatment (LE, 1a; GR, A) [17]: in case of renal abscess, percutaneous or surgical drainage, and in infected hydronephrosis, internal drainage (double J-DJ or mono J- MJ) or percutaneous nephrostomy.

If possible, specific treatment of the diagnosed infection should be started as soon as possible.

Empirical antimicrobial therapy effective against both Gram-positive and Gram-negative bacteria should be initiated. A calculated parenteral antibiotic should be reassessed once culture results become available, usually within 48–72 h.

In case of *E. coli* and other Enterobacteriaceae isolation, a third-generation cephalosporin or piperacillin in combination with a beta-lactamase inhibitor or fluorquinolone with propensity to achieve high urinary concentration (e.g. ciprofloxacin, levofloxacin) should be used. A combination therapy with an aminoglycoside or a carbapenem may be essential in areas with high rate of fluoroquinolone resistance. Reserve antibiotics such as imipenem or meropenem if a difficult resistance situation is suspected [18].

References

1. Foxman B (2002) Epidemiology of urinary tract infections: incidence, morbidity and economic costs. Am J Med 113(Suppl. 1A):5S–13S
2. Gupta K, Hooton TM, Naber KG et al (2011) International clinical practise guidelines for the treatment of acute uncomplicated cystitis and pyelonephritis in women: a 2010 update by the infectious diseases Society for Microbiology and Infectious Diseases. Clin Infect Dis 52:103
3. Stamm WE (1997) Urinary tract infections in young men. In: Bergan T (ed) Urinary tract infections. Kager, Basel, pp 46–47
4. Kunin C (1997) Urinary tract infections, in detection, prevention and management. Lea & Febiger, Philadelphia
5. Gupta K et al (2007) Short-course nitrofurantoin for the treatment of acute uncomplicated cystitis in women. Arch Intern Med 167(20):2207–2212
6. Lecomte F et al (1997) Single-dose treatment of cystitis with fosfomycin trometamol (Monuril): analysis of 15 comparative trials on 2,048 patients. G Ital Ostet Ginecol 19:399–404
7. Nicolle LE (2000) Pivmecillinam in the treatment of urinary tract infections. J Antimicrob Chemother 46(Suppl 1):35–39. discussion 63-5
8. Czaja CA, Scholes D, Hooton TM, Stamm WE (2007) Population-based epidemiologic analysis of acute pyelonephritis. Clin Infect Dis 45:273
9. Funfstuck R et al (2012) Urinary tract infection in patients with diabetes mellitus. Clin Nephrol 77(1):40–48
10. Naber KG et al (2008) Surveillance study in Europe and Brazil on clinical aspects and antimicrobial resistance epidemiology in female with cystitis (ARESC): implication for empiric therapy. Eur Urol 54(5):1164–1175

11. Scholes D et al (2005) Risk factors associated with acute pyelonephritis in healthy women. Ann Intern Med 142(1):20–27

12. Cattel WR (1992) Urinary tract infection and acute renal failure. In: Raine AE (ed) Advanced renal medicine. Oxford University Press, Oxford, pp 302–313

13. Fulop T (2012) Acute pyelonephritis workup. https://emedicine.medscape.com/article/245559-workup

14. Wagenlehner FM, Weidner W, Naber KG (2007) Pharmacokinetic characteristics of antimicrobials and optimal treatment of urosepsis. Clin Pharmacokinet 46(4):291–305

15. Bone RC et al (1992) Definitions for sepsis and organ failure and guidelines for the use of innovative therapies in sepsis. The ACCP/SCCM consensus conference committee. American College of Chest Physicians/Society of Critical Care Medicine. Chest 101(6):1644–1655

16. Levy MM et al (2003) 2001 SCCM/ESICM/ACCP/ATS/SIS international sepsis definitions conference. Crit Care Med 31(4):1250–1256

17. Grabe M, Bartoletti R, Bjerklund-Johansen TE et al (2014) Guidelines on urological infections. European Association of Urology Available at: http://uroweb.org/wp-content/uploads/19-Urological-infections_LR2.pdf

18. Safdar N, Handelsman J, Maki DG (2004) Does combination antimicrobial therapy reduce mortality in gram-negative bacteraemia? A meta-analysis. Lancet Infect Dis 4:519–527

Antonio Maria Granata
and Ai Ling Loredana Romanò

The male reproductive tract consists in external structures such as the penis, scrotum, testis, and internal structures including the prostate gland, epididymis, vas deferens, and seminal vesicles.

Male reproductive tract infections (MRTIs) are very common diseases of the genital system. These infections are caused by bacteria, virus, or other organisms and can be either endogenous, iatrogenic, or sexually transmitted. All those infections have a higher incidence after urologic procedures, such as prostatic biopsy, indwelling, or intermittent catheter. Chronic infections of epididymis and prostate are frequently associated with urine voiding dysfunctions that cause high pressure and reflux in genital duct.

5.1 Epididymitis and Orchitis

Inflammation of epididymis and testes generally results from infection; epididymitis is the most common infection, but in some case when inflammation spreads to the adjacent testicle, orchitis can develop. Isolated orchitis is rare and is gener-

ally associated with mumps infection in prepubertal boys (13 years or younger).

The incidence can be described with a bimodal distribution, occurring in young adults with the peak incidence between 16 and 30 years of age; the other peak incidence is present in 51–70 years of age.

In epididymitis, the most usual route of infection is the retrograde ascent of pathogens, and bacteria are frequently responsible, with different age distribution: in the first age group (16–30 years), the most common pathogens are sexually transmitted, such as *Chlamydia trachomatis*, *Ureaplasma urealyticum*, and *Neisseria gonorrhoeae*. In the second group (51–70 years), the primary pathogens are coliform bacteria, coming from urinary tract, and the infections are frequent consequence of voiding dysfunctions. *Escherichia coli* is the most frequent causative pathogen; nevertheless other common microbial agents are *Haemophilus i.*, *Proteus mirabilis*, *Klebsiella pneumoniae*, and *Pseudomonas aeruginosa*.

Mycobacterium tuberculosis, fungi, and virus, including cytomegalovirus, are uncommon causative agent but have to be strongly considered in HIV patients.

Epididymitis and orchitis are classified as acute or chronic processes according to the onset and clinical course. Epididymitis is almost always unilateral and relatively acute in onset. In young males it is frequently associated with sexual activity and infection of the consort. The majority of cases in sexually active males aged

A.M. Granata (✉) • A.L.L. Romanò
Urology Department, ASST FBF Sacco—Ospedale
Luigi Sacco, Via G.B. Grassi 74, Milan 20157, Italy
e-mail: antonio.granata@asst-fbf-sacco.it; ailing.
romano@asst-fbf-sacco.it

© Springer International Publishing AG 2018
M. Tonolini (ed.), *Imaging and Intervention in Urinary Tract Infections and Urosepsis*,
https://doi.org/10.1007/978-3-319-68276-1_5

<35 years are due to sexually transmitted organisms, whereas in elderly patients, it is usually due to common urinary pathogens.

Epididymitis causes pain and swelling, which begins in the tail of the epididymis and may spread to involve the rest of the epididymis and testicular tissue. The spermatic cord is usually tender and swollen.

History and physical examination are thus very important to achieve a diagnosis, especially to exclude sperm cord torsion.

The differential diagnosis between epididymitis and testicular torsion is one of the most frequent problems for the urologist attending the emergency room, because torsion is a surgical emergency and the likelihood of testicular salvage decreases as the duration of torsion increases.

The microbial aetiology of epididymitis can sometimes be determined by examination of a urethral swab and/or a urine culture [1].

Fluoroquinolones with activity against *C. trachomatis* (e.g. ofloxacin and levofloxacin) should be the drugs of first choice. If *C. trachomatis* has been detected, treatment could also be continued with doxycycline, 200 mg/day, for a total of at least 2 weeks, and the sexual partner should also be treated [2]. In abscess-forming epididymitis or orchitis, or in patients not responding to antibacterial treatment during the first 72 h, surgery should be considered [3]. In severe cases an abscess involving the testis may even require orchiectomy.

Chronic epididymitis can sometimes be the first clinical manifestation of urogenital tuberculosis.

Complications in epididymo-orchitis include abscess formation, testicular infarction, testicular atrophy, reactive hydrocele, development of chronic epididymal induration, and infertility.

5.1.1 Imaging

In the differential diagnosis of sperm cord torsion, to improve diagnostic accuracy and avoid unnecessary surgery, color Doppler ultrasonography has become the preferred imaging technique for evaluating the acute scrotum.

The color Doppler equipment should be calibrated to demonstrate blood flow in the normal testis. For flow measurements, the Doppler cursor must be positioned within the testis. When normal or increased flow is demonstrated, torsion is excluded. Conversely, in epididymitis and orchitis, hypervascularization of both epididymis and testis is commonly found [4].

5.2 Prostatitis and Infections of Seminal Vesicles

The most used classification of prostatitis was published in 1999 by the National Institutes of Health (NIH) and includes four categories: acute, chronic bacterial prostatitis, chronic pelvic pain syndrome (CPPS), and asymptomatic inflammatory prostatitis.

Acute prostatitis and chronic bacterial prostatitis are defined by documented bacterial infections of the prostate. The isolation of bacteria allows the differentiation of chronic prostatitis from CPPS and asymptomatic inflammatory prostatitis. According to the duration of symptoms, prostatitis is considered chronic when symptoms persist for at least 3 months [5].

Bacterial prostatitis may be caused by ascending infection through the urethra, refluxing urine into prostate ducts, or direct extension or lymphatic spread from the rectum.

Approximately 80% of the pathogens are Gram-negative organisms (e.g., *Escherichia coli*, *Enterobacter*, *Serratia*, *Pseudomonas*, *Enterococcus*, and *Proteus* species) [6]. Sexually transmitted agents like *Neisseria gonorrhoeae* and *Chlamydia trachomatis* can also cause prostatitis.

In HIV-infected patients, viral and granulomatous prostatitis may be present, caused by virus as *Cytomegalovirus* (CMV), *Mycobacterium tuberculosis*, or fungi, such as *Candida albicans* [7, 8].

As described in epididymitis, sexually transmitted agents are frequently encountered in young patients, coliform bacteria in older man with voiding dysfunctions.

The process that leads to a chronic bacterial prostatitis can include an insufficient initial therapy or, often, some concomitant voiding dysfunction problem; *E. coli* is responsible for 75–80% of chronic bacterial prostatitis cases; *Enterococci, Pseudomonas, Chlamydia trachomatis, Ureaplasma urealyticum,*and *Trichomonas vaginalis* are usually isolated in the remainder of cases.

Patients with acute bacterial prostatitis can manifest with fever, perineal pain, lower urinary tract symptoms, and spontaneous urethral discharge. Conversely, those with chronic bacterial prostatitis typically have no systemic symptoms but sovrapubic, testicular, or perineal pain and lower urinary tract symptoms [9].

Digital rectal examination in patients with acute bacterial prostatitis may reveal a tender, hot, and painful gland. Prostatic massage should be avoided to reduce the risk of bacterial spreading.

The most important investigation for bacterial identification in acute prostatitis is the urine culture. In chronic bacterial prostatitis, a Meares-Stamey test analyzing segmented urine and of expressed prostatic secretion (EPS) is needed [10].

Pyospermia and hematospermia in men in endemic regions or with a history of tuberculosis should be investigated for urogenital tuberculosis [8].

Patients with acute bacterial prostatitis who appear acutely ill or with have evidence of sepsis require hospital admission for parenteral antibiotics and supportive care [6]. Antibiotic therapy should initially include parental bactericidal agents such as broad-spectrum penicillin derivatives, third-generation cephalosporins with or without aminoglycosides, or fluoroquinolones. Patients without toxic symptoms can be treated on an outpatient basis with a 14- to 28-day course of oral antibiotics, usually a fluoroquinolone or trimethoprim-sulfamethoxazole.

In cases of prostatic abscess, it has to be drained under local anesthesia either transrectally or transperineally.

For the chronic bacterial prostatitis, a 4- to 6-week of antibiotic therapy is indicated.

Fluoroquinolones provide relief in about 50% of patients, and treatment is more effective if treatment starts earlier in the course of symptoms [10].

5.2.1 Imaging

Suprapubic ultrasonography is routinely used to assess volume of retained urine in cases of prostatitis associated with significant voiding dysfunction.

On transrectal ultrasonography (TRUS), a hypoechoic halo in the periurethral region and a heterogeneous echo pattern can often be seen. However, it is not so reliable for the diagnosis of prostatitis; thus it is not routinely indicated in patients with acute prostatic symptoms. Moreover during an episode of acute prostatitis, transrectal ultrasonography can be very painful; thus it has to be definitely avoided.

Imaging has indeed a very important role when an abscess is suspected [11]. A TRUS in many can be sufficiently accurate and can be used during a perineal drainage.

In other situations, magnetic resonance imaging (MRI) is helpful, for example, in case of immunodeficient patients with unclear perineal symptoms.

5.3 Fournier's Gangrene

The scrotum can be frequently involved during orchitis and epididymitis, and in these cases the cutaneous and subcutaneous infection responds to a basic antibiotic therapy.

The crucial differential diagnosis is Fournier's gangrene, an aggressive and frequently fatal category of necrotizing fasciitis, characterized by a polymicrobial soft tissue infection of the perineum, perianal region, and external genitalia. Fournier's gangrene remains rare, but its incidence is increasing with an ageing population, higher prevalence of diabetes, and emergence of multiresistant pathogens [12].

Risk factors include immunosuppression, diabetes, obesity, and malnutrition. Fournier's gangrene is typically polymicrobial in origin, including different bacteria such as *S. aureus*, *Streptococcus* sp., *Klebsiella* sp., *E. coli*, and anaerobes. These organisms secrete endotoxins causing tissue necrosis and severe cardiovascular impairment. Subsequent inflammatory reaction by the host contributes to multi-organ failure and death if untreated.

The typical patient with Fournier's gangrene is an elderly man in his sixth or seventh decade of life with comorbid diseases; at the presentation there is intense pain and tenderness in the genitalia, fever, edema, or erythema of the scrotal skin, until clear necrotic areas evidence. Crepitus on palpation and a foul-smelling exudate can be present in more advanced disease [13].

Systemic effects of this process vary from local tenderness with no toxicity to florid septic shock.

The degree of internal necrosis is usually vastly greater than suggested by external signs, and consequently, adequate, repeated surgical debridement is necessary to save the patient's life. Consensus from case series suggests that surgical debridement should be early (<24 h) and complete, because delayed and/or inadequate surgery results in higher mortality. Concurrent parenteral antibiotic treatment should be given that covers all causative organisms and can penetrate inflammatory tissue. This can then be refined following surgical cultures. The benefit of pooled immunoglobulin therapy and hyperbaric oxygen remains uncertain and should not be used routinely. With aggressive early surgical and medical management, survival rates are >70% depending upon patient group and availability of critical care. Following resolution, reconstruction using skin grafts can be necessary [10].

5.3.1 Imaging

Fournier's gangrene is a serious emergency and the role of radiologist is pivotal. The differential diagnosis between severe orchitis involving the scrotum and necrotizing fasciitis benefits from computed tomography (CT), which should be considered the imaging study of choice. Indeed the presence of subcutaneous air, due to the anaerobic bacteria, is very suggestive of Fournier's gangrene, especially in the presence of an appropriate clinical history.

References

1. Pilatz A et al (2015) Acute epididymitis revisited: impact of molecular diagnostics on etiology and contemporary guideline recommendations. Eur Urol 68:428
2. Pickard R, Bartoletti R et al (2016) Acute infective epididimytis. European Association of Urology (EAU). Urological Infections Guidelines. Available at: http://uroweb.org/wp-content/uploads/EAU-Guidelines-Urological-Infections-2016-1.pdf
3. Banyra O, Shulyak A (2012) Acute epididymo-orchitis: staging and treatment. Cen Eur J Urol 65(3):139–143
4. Nicholson A et al (2010) Management of epididymo-orchitis in primary care: results from a large UK primary care database. Br J Gen Pract 60:407
5. Krieger JN, Nyberg L Jr, Nickel JC (1999) NIH consensus definition and classification of prostatitis. JAMA 282:236–237
6. Gill BC, Shoskes DA (2016) Bacterial prostatitis. Curr Opin Infect Dis 29(1):86–91
7. Mastroianni A, Coronado O, Manfredi R, Chiodo F, Scarani P (1996) Acute cytomegalovirus prostatitis in AIDS. Genitourin Med 72(6):447–448
8. Gebo KA (2002) Prostatic tuberculosis in an HIV infected male. Sex Transm Infect 78(2):147–148
9. Wagenlehner FM et al (2013) National Institutes of Health chronic prostatitis symptom index (NIH-CPSI) symptom evaluation in multinational cohorts of patients with chronic prostatitis/chronic pelvic pain syndrome. Eur Urol 63(5):953–959
10. Grabe M, Bartoletti R, et al (2015) Prostatitis and chronic pelvic pain syndrome. Guidelines on urological infections-limited update March 2015. European Association of Urology (EAU). Available at: https://uroweb.org/wp-content/uploads/19-Urological-infections_LR2.pdf
11. de la Rosette JJ, Giesen RJ et al (1995) Automated analysis and interpretation of transrectal ultrasonography images in patients with prostatitis. Eur Urol 27(1):47–53
12. Singh A, Ahmed K, Aydin A, Khan MS, Dasgupta P (2016) Fournier's Gangrene. A clinical review. Arch Ital Urol Androl 88(3):157–164
13. Pernetti R, Palmieri F, Sagrini E et al (2016) Fournier's Gangrene: clinical case and review of the literature. Arch Ital Urol Androl 88(3):237–238

Nothing Is Simple in Acute Pyelonephritis: A Pragmatic, Semantic Nephrologist's View

Giorgina Barbara Piccoli and Francesca Ragni

Acute pyelonephritis (APN), first described in Egyptian medicine, has been known for over two millennia [1]. Descriptions of the risk of death due to sepsis and of evolution into subacute forms ultimately resulting in uraemia and death are over 200 years old [1]. Yet there is still much that needs to be known about this life-threatening and relatively widespread condition, and, as this short nonsystematic, critical review will discuss, nothing is simple in APN.

Firstly, we lack a clear, standard definition, whereas APN is currently seen both as a parenchymal disease, defined by imaging, and as an upper urinary tract infection, defined on clinical bases.

Secondly, while in children APN is considered a parenchymal disorder, which may be linked with vesicoureteral reflux, in adults it is seen as an upper urinary tract disorder, not necessarily requiring imaging confirmation.

Thirdly, the relationship with predisposing factors is complex. This confusion is reflected in the current terminology: the adjectives complicated and noncomplicated pyelonephritis define the presence of predisposing factors and not the effect of a severe disease. The issues of pregnancy in adults, of reflux in children, and of kidney transplantation are also a part of this complex series of factors.

Fourthly, partly as a consequence of the previous points, the outcomes of treatment and, consequently, treatment schedules change remarkably. Should we be concerned about kidney scars? Do we need to look for them?

This review will discuss these open questions with particular regard to their practical implications, leaving the pathogenetic issues and treatment schedules to the chapters which deal specifically with these topics.

6.1 What Is APN?

Unlike the classic "orphan diseases", which are too rare to have a fully acknowledged "parent", i.e. caregiver, acute pyelonephritis probably has too many "parents" to be fully and satisfactorily managed by any of them. In fact, this relatively common disease is managed differently in different parts of the world, to some extent as an effect of the different intervenients in its management, while in Italy "noncomplicated" or primary APN is often man-

G.B. Piccoli (✉)
Dipartimento Scienze cliniche e biologiche, Università di Torino, Regione Gonzole, Orbassano, TO 10100, Italy

Nephrologie, Centre Hospitalier Le Mans, Le Mans, France
e-mail: gbpiccoli@yahoo.it

F. Ragni
AOU San Luigi SCDU Urologia, AOU San Luigi, Regione Gonzole, Orbassano, TO 10100, Italy
e-mail: francesca_ragni@yahoo.it

© Springer International Publishing AG 2018
M. Tonolini (ed.), *Imaging and Intervention in Urinary Tract Infections and Urosepsis*,
https://doi.org/10.1007/978-3-319-68276-1_6

aged by nephrologists and complicated APN by the urologists; in Germany urology is the main setting of care, while in other parts of the world, the disease is treated in internal medicine, emergency medicine or infectious diseases, while paediatricians are the main interveners in children [2–7]. No wonder, therefore, that management, approaches and focus are different, as this book itself also shows.

The main focus for infectious disease and internal medicine specialists is healing the active pyelonephritis lesions; urologists are more concerned about predisposing factors and nephrologists with long-term consequences. As a further result, the imaging employed may vary according to the setting of care, while nephrologists are principally interested in kidney scar development and will tend to focus not only on defining the initial disease but also on determining whether there is residual damage (kidney scars), a focus shared with paediatricians and internal medicine and infectious disease specialists which are more concerned with the severity of the disease and may limit imaging to clinically severe cases and to the initial diagnostic phase [8–12]. Conversely, paediatricians and urologists are more prone to investigate the presence of predisposing factors and more frequently ask for a search for vesicoureteral reflux, even in the absence of a true reflux nephropathy, characterised by ureteric dilatation and tortuosity [8, 13–15].

The issue is still open and will probably remain so; indeed, more than 20 years ago, in a well-grounded, lucid paper that is still pertinent to the issues we currently face, Talner commented on the lack of agreement on the terminology of APN and, as a consequence, on the lack of univocal diagnostic definitions of this disease [16]. Since in medicine, the lack of a definition is a lack of a diagnosis and the lack of a diagnosis often means a lack of agreement on treatment, this problem is not only a semantic one. In fact it may be one of the reasons for the lack of conformity in diagnostic and therapeutic approaches to a disease that has been known to medicine for over two millennia [17].

According to the most commonly found, simple (possibly simplistic), "classic" textbook definition, acute pyelonephritis (APN) is a severe infectious disease involving the pelvis, calices and kidney parenchyma [17–20]. Such a definition obviously implies demonstrating the involvement of the kidney parenchyma by imaging or by a renal biopsy, as will be further discussed. According to this morphologic definition, there are two different types of involvement of the upper urinary tract: pyelonephritis, in which there is a demonstrated involvement of the renal tissue; and cystopyelitis, in which the infection, which has a superimposable clinical presentation, is limited to the renal pelvis and no sign of parenchyma involvement is found at imaging [17].

This classic morphologic definition has the advantage of distinguishing between two types of lesions that, in spite of a similar presentation, can have a different clinical course—more severe in the presence of parenchyma involvement, with severity that may be proportional to the extension of that involvement and to the presence of abscessed lesions. However, the drawback of the morphologic definition is that it requires a "second-line" imaging test (contrast-enhanced CT scan, nuclear magnetic resonance—MRI—or renal scintigraphy), since renal ultrasound, which is relatively inexpensive and easily available and is therefore of pivotal importance for the demonstration of mechanic predisposing factors (obstruction, malformation, ectopic kidney, dilatation), is not reliable in distinguishing the parenchymal lesions of pyelonephritis unless they are abscessed [21–24].

Therefore, faced with the pressure of cost constraints, at least for adult patients, the most commonly used definitions are solely clinical, based on the classic tetrad of fever, costovertebral tenderness, positive urinary culture and lower urinary tract symptoms. The term upper urinary tract infection encompasses both of the forms mentioned above (cystopyelitis and acute pyelonephritis) and proposes clinical triage at referral and response to empiric treatment after referral as selection criteria for which cases should undergo imaging evaluation [25–31]. These selection criteria mainly include the severity of the initial presentation, the lack of rapid response to therapy or a short-term relapse of a symptomatic infection. Both approaches have a strong logic, and both can prove effective. However, in the absence of a comparison between a morphologic and a clinical approach to APN, the choice relies on organisation, opinions and health-care differences, as will be further discussed.

6.2 What Happens When APN Is Diagnosed in Late Adolescents?

There is general agreement on the use of a morphologic definition of APN in children and on the importance of detecting kidney scars [32–36]. This policy depends largely on the close link between vesicoureteral reflux and APN in children, a relationship so close that it has led some authors to propose that the development of APN is proof of the presence of an at least intermittent vesicoureteral reflux. In this context, the presence of kidney scars is the most important predictor of the development of further scars and of functional impairment or hypertension in adulthood; hence, the usual policy includes not only the confirmation of parenchymal involvement at baseline but also a control, usually after 6 months, with an imaging technique [32–36].

However, at least theoretically, at follow-up, MAG 3 furosemide scan makes it possible to identify ureteral dysfunction, which represents a risk factor for recurrent infections. Furthermore, since the focus is on the development of kidney scars, some authors hold that the most important imaging is the one done at follow-up and suggest performing the latter only in patients rapidly responding to their antibiotic treatment [36].

Conversely, in adults, the most commonly chosen definition is the clinical one, which does not require imaging for a differential diagnosis of parenchyma involvement and limits the first approach to ultrasound, allowing us to discriminate between upper urinary tract infections with or without mechanical predisposing factors; the availability of contrast-enhanced techniques, which may identify pyelonephritis foci, has increased interest in the use of this approach [37–40].

As previously mentioned, the advantages of this pragmatic approach are largely context related, are probably more sound in settings in which the prevalence of less severe forms is higher (generally those where patients are admitted to the hospital before starting antibiotic treatment) and are probably less sound in settings, such as Italy or in some Asian countries, in which referral to the hospital usually follows a lack of response to an empiric antibiotic treatment (self-prescribed or prescribed by a family physician) [7, 41–45].

This hypothesis is borne out by northern Italian studies, which demonstrate that referral to the emergency ward usually occurs after failure to control symptoms with an empiric antibiotic treatment, altering, as a consequence, the classical APN tetrad, in which lower urinary tract symptoms are often absent and urinary cultures often test negative and parenchymal lesions are prevalent. On the account of these data, the same groups strongly suggest performing adequate imaging at presentation and at least at the end of follow-up [7, 23, 24, 43].

A simple way to assess the interest in first-line imaging in each setting is to analyse how many of the patients referred would meet the selection criteria for the randomised controlled trials (RCTs) which are the bases of our current guidelines. In particular, since, in the absence of imaging, the success of therapy is usually measured upon the negativisation of the patient's urinary cultures, the current guidelines cannot be implemented in settings in which most of the patients had a negative urinary culture and/or had already been treated with antibiotics before referral, as a previous study done by our group demonstrated to be the case in northern Italy [23, 42, 43]. In this setting, the number of patients that, at referral to the hospital, would have been enrolled in one of the RCTs on which the current guidelines are based was less than 20%, thus clearly demonstrating the impossibility of implementing the upper urinary tract approach in our setting.

6.3 Complicated or "Complicating" Pyelonephritis?

The term complicated is usually employed to identify the "secondary" forms of APN. These include malformations and vesicoureteral reflux, as well as obstructions, the most feared and extreme outcome of pyelonephritis. Conversely, noncomplicated pyelonephritis usually describes the forms, typical of young women in childbearing age, in which no predisposing mechanical or systemic factor is identified [16, 17, 37, 39, 45, 46]. According to this definition, complicated forms encompass also APN in kidney graft and APN in pregnancy. While this distinction is still the main reference, the presence of renal abscesses is considered by some authors as a factor defining a "complicated APN", considering, this time, the adjective complicated linked to the disease process itself.

The epidemiology of APN varies according to age and sex.

As previously mentioned, in children, APN is often, even if possibly not always, the result of vesicoureteral reflux; hence, it's more often "complicated" in this age group [32–36]. Conversely, noncomplicated APN is almost exclusively a disease of women, in particular those of childbearing age. The rarity of APN in young men has led some experts to conclude that by definition APN in a male subject is "complicated" [41–43].

In elderly males, prostatic hypertrophy is the most common cause of APN, while in postmenopausal women, tissue atrophy and uterine prolapse are frequent concomitants [47–49].

The absence or presence of predisposing factors conditions the choice of therapeutic approaches employed to correct them. Their severity and complexity ultimately determine the therapeutic response. In this regard, imaging is subordinated to the underlying problem (Table 6.1).

Table 6.1 Indications, advantages and limits of the most widely used imaging tests in acute pyelonephritis. A nephrological view

Imaging test	Potential indications and advantages	Limitations
Ultrasound (US)	Easily available, inexpensive, often feasible in the emergency room. Indicated in all cases, to distinguish between complicated and noncomplicated APN. Can also detect abscessualised lesions	Not able to distinguish between normal parenchyma and non- abscessed lesions
Contrast-enhanced US	Does not involve for radiation, often feasible in the emergency room. A good choice in experienced hands	Relatively high cost, operator dependent, no standardisation and lack of agreed assessment of sensibility and specificity
CT scan with contrast media	First gold standard imaging technique. Rapidly available in most settings; may be of use in particular in cases in which a further surgical approach is foreseen (complicated APN). Can be the first choice where MRI is not available, in particular in elderly women or in males, in which complicated APN is expected and radioprotection is less crucial	Ionising radiation exposure; need for contrast media. Limitations in allergic patients. Use only when absolutely necessary for women of childbearing age
Magnetic resonance imaging (MRI) with contrast media	At least comparable to CT scan in terms of sensibility and specificity. No need for ionising radiations and, therefore, first choice for women of childbearing age	Need for gadolinium-enhanced media. Not feasible in claustrophobic patients. Expensive, not always readily available. Long test, not easy to use with children
Magnetic resonance imaging (MRI) without contrast media including diffusion-weighted imaging (DWI)	Less experience but results probably similar to those obtained using MRI with contrast media in terms of sensibility and specificity. No need for ionising radiations, so the first choice for women of childbearing age and for pregnant women	Not feasible for claustrophobic patients. Expensive, not readily available. Relatively long test, not easy to use with children. As in all relatively new techniques, results may depend on radiologist's experience
DMSA scintigraphy	First choice for children, provides useful information on parenchymal involvement. Feasible with assistance; does not require nephrotoxic media	Exposure to ionising radiations; not able to distinguish between recent, healed and new lesions
MAG 3 scintigraphy	Can provide useful information on "minor" predisposing factors, including ureteral dyskinesia	Nonstandardised. Exposure to ionising radiations; not able to distinguish between recent, healed and new lesions

Conversely, in noncomplicated APN, some groups, like ours, grade the duration of therapy on the extension of the parenchymal involvement and on the type of lesions, suggesting longer treatment in the case of large or abscessualised lesions.

In fact, how long healing takes is not fully understood: an adequate antibiotic therapy is able to resolve the main symptoms of fever and pain within a few days, and complete normalisation of C-reactive protein and of other inflammatory markers occurs on the average within 1 week. Normalisation of imaging takes a much longer time, however: about 4 weeks in the case of non-abscessed lesions and up to 8 weeks in the case of abscessed lesions. The persistence of pathogens in the lesions detected at imaging has not been demonstrated, since kidney biopsy is not performed in such a setting. The long therapeutic schedules proposed by some groups, including ours, are based on the logical, but never demonstrated hypothesis that healing of the lesions found with imaging is synonymous with complete healing, and continue the treatment up to radiological healing [10, 17, 44].

6.4 Why Should We Be Concerned About Kidney Scars?

The life-threatening risks of Gram-negative sepsis, occurring either during the acute phase or as a result of kidney abscesses, are still matters of concern but are usually clustered in the first disease phases, in which patients are often managed in an emergency setting. The interest of the nephrologist is instead focused on the long-term sequelae of APN, namely, on parenchymal kidney scars at the sites of infectious foci [50–59].

The interest in kidney scars is due to the postulate that they may have a detrimental effect on renal function, play a role in the pathogenesis of secondary hypertension and represent a risk factor for pregnancy outcomes.

The development of kidney scars is likely to mark the relevance and severity of the predisposing conditions in complicated pyelonephritis and is generally linked with abscessualised lesions in the case of noncomplicated APN.

In the case of noncomplicated APN, the hypotheses followed by the Italian school, their limits and the therapeutic choices followed by our group are depicted in Tables 6.2 and 6.3.

While in the absence of randomised trials and in the presence of very few observational studies assessing the outcomes of kidney scars, no conclusion is possible, the meta-analysis of the few randomised studies that have been done (Tables 6.2 and 6.3) suggests an advantage of longer treatment in controlling the incidence of renal scars.

A further open question regards the long-term effect of kidney scars [50–59].

Noncomplicated pyelonephritis is typically a disease of the young, and long-term data on the effect of pyelonephritis scars are lacking. On account of the redefinition of chronic kidney disease, which encompasses not only kidney function impairment but also any anomaly of blood or urine composition and all the permanent lesions involving the renal parenchyma, APN scars indicate the presence of CKD. They probably represent a risk factor for adverse pregnancy-related outcomes and may require long-term follow-up. Hence, in the absence of sound evidence of the absence of long-term effects of kidney scars, evidence that it is probably unrealistic to expect, the nephrology approach focuses on prevention of kidney scars, balancing the risk involved with the side effects of a long-term antibiotic treatment.

6.5 What This Review Does Not Address: Some Notes on Pregnancy and Kidney Transplantation

This short review seeks to help clinicians understand and evaluate the different definitions of APN. It did not address the issue of chronic pyelonephritis, which we considered to be the result of subsequent APN episodes, and it did not consider APN in pregnancy and after kidney transplant, which have similar features but different limitations in terms of diagnostic techniques (in pregnancy only ultrasound is considered fully safe; care for avoiding nephrotoxicity is a must

Table 6.2 Papers analysing kidney scar development in adults

Author	Year	Country	Scope of the work	Case (controls) imaging
Kim JS	2014	Korea	Relationship between uncommon CT findings and clinical aspects in patients with acute pyelonephritis	125 patients; CT scans at diagnosis
Piccoli GB	2011	Italy (San Luigi)	The clinical and imaging presentation of acute "noncomplicated" pyelonephritis: a new profile for an ancient disease	119 patients; CT and MR scans at diagnosis and over follow-up
Martina MC	2010	Italy (Molinette)	Dynamic MR in acute pyelonephritis	125 patients; MR scans at diagnosis and over follow-up
Piccoli GB	2006	Italy (Molinette)	Development of kidney scars after acute uncomplicated pyelonephritis: relationship with clinical, laboratory and imaging data at diagnosis	58 patients; CT or MR scans
Piccoli G	2005	Italy (Molinette)	Acute pyelonephritis; a new approach to an old clinical entity	54 patients; CT or MR scans
Raz R	2003	Israel	Long-term follow-up of women hospitalised for acute pyelonephritis	63 patients clinical diagnosis, scintigraphy over follow-up
Bailey RR	1996	New Zealand	DMSA renal scans in adults with acute pyelonephritis	81 patients (73 women) clinical diagnosis, scintigraphy and US at diagnosis and over follow-up
Fraser IR	1995	Australia	A prospective study of cortical scarring in acute febrile pyelonephritis in adults: clinical and bacteriological characteristics	164 patients (142 female); IVU, CT scan and scintigraphy at diagnosis. Only CT and scintigraphy at follow-up
Tsugaya M	1992	Japan	Renal cortical scarring in acute pyelonephritis	14 patients (13 women and 1 man aged from 18 to 70); CT scans and IVU
Soulen MC	1989	USA	Sequelae of acute renal infections: CT evaluation	65 patients; CT scan at diagnosis and over follow-up; 17 of 65 had undergone more than one CT examination
Sandberg T	1989	Sweden	Selective use of excretory urography in women with acute pyelonephritis	103 patients; excretory urography at follow-up
Meyrier A	1989	France	Frequency of development of early cortical scarring in acute primary pyelonephritis	55 patients; CT scan at diagnosis and 27 over follow-up. 44 cases with kidney lesions
Huland H	1982	Germany	Renal scarring after symptomatic and asymptomatic upper urinary tract infection: a prospective study	17 patients with UTI and recurrent pyelonephritis; voiding cystography and excretory urography at follow-up. No patients had vesicoureteral reflux, obstructive uropathy, neurogenic bladder or nephrolithiasis

CT computed tomography, *MR* magnetic resonance, *US* ultrasonography, *IVU* intravenous urography, *UTI* urinary tract infection
Piccoli G. Molinette: partial duplicate with Piccoli GB 2006

Table 6.3 Incidence of kidney scars after APN in adults

Author	Year	Cases	% Previous	% Abscessed	% New scars	Scar definition
Kim JS	2014	125	8%	16%	n.r.	n.a.
Piccoli GB	2011	119	15.1%	39.5%	n.r.	n.a.
Martina MC	2010	125	23.2%	32.5%	16.5%	Parenchymal retraction, deformation of renal contour and constant signal hypo-density both at baseline and on delayed post-contrast scans
Piccoli GB	2006	58	6.9%	15.5%	29.3%	Scarring is visible as renal parenchymal atrophy
Piccoli G	2005	54	n.r.	n.r.	22.2%	Scars appear as diffuse or sharp indentation of the kidney's contour with thinning of cortex
Raz R	2003	63	n.r.	n.r.	46%	Scar: if a cortical uptake defect or diffuse hypo-activity is present
Bailey RR	1996	81	6% (All with reflux nephropathy)	n.r.	n.r.	n.a.
Fraser IR	1995	164	n.r.	n.r.	25.5%	n.a.
Tsugaya M	1992	14	n.r.	n.r.	42.9%	Scar: presence of renal parenchymal atrophy
Soulen MC	1989	17	29.4%	58.82%	All new scars: 41.18%	n.a.
Sandberg T	1989	103	n.r.	n.r.	13.6%	Localised renal parenchymal reduction with or without deformation of the adjacent calyx
Meyrier A	1989	55	n.r.	n.r.	37%	n.a.
Huland H	1982	17	11.7%	n.r.	0%	n.a.

after kidney transplantation) and nephrotoxic or potentially teratogenic agents.

Nor does the review deal with the problem of infections in the renal cysts, discussed elsewhere in this book, or rare infections, such as emphysematous APN and tuberculosis. We refer readers interested in these topics to other chapters in the book (*insert*).

6.6 Conclusions: Why We Need Further Research

APN is an ancient disease, yet much remains to be learned about it.

While we know something about it, namely, the pathogens that cause it, the imaging that is required to make a diagnosis and what short-term follow-up should be, we know less about the long-term effect of kidney scars, how long treatment should continue and what the effect of treatment duration on kidney scars is. The nephrologist's conclusions can thus be summarised into two sentences.

Do not think that we know everything there is to know about APN. Before applying guidelines, test the inclusion and exclusion criteria of the main RCTs with the data available for each population.

A prospective randomised trial is probably needed to asses duration of therapy in a setting in which imaging is done at referral and before stopping therapy, with at least a medium-term outcome, i.e. kidney scars.

Further studies are clearly needed and many mysteries remain to be solved before we fully understand this ancient disease.

References

1. Thiemich M (1910) Über die eitrigen Erkrankungen der Nieren und Harnwege im Säuglingsalter. Jahr Kinderheilkd 72:243
2. Subcommittee on Urinary Tract Infection, Steering Committee on Quality Improvement and Management, Roberts KB (2011) Urinary tract infection: clinical practice guideline for the diagnosis and management of the initial UTI in febrile infants and children 2 to 24 months. Pediatrics 128(3):595–610
3. Roberts KB (2012) Revised AAP guideline on UTI in febrile infants and young children. Am Fam Physician 86(10):940–946
4. Sigler M, Leal JE, Bliven K, Cogdill B, Thompson A (2015) Assessment of appropriate antibiotic prescribing for urinary tract infections in an internal medicine clinic. South Med J 108(5):300–304
5. Kang C, Kim K, Lee SH, Park C, Kim J, Lee JH, Jo YH, Rhee JE, Kim DH, Kim SC (2013) A risk stratification model of acute pyelonephritis to indicate hospital admission from the ED. Am J Emerg Med 31(7):1067–1072
6. Gupta K, Hooton TM, Naber KG, Wullt B, Colgan R, Miller LG, Moran GJ, Nicolle LE, Raz R, Schaeffer AJ, Soper DE, Infectious Diseases Society of America; European Society for Microbiology and Infectious Diseases (2011) International clinical practice guidelines for the treatment of acute uncomplicated cystitis and pyelonephritis in women: a 2010 update by the Infectious Diseases Society of America and the European Society for Microbiology and Infectious Diseases. Clin Infect Dis 52(5):e103–e120
7. Giacchino F, Piccoli G, Colla L, Fenoglio R, Marazzi F, Amore A, Rollino C, Stratta P, Vella Maria C, Deluca A, Boero R, Chiarinotti D, Licata C, Cravero R, Bainotti S, Manes M, Marcuccio C, Brezzi B, Filippo M, Pignone E, Reinero R, Radin E, Tamagnone M (2014) Acute pyelonephritis and renal abscesses in piedmont and Aosta Valley. G Ital Nefrol 31(4): pii: gin/31.4.10
8. Bailey RR, Lynn KL, Robson RA, Smith AH, Maling TM, Turner JG (1996) DMSA renal scans in adults with acute pyelonephritis. Clin Nephrol 46(2):99–104
9. Craig WD, Wagner BJ, Travis MD (2008) Pyelonephritis: radiologic-pathologic review. Radiographics 28:255–276
10. De Pascale A, Piccoli GB, Priola SM, Rognone D, Consiglio V, Garetto I, Rizzo L, Veltri A (2013) Diffusion-weighted magnetic resonance imaging: new perspectives in the diagnostic pathway of non-complicated acute pyelonephritis. Eur Radiol 23:3077–3086
11. Kim JS, Lee S, Lee KW, Kim JM, Kim YH, Kim ME (2014) Relationship between uncommon computed tomography findings and clinical aspects in patients with acute pyelonephritis. Korean J Urol 55(7):482–486
12. Campos-Franco J, Macia C, Huelga E, Diaz-Louzao C, Gude F, Alende R, Gonzalez-Quintela A (2017) Acute focal bacterial nephritis in a cohort of hospitalized adult patients with acute pyelonephritis. Assessment of risk factors and a predictive model. Eur J Intern Med 39:69–74
13. Mola G, Wenger TR, Salomonsson P, Knudsen IJD, Madsen JL, Møller S, Olsen BH, Vinicoff PG, Thorup J, Cortes D (2017) Selective imaging modalities after first pyelonephritis failed to identify significant urological anomalies, despite normal antenatal ultrasounds. Acta Paediatr 106(7):1176–1183. https://doi.org/10.1111/apa.13894. [Epub ahead of print]
14. Pinthus JH, Oksman Y, Leibovitch I, Goshen E, Dotan ZA, Schwartz A, Ramon J, Zwas ST, Mor Y (2005) The role of indirect radionuclide cystography during the acute phase of pyelonephritis in young women. BJU Int 95(4):619–623
15. Kim SB, Yang WS, Ryu JS, Song JH, Moon DH, Cho KS, Park JS, Hong CD (1994) Clinical value of DMSA planar and single photon emission computed tomography as an initial diagnostic tool in adult women with recurrent acute pyelonephritis. Nephron 67(3):274–279
16. Talner LB, Davidson AJ, Lebowitz RL, Dalla Palma L, Goldman SM (1994) Acute pyelonephritis: can we agree on terminology? Radiology 192:297–305
17. Piccoli GB, Consiglio V, Colla L, Mesiano P, Magnano A, Burdese M, Marcuccio C, Mezza E, Veglio V, Piccoli G (2006) Antibiotic treatment for acute "uncomplicated" or "primary" pyelonephritis: a systematic, semantic revision. Int J Antimicrob Agents 28(Suppl 1):S49–S63
18. Heptinstall RH (1992) Pathology of the kidney. In: Heptinstall RH (ed) Pyelonephritis: pathologic features. Little Brown, Boston, pp 1489–1561
19. Hooton TM, Stamm WE (1997) Diagnosis and treatment of uncomplicated urinary tract infection. Infect Dis Clin N Am 11:551–581
20. Lichtenberger P, Hooton TM (2008) Complicated urinary tract infections. Curr Infect Dis Rep 10:499–504
21. Martina MC, Campanino PP, Caraffo F, Marcuccio C, Gunetti F, Colla L, Cassinis MC, Gandini G (2010) Dynamic magnetic resonance imaging in acute pyelonephritis. Radiol Med 115(2):287–300
22. Meyrier A (1990) Quels examens radiologiques demander devant une pyelonephrite aigue? Ann Med Interne 141(1):5–7

23. Piccoli GB, Consiglio V, Deagostini MC, Serra M, Biolcati M, Ragni F, Biglino A, De Pascale A, Frascisco MF, Veltri A, Porpiglia F (2011) The clinical and imaging presentation of acute "non complicated" pyelonephritis: a new profile for an ancient disease. BMC Nephrol 12:68

24. Piccoli G, Colla L, Maass J, Stratta P, Bianchi C, Burdese M, Mesiano P, Marcuccio C, Mezza E, Mazzucco G, Piccoli GB (2005) Acute pyelonephritis: a new approach to an old clinical entity. J Nephrol 18:474–496

25. Groen J, Pannek J, Castro Diaz D, Del Popolo G, Gross T, Hamid R, Karsenty G, Kessler TM, Schneider M, 't Hoen L, Blok B (2016) Summary of European Association of Urology (EAU) guidelines on Neuro-urology. Eur Urol 69(2):324–333

26. Johansen TE (2004) The role of imaging in urinary tract infections. World J Urol 22(5):392–398

27. Spoorenberg V, Hulscher ME, Akkermans RP, Prins JM, Geerlings SE (2014) Appropriate antibiotic use for patients with urinary tract infections reduces length of hospital stay. Clin Infect Dis 58(2):164–169

28. Wu HC, Chang CH, Lai MM, Lin CC, Lee CC, Kao A (2003) Using Tc-99m DMSA renal cortex scan to detect renal damage in women with type 2 diabetes. J Diabetes Complicat 17(5):297–300

29. Kranz J, Schmidt S, Lebert C, Schneidewind L, Vahlensieck W, Sester U, Fünfstück R, Helbig S, Hofmann W, Hummers E, Kunze M, Kniehl E, Naber K, Mandraka F, Mündner-Hensen B, Schmiemann G, Wagenlehner FME (2017) Epidemiology, diagnostics, therapy, prevention and management of uncomplicated bacterial outpatient acquired urinary tract infections in adult patients: update 2017 of the interdisciplinary AWMF S3 guideline. Urologe A 56(6):746–758. https://doi.org/10.1007/s00120-017-0389-1. [Epub ahead of print]

30. Demonchy E, Dufour JC, Gaudart J, Cervetti E, Michelet P, Poussard N, Levraut J, Pulcini C (2014) Impact of a computerized decision support system on compliance with guidelines on antibiotics prescribed for urinary tract infections in emergency departments: a multicentre prospective before-and-after controlled interventional study. J Antimicrob Chemother 69(10):2857–2863

31. Colgan R, Williams M, Johnson JR (2011) Diagnosis and treatment of acute pyelonephritis in women. Am Fam Physician 84(5):519–526

32. Shaikh N, Ewing AL, Bhatnagar S, Hoberman A (2010) Risk of renal scarring in children with a first urinary tract infection: a systematic review. Pediatrics 126:1084–1091

33. Karavanaki KA, Soldatou A, Koufadaki AM, Tsentidis C, Haliotis FA, Stefanidis CJ (2017) Delayed treatment of the first febrile urinary tract infection in early childhood increased the risk of renal scarring. Acta Paediatr 106(1):149–154

34. Bayram MT, Kavukcu S, Alaygut D, Soylu A, Cakmakçý H (2014) Place of ultrasonography in predicting vesicoureteral reflux in patients with mild renal scarring. Urology 83(4):904–908

35. Oh MM, Kim JW, Park MG, Kim JJ, Yoo KH, Moon du G (2012) The impact of therapeutic delay time on acute scintigraphic lesion and ultimate scar formation in children with first febrile UTI. Eur J Pediatr 171(3):565–570

36. Doganis D, Siafas K, Mavrikou M, Issaris G, Martirosova A, Perperidis G, Konstantopoulos A, Sinaniotis K (2007) Does early treatment of urinary tract infection prevent renal damage? Pediatrics 120(4):e922–e923

37. Fontanilla T, Minaya J, Cortés C, Hernando CG, Arangüena RP, Arriaga J, Carmona MS, Alcolado A (2012) Acute complicated pyelonephritis: contrast-enhanced ultrasound. Abdom Imaging 37(4): 639–646

38. Carnell J, Fischer J, Nagdev A (2011) Ultrasound detection of obstructive pyelonephritis due to urolithiasis in the ED. Am J Emerg Med 29(7):843.e1–843.e3

39. Chen KC, Hung SW, Seow VK, Chong CF, Wang TL, Li YC, Chang H (2011) The role of emergency ultrasound for evaluating acute pyelonephritis in the ED. Am J Emerg Med 29(7):721–724

40. Dell'Atti L, Borea PA, Ughi G, Russo GR (2010) Clinical use of ultrasonography associated with color Doppler in the diagnosis and follow-up of acute pyelonephritis. Arch Ital Urol Androl 82(4):217–220

41. Piccoli GB, Colla L, Burdese M, Marcuccio C, Mezza E, Maass J, Picciotto G, Sargiotto A, Besso L, Magnano A, Veglio V, Piccoli G (2006) Development of kidney scars after acute uncomplicated pyelonephritis: relationship with clinical, laboratory and imaging data at diagnosis. World J Urol 24(1): 66–73

42. Piccoli GB, Cresto E, Ragni F, Veglio V, Scarpa RM, Frascisco M (2008) The clinical spectrum of acute "uncomplicated" pyelonephritis from an emergency medicine perspective. Int J Antimicrob Agents 31S:S46–S53

43. Rollino C, Beltrame G, Ferro M, Quattrocchio G, Sandrone M, Quarello F (2012) Acute pyelonephritis in adults: a case series of 223 patients. Nephrol Dial Transplant 27:3488–3493

44. Kim Y, Seo MR, Kim SJ, Kim J, Wie SH, Cho YK, Lim SK, Lee JS, Kwon KT, Lee H, Cheong HJ, Park DW, Ryu SY, Chung MH, Pai H (2017) Usefulness of blood cultures and radiologic imaging studies in the Management of Patients with community-acquired acute pyelonephritis. Infect Chemother 49(1): 22–30

45. Oh SJ, Je BK, Lee SH, Choi WS, Hong D, Kim SB (2016) Comparison of computed tomography findings between bacteremic and non-bacteremic acute pyelonephritis due to Escherichia coli. World J Radiol 8(4):403–409

46. Yu M, Robinson K, Siegel C, Menias C (2017) Complicated genitourinary tract infections and mimics. Curr Probl Diagn Radiol 46(1):74–83

47. Wi YM, Kim SW, Chang HH, Jung SI, Kim YS, Cheong HS, Ki HK, Son JS, Kwon KT, Heo ST, Yeom JS, Ko KS, Kang CI, Chung DR, Peck KR, Song JH (2014) Predictors of uropathogens other than *Escherichia coli* in patients with community-onset acute pyelonephritis. Int J Clin Pract 68(6):749–755

48. Mody L, Juthani-Mehta M (2014) Urinary tract infections in older women: a clinical review. JAMA 311(8):844–854

49. Matthews SJ, Lancaster JW (2011) Urinary tract infections in the elderly population. Am J Geriatr Pharmacother 9(5):286–309

50. Fraser IR, Birch D, Fairley KF, John S, Lichtenstein M, Tress B (1995) Kincaid-Smith a prospective study of cortical scarring in acute febrile pyelonephritis in adults: clinical and bacteriological characteristics. Clin Nephrol 43(3):159–164

51. Huland H, Busch R, Riebel T (1982) Renal scarring after symptomatic and asymptomatic upper urinary tract infection: a prospective study. J Urol 128(4):682–685

52. Leroy S, Fernandez-Lopez A, Nikfar R, Romanello C, Bouissou F, Gervaix A, Gurgoze MK, Bressan S, Smolkin V, Tuerlinckx D, Stefanidis CJ, Vaos G, Leblond P, Gungor F, Gendrel D, Chalumeau M (2013) Association of procalcitonin with acute pyelo-nephritis and renal scars in pediatric UTI. Pediatrics 131(5):870–879. Date of Publication: May 2013

53. Meyrier A, Condamin MC, Fernet M, Labigne-Roussel A, Simon P, Callard P, Rainfray M, Soilleux M, Groc A (1989) Frequency of development of early cortical scarring in acute primary pyelonephritis. Kidney Int 35(2):696–703

54. Meyrier A (1990) Long-term risks of acute pyelone-phritis. Nephron 54:197–201

55. Meyrier A, Condamin MC (1990) Les forms atypiques des pyelonephritis aigues primitives. Rev Pract 40(14):1275–1278

56. Meyrier A, Guibert J (1992) Diagnosis and drug treat-ment of acute pyelonephritis. Drugs 44(3):356–367

57. Raz R, Sakran W, Chazan B, Colodner R, Kunin C (2003) Long-term follow-up of women hospi-talized for acute pyelonephritis. Clin Infect Dis 37(8):1014–1020

58. Soulen MC, Fishman EK, Goldman SM (1989) Sequelae of acute renal infections: CT evaluation. Radiology 173(2):423–426

59. Tsugaya M, Hirao N, Sakagami H, Ohtaguro K, Washida H (1992) Renal cortical scarring in acute pyelonephritis. Br J Urol 69(3):245–249

Part II

Imaging of Upper Urinary Tract Infections

Ultrasound of Upper Urinary Tract Infections

7

Emilio Quaia, Antonio G. Gennari, and Maria A. Cova

7.1 Introduction

Urinary tract infection (UTI) is the most common bacterial infection. It accounts for 8.6 million visits in the ambulatory care setting in the United States [1]. Women are at higher risk for UTI, with a self-reported annual incidence of 12%, and by the age of 32, half of them have suffered at least one UTI [1]. Moreover UTI recurrence is high. Most UTI infections are acute cystitis that regress rapidly with proper antibiotic therapy. Luckily acute pyelonephritis is much less common than cystitis, with a peak annual incidence of 25 cases per 10,000 women 15–34 years of age [1]. Incidence of UTI in men younger than 60 years of age is rare, but after 85, incidence duplicates but still remains half that of women. UTI is the most common cause of bacteraemia in older men [2]. UTI is really common also in children. Infection is initiated when potential pathogens migrate from the bowel lumen to urethra and ascend to the kidneys. Risk factors are different for women (sexual intercourse, use of spermicides, previous urinary tract infection and a new sex partner) and men (benign prostatic hyperplasia and increased ratio of catheterization). It is mandatory to differentiate uncomplicated UTI (episodes of acute cystitis and pyelonephritis in healthy premenopausal, non-pregnant woman, with no history suggesting abnormalities of urinary tract) and complicated UTI (all the other cases). Usually imaging is not required for diagnosis and treatment of uncomplicated UTI in adult patients. Moreover patients with conditions predisposing to infections (immunocompromised or diabetic patients) may benefit from early imaging. Imaging is used to detect disease and define its nature and extent and reveal predisposing conditions and complications.

7.2 Imaging Modalities

Several imaging modalities have been used to image UTIs in the past decades. Even though we will later discuss each technique, ultrasound (US) is the modality of choice for initial evaluation in children. Children should be scanned both in supine and prone position. Computed tomography (CT) and magnetic resonance (MR) are inacceptable for routine use. Even though the usage of CT is common in adult medicine, we highly

E. Quaia (✉)
Edinburgh Imaging facility, Queen's Medical Research Institute, University of Edinburgh, 47 Little France Crescent, Edinburgh EH16 4TJ, UK
e-mail: equaia@exseed.ed.ac.uk

A.G. Gennari • M.A. Cova
Department of Radiology, Cattinara Hospital, University of Trieste, Strada di Fiume 447, Trieste 34149, Italy

© Springer International Publishing AG 2018
M. Tonolini (ed.), *Imaging and Intervention in Urinary Tract Infections and Urosepsis*,
https://doi.org/10.1007/978-3-319-68276-1_7

recommend US as a first-line imaging modality also in adults since it is inexpensive, immediate, painless, widely available and radiation-free. CT and MR should be used as a second-line imaging modality in complicated patients.

7.2.1 Plain Film

Abdominal radiography is a rapid and relatively inexpensive examination, so it was used as a part of the initial examination study in patients with suspected pyelonephritis. However abdominal radiography had low sensitivity and specificity. Moreover it became the initial step of every excretory urographic study, but the successive use of CT overcame that of plain films in almost all institutions. The CT scout radiography allows the detection of urinary calcifications and gas but has several drawbacks including the unreliable differentiation of abdominal gas from the presence of gas in the UT and the difficult detection of small urinary calcification superimposed on normally calcified structures such as vertebral transverse process [3].

7.2.2 Intravenous Urography

Intravenous urography (IVU) had a well-established role in the evaluation of the UT; in fact it allows the visualization of the kidneys, ureters and bladder after the intravenous injection of contrast medium. Kidneys contrast medium removal (filtration) from the blood stream and excretion in the UT enable the opacification of the structures mentioned above and to image them thanks to several plain films taken at predefined image intervals as the contrast flows through the different portions of the UT. The possible imaging findings in positive IVU were a diffuse oedema and an enlargement of the affected kidneys, a delayed and attenuated nephrogram, a retarded filtration and excretion of the contrast medium which determine an effacement or a delayed filling of the renal collecting system with decreased opacity and a dilatation of the renal collecting system [4].

Nowadays IVU has increasingly been replaced by computed tomography urography (CTU) even though there is a paucity of comparative studies between the two techniques [5]. Referring physician is pleased by the large amount of data CTU provides not only on UT but also on other abdominal organs and structures, and patients prefer CTU due to the absence of preparatory bowel cleansing. Two major drawbacks are costs and radiation dose: CTU undoubtedly costs more and exposes patients to a higher dose (10–35 mSv) compared to IVU (5 mSv), but CTU data should be critically reviewed on the basis of the number of phased used, newest low kilovolt (kV) and milliampere second (mAs) protocol and automatic tube-current modulation. In conclusion literature suggests that a dose reduction is feasible technically, but exam protocols should be tailored on patient's characteristics and clinical problems [5].

7.2.3 Ultrasonography

US is an inexpensive, repeatable, widely available, radiation-free imaging technique, based on properties of acoustic physic. Its widespread use makes it essential in the initial evaluation of the kidneys. Moreover, in urological pathologies, US frequently confirm clinical suspicion or even lead to final diagnosis. In US high-frequency ultrasound waves are generated within the probe, where an electric field is applied to an array of piezoelectric crystals causing them to vibrate, thus generating ultrasound waves. After being generated, waves are sent in the tissues where they interact with multiple human body surfaces being attenuated, reflected and/or refracted. The retuned echoes (to the probe) are reconverted to electrical impulses and generate images. Given the assumptions of a constant waves' speed within human tissues (1540 m/s) and constant attenuation and waves' straight path, different echo times are used to characterize (define the echogenicity) and localize different tissue types; the same assumptions lead also to artefact formation. Ring-down artefact (typical of air presence) occurs when US beam encounters fluid, trapped within a tetrahedron of air bubbles. It determines a repeated vibration of the air-fliud system creating a continuous echo transmitted back to the probe. A bright reflector with a continuous bright line extending posteriorly is the way this artefact is displayed [6]. Shadowing artefact is characterized by a signal void behind a high attenuating zone. In fact when the ultrasound beam encounters an area with an extremely higher attenuation, compared to the neighbouring tissues, most of the echoes are reflected, so the echoes returning from structures beyond are highly attenuated as well. Bones and calcified structures such as nephrolithiasis typically present shadowing [6].

US-Doppler imaging utilizes Doppler effect (calculating frequency shift) to imagine moving structures, usually blood, within a region of interest. Structures can be imaged, quantitatively and qualitatively, as moving towards the probe or away from it. US-Doppler imaging is helpful in vessel imaging as well as in the definition of the vascularization of a specific tissue area. Anyhow even US-Doppler imaging has its own artefact. In twinkling artefact, which is typically associated with rough hyperechoic, irregular surfaces, an alternating scintillation of colours on US-Doppler imaging is displayed beneath the hyperechoic structure. It is commonly referred to a form of intrinsic noise related to the multiple internal reflections of the incident ultrasound beam on multiple cracks, which broaden the spectrum. This phenomenon may aid in detection of renal calculi.

A proper and detailed US examination of kidneys starts with patient in supine position. At first renal length (longitudinal axis) and cortical thickness should be analysed. Even though normal right kidney mean longitudinal diameter is 10.74 ± 1.35 cm, and left kidney mean longitudinal diameter is 11.10 ± 1.15 cm, length should be related to patient's height and phenotype. Normal renal anatomy is arranged in an outer echogenic cortex, echo-poor pyramids and the sinus. Ribs sometimes obscure some portion of kidneys. In such cases the sonographer should find a proper acoustic window locating the probe between ribs or asking the patient to breathe deeply in order to rise them up.

The recent widespread use of contrast-enhanced ultrasorography (CEUS) raised concern to an otherwise old technique; in fact at first it was described in 1968. CEUS is based on microbubble-based contrast agents (3–10 μm) composed of a shell of biocompatible materials (lipids and proteirs) filled with gas (air, perfluorocarbon or sulphur hexafluoride), each of the components determine specific physical and mechanical properties. Particularly the biocompatible shell affects their capability to oscillate. In CEUS the US beam interacts with microbubbles in several different ways: at high acoustic power, microbubbles are destructed, while at low acoustic power, they produce a sound with the same frequency (f0) of the insonating beam (Fig. 7.1). At their resonant frequency, higher than the latter one, a non-linear vibration is produced, so harmonic (2f0, 3f0, etc.) and subharmonic (f0/2, f0/3, etc.) peaks are generated after the first resonance frequency peak. The mechanism underlying US contrast medium is completely different from other types of contrast media; in fact microbubbles are confined within vascular, so they do not pass in the interstice.

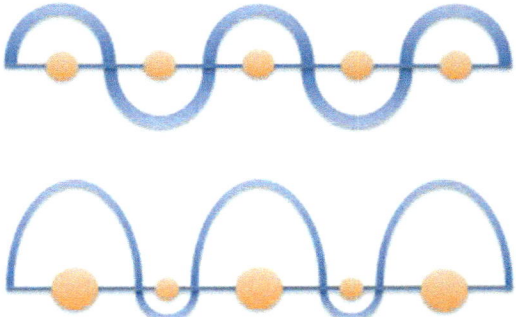

Fig. 7.1 At low acoustic power (10-20 Kilo Pascal) microbubbles mantains the same radius after compression and relaxation so produce a sound with the same frequency of the insonating bram (higher portion of the image). At higher iacoustic power (40-50 Kilo Pascal) microbubbles interact with the US beam expanding and contracting in a non-linear mode (lower portion of the image). Both of these characteristics has been used to obtain CEUS images

Sonoelastography (SE) is an ultrasound technique to image the relative elastic/mechanical properties of soft tissue. Tissue could be imaged using strain elastography or shear-wave elastography. In strain elastography tissue is manually compressed with the probe. Speckle tracking is used to image speckle displacement, which is correlated to tissue displacement. Harder materials are deformed less, so speckle are more stable, contrary softer materials are easier to compress and speckle are displaced more. Shear-wave elastography uses US beam both to compress tissues at a specific depth and to image the propagation of shear-wave displacement in the tissue. The US equipment produce a push pulse which compress parenchyma generating low-frequency waves (low than 1000 Hz) radiating in a plane perpendicular to the image plane. Shear waves are then imaged using real-time Doppler or time of flight techniques. A specific vendor has also developed an innovative way to image larger tissue portion. Multiple push pulse are sent at different depth creating a conical wavefront that is used to image mechanical properties of larger sampled areas. However each technique has its own advantages and drawbacks. Strain elastography is simpler and cheaper, but tissue compression is subjective and deeper organs are difficult to evaluate. Moreover strain elastography is nonquantitative. It may only express the ratio of stiffness/elasticity of the pathological portion to the normal one. Shear-wave elastography does not necessitate compression, and it is more quantitative; anyhow quantitative results of different vendors are not comparable, and renal parenchymal complexity modifies shear-wave propagation. Kidneys have a very complex architecture with a multitude of tubules parallel to the papilla axis. Shear-wave velocity reduces encountering tubules and vascular structures thus altering elasticity values.

7.3 Acute Infection

7.3.1 Pyelonephritis

Pyelonephritis is defined as an infection of the renal parenchyma, calyces and renal pelvis and represents a potentially organ- and/or life-threatening infection. Usually, renal infection is caused by direct bacterial infection throughout two different routes: ascending the UT (most common) and via the bloodstream (less common). Therefore in ascending pyelonephritis, the medulla is firstly involved; contrary haematogenous spread is first seen as cortical, even though, after 48, this distinction is not feasible. Moreover in haematogenous spread, both kidneys are typically involved. Common pathogens in ascending forms are *Escherichia coli* and *Enterococcus faecalis*, two bowel organisms that frequently infect UT. Streptococci and staphylococci are the most involved organisms in haematogenous diffusion [7]. In younger patients pyelonephritis is more frequent in women [7]. Common symptoms are fever, chills, leukocytosis, unilateral or bilateral flank pain, dysuria and urinary frequency and urgency. Infrequently gastrointestinal symptoms may be seen such as abdominal pain, nausea, vomiting and diarrhoea. Elevated C-reactive protein, elevated erythrocyte sedimentation rate and leukocytosis with a neutrophilic shift are common findings at blood tests. Other typical findings are pyuria, granular or leukocyte casts, bacteriuria and positive urinary cultures. Sometimes blood cultures and urine cultures share the same bacteria. If untreated pyelonephritis often leads to renal scaring, so timely diagnosis and management is such important on patients' outcomes. At gross pathology involved kidneys are generally enlarged and display whitish patchy areas of varying size alternating to spared parenchyma. Thin yellow streaks crossing through the medulla representing collecting ducts filled with pus may also be seen [7]. On sectioning, diffuse involvement of parenchymal surface by microabscesses may be present [7]. In cases associated with urinary obstruction, renal pelvis and calices may be dilated. Sometimes, severe infection may lead to papillary necrosis. At microscopy evaluation acute bacterial pyelonephritis is characterized by prominent neutrophilic inflammation of the renal tubules, typically sparring glomeruli and vessels [7]. There is an associated destruction of tubular basement membranes, resulting in inflammation spilling into the renal interstitium. Parenchymal involvement is often patchy, with alternating areas of intense inflammation and relatively normal-appearing zones [7].

Abdominal radiograph is a rapid, inexpensive examination that was routinely obtained as the first component of IVU. However the widespread use of CT has overtaken that of radiography. Moreover the information derived from abdominal radiograph were scarce: urinary tract gas and calcifications. IVU helped in delineating the anatomy of the UT and pelvicalyceal system. Renal enlargement, striated or delayed nephrogram, delayed calyceal appearance and dilatation or effacement of the collecting system were typical findings of acute renal infection. However only a paucity of patients had abnormal IVU findings and there was a low parenchymal detail; therefore other imaging techniques are preferred. Even though US is negative in a vast majority with suspected pyelonephritis, it is frequently used as a first-line diagnostic tool. Interstitial nephritis is not visible on routine greyscale images. Positive US findings are renal enlargement, loss of renal sinus fat due to oedema, congenital anomalies, hydronephrosis and modifications in renal echogenicity and corticomedullary differentiation system [3, 8]. The latter finding could represent haemorrhage (hyperechoic), oedema (hypoechoic) or abscess formation (Fig. 7.2). Colour Doppler improves sensitivity to parenchymal abnormality as most pyelonephritic lesions are ischaemic, and power Doppler helps in evaluating of hypoperfused areas. Several pitfalls are associated with US kidney evaluation such as differentiations of calcification from intraparenchymal or collecting system gas (manifested, respectively, as "clean" shadowing and "dirty" shadowing with echoes and reverberations) and identification of perinephric extension of infection system. The urinary bladder should always be imaged in a US evaluation for suspected pyelonephritis. Newer applications such as tissue harmonic and US contrast agents may enhance sensitivity. With tissue harmonic imaging, pyelonephritic lesions were commonly seen as focal or segmental, patchy, hypoechoic areas extending from the medulla to the renal capsule [3]. CT is the modal-

ity of choice in acute bacterial pyelonephritis. In fact it is superior to US providing detailed anatomic and physiologic information allowing the definition of both extrarenal and intrarenal pathologic conditions. However CEUS is an alternative that has been proven to be equally accurate in the detection of acute pyelonephritis [9] even though there is a paucity of literature and EFSUMB 2008 guidelines do not include complicated pyelonephritis as an indication for CEUS [10]. Parenchymal enhancement after microbubble injection is evaluated continuously. Anyhow two major phases could be considered: a cortical phase, in which there is a pronounced enhancement of the cortex (15–30 s after contrast injection), and a parenchymal phase, in which both the cortex and medullae enhance (25 s–4 min after contrast injection). Parenchymal phase may also be divided into early parenchymal phase (25 s–1 min) and late parenchymal phase (after 1 min) [11]. Typical CEUS features of pyelonephritis are a cortical or corticomedullary focal wedge-shaped or round lesion, less enhancing compared to the surrounding parenchyma [11] (Fig. 7.2), but CEUS may also demonstrate normal parenchymal enhancement. However microbubbles are not nephrotoxic so it is safe to use them, even in patients with marginal renal function as a first-line exam. US elastography has not been used yet to differentiate areas of nephritis from surrounding healthy parenchyma. However infection and inflammation determine tissue oedema and urine flow blockage due to tubular obstruction, so renal stiffness increases (Fig. 7.2). Moreover abscess formation leads to colliquation, so during early stages, when abscess cavity is not still formed, parenchyma may show reduced tissue stiffness values compared to nephritis areas. Even though its clinical utility in acute pyelonephritis is debated, alteration at renal cortex scintigraphy may be seen and may last for at least 3 months after infections. Early scintigraphic findings usually do not predict the late outcome [12]. That is why renal cortex scintigraphy is advocate in the detection of post-pyelonephritis renal scarring, even though there is no consensus between authors on the correct timing. Moreover

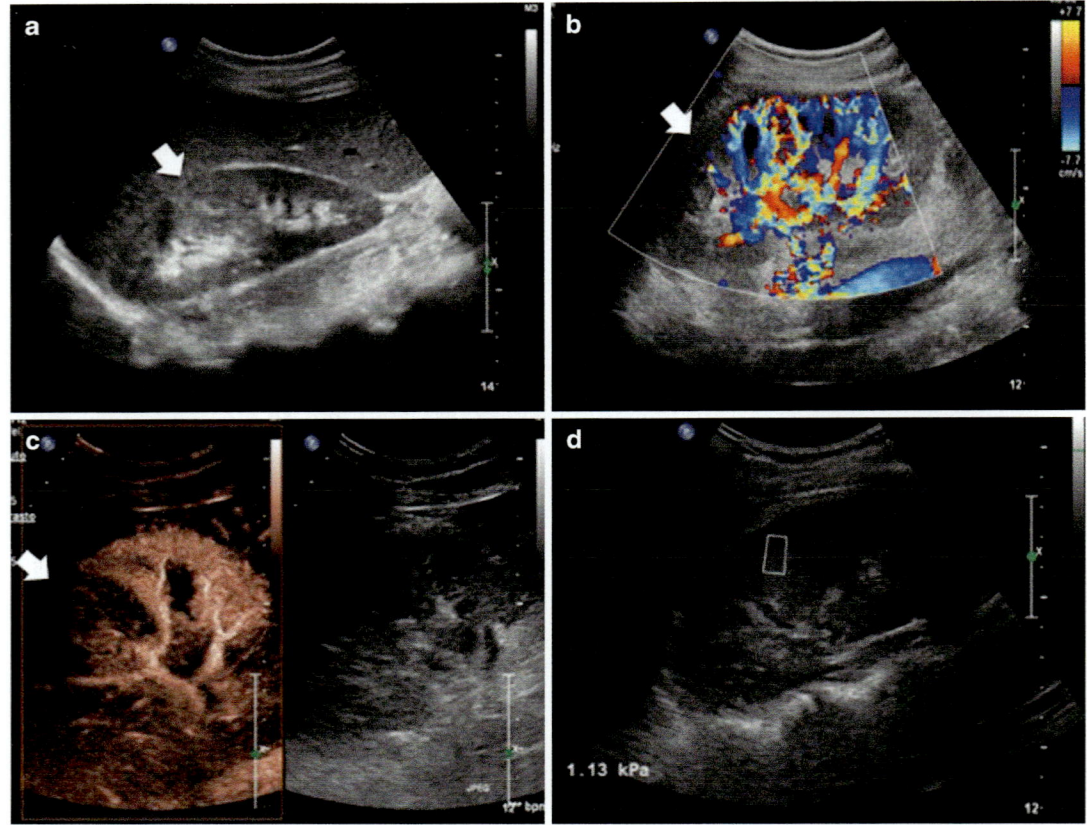

Fig. 7.2 US findings in a female patient with fever, chills, and right flank pain in who right kidney pyelonephritis was suspected. A paracoronal US scan (**a**) showing an enlarged hyperechoic area (*arrow*) of parenchyma in which there is loss of corticomedullary differentiation. The correspond-ing color-Doppler findings (**b**) are an ischaemic area (*arrow*). CEUS (**c**) and SE (**d**) enhance diagnostic confi-dence confirming that the area has no enhancement (*arrow* in **c**) after microbubbles injection and is stiffer compared to the adjacent renal structures (*white box* in **d**)

renal cortical scintigraphy using 99mTc-DMSA has proved to be more sensitive than US and IVU and as accurate as CT and MRI in the diagnosis of acute pyelonephritis [13].

7.3.2 Pyonephrosis and Hydronephrosis

As detailed previously, hydronephrosis, a dis-tention and dilatation of renal pelvis and caly-ces, caused by an obstruction of the free urine flow, is a predisposing factor for UTI and per-manent renal dysfunction. It may be unilateral or bilateral. The distention of both the ure-ter and the renal pelvis and calices is defined hydroureteronephrosis. Pyonephrosis repre-sents an infected, obstructed and frequently enlarged, collecting system [3]. Symptoms are non-specific and similar to those of other UTI and include fever, chills and flank pain. It should be suspected in patients with known UT obstruction associated with flank pain and fever. Early diagnosis is mandatory because direct, immediate intervention is crucial. When pyonephrosis is left untreated, renal func-tion deteriorates rapidly and permanently [3]. Moreover patients frequently develop septic shock. Pyonephrosis may be caused by a broad spectrum of pathologic conditions. Pathogens reach the collecting system through ascending infection or haematogenous spread. There are wide predisposing risk factors such as obstruction due to calculi, ureteropelvic junction obstruction, tumours, complications from pyelonephritis or strictures and immunosuppression (diabetes, steroids, acquired immunodeficiency syndrome).

In the past IVU was an important clinical tool in pyonephrosis in the detection of obstructive uropathy. US is valuable in the identification of pelvicalyceal system dilatation, echogenic debris, fluid-fluid levels within the collecting system and occasionally gas. The presence of debris is the most reliable sign of pyonephrosis. Furthermore US can detect calculi at the vesicoureteric junction, but the detection of ureteric calculi is more challenging [3, 8]. It is thought that the evaluation of vascular resistive indices ameliorates sensitivity, but there has been paucity of studies. Drainage of the infected collecting system can be accomplished under CT, US or fluoroscopic guidance, placing a percutaneous nephrostomy. Drainage decompresses the collecting system, allowing better renal plasma flow and delivery of antibiotics to both parenchyma and urine.

7.3.3 Emphysematous Pyelonephritis

Emphysematous pyelonephritis (EPN) refers to a unilateral, fulminant, necrotizing, gas forming, infection of the renal parenchyma and the perinephric tissues [14]. Renal emphysema and pneumonephritis are other terms that have been used to describe this condition; contrary emphysematous pyelitis is the presence of gas in the renal pelvis alone, without parenchymal involvement. EPN is a rare and often life-threatening condition that usually occurs in uncontrolled diabetic patients, more frequently in women [8]. Mortality is high, and without early therapeutic intervention, the condition generalizes to fulminant sepsis, and urgent nephrectomy is mandatory. *Escherichia coli*, *Enterobacter*, *Klebsiella pneumoniae* and *Proteus mirabilis* account for

most of the reported cases, with *Escherichia coli* accounting for 60% [14]. Severely damaged, ischaemic kidneys in uncontrolled diabetic patients are the substrate on which pathogenic bacteria form gas causing mixed acid fermentation in a hyperglycaemic environment. The subsequent evolution is tissue destruction, purulent infection and inhibition of removal of locally produced gas [14].

In about 70% of patients, an abnormal collection of gas, either mottled gas within the renal fossa or crescentic collection within the Gerota fascia, could be detected in up to 85% of patients [3, 8]. US demonstrates an enlarged kidney with hyperechoic nondependent foci within the renal parenchyma or the collecting system that present distal shadowing reverberation. This characteristic feature helps in the distinction from renal calculi. Nevertheless US ability to correctly characterize EPN is low due to the presence of adjacent bowel gas or calculi that may confuse the interpretation.

7.3.4 Emphysematous Pyelitis

In emphysematous pyelitis (EP), the presence of gas is limited to the renal excretory system. It is a very rare and benign condition with a low overall mortality rate as compared to EPN. Thus, it is mandatory to distinguish between these two entities because of the prognostic differences and different clinical management. As in EPN, also in EP, gas production in the excretory system is secondary to acute bacterial infection [10]. EP is frequently associated with diabetes mellitus and obstruction of the UT. The diagnosis is frequently delayed due to the non-specificity of symptoms, similar to the clinical presentation of uncomplicated acute pyelonephritis [10].

Abdominal radiography demonstrates gas outlining the pelvicalyceal system and ureters. However, abdominal radiography sensitivity is low (33%), due to difficulty in differentiating renal gas from air in overlying loops of bowel [10]. At US high-amplitude nondependent flat echoes are typically within the renal sinus or calices but could be mistaken with calculi or the surrounding intra bowel air.

7.3.5 Renal Abscess

Renal abscess may result from an untreated or inadequately treated acute pyelonephritis that progress to tissue necrosis and liquefaction or from haematogenous spread of bacteria from a primary extrarenal focus of infection. Renal abscess has to be suspected when appropriate pyelonephritis therapy does not lead to clinical response [3]. Moreover immunocompromised, diabetic patients and those with UT obstruction are at greater risk. Gram-negative pathogens are more frequently encountered in ascending infections; conversely gram-positive organisms, such as *Staphylococcus aureus*, are associated with haematogenous spreading [8]. Severe renal parenchymal involvement and corticomedullary abscess could reach the renal capsule and perforate it, forming a perinephric abscess that is contained by Gerota fascia. If the UT is unobstructed, renal abscesses often drain spontaneously into the calyces and ureter [8]. It has to be kept in mind that pancreatitis, diverticulitis and Crohn's disease may also reach the perirenal space and produce similar appearances.

At US abscess appears as hypoechoic mass with borders that become more defined as the abscess encapsulates (Fig. 7.3). Sometimes in the cavity internal echoes, representing debris, and hyperechogenic foci with acoustic shadowing,

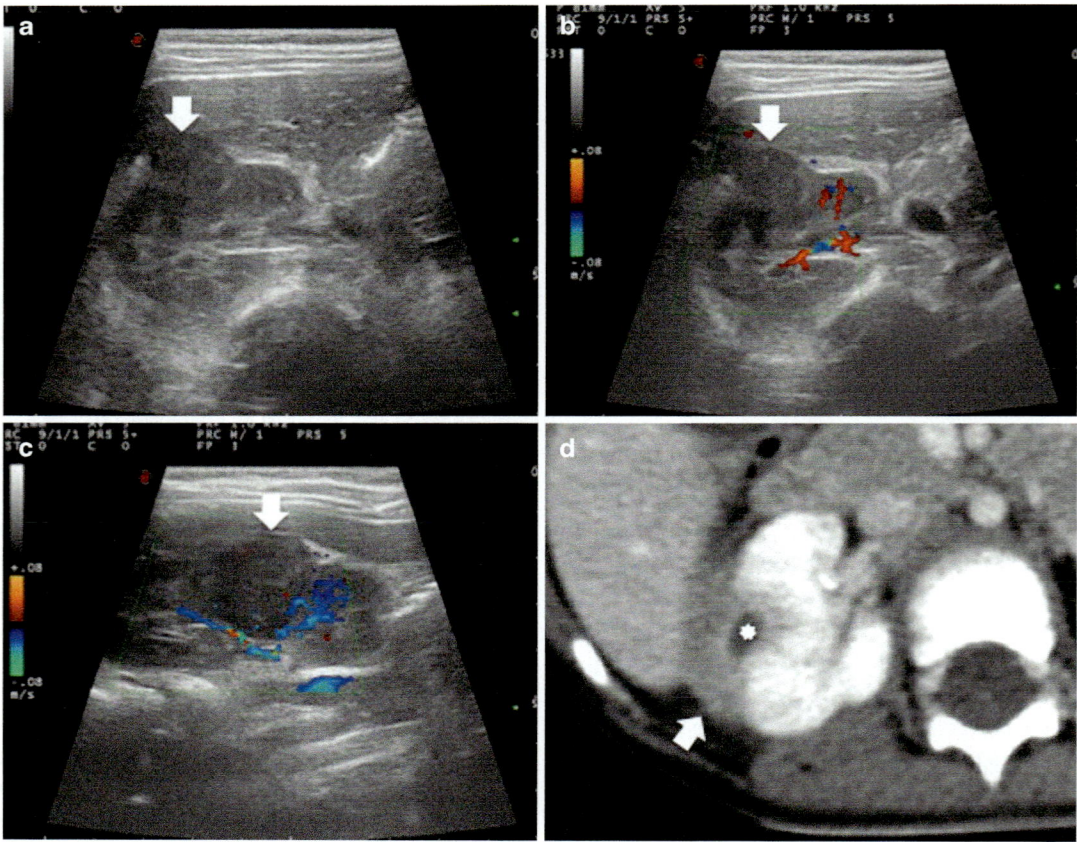

Fig. 7.3 US (**a**, **b**, **c**) and CT (**d**) findings in a young female patient, with known right kidney pyelonephritis, irresponsive to antibiotic treatment. A para-axial US scan demonstrating a bulky hypoechoic mass (*arrow*) arising from the right renal parenchyma protruding within the fat tissue of perirenal space. A para-axial (**b**) and a paracoronal (**c**) color-Doppler evaluation, showing the lack of flow signal in the mass (*arrow*). Axial contrast enhanced CT scan at nephroparenchymal phase confirms (*arrow*) the presence of an abscess, revealing a hypodense area (*) delimited by a hyperdense rim, and the involvement of the surrounding fat tissue

suggestive of air, may also be seen. Debris are movable with patient decubitus. Loculation and septations are other possible imaging findings. Typically there is no internal flow on colour Doppler images [3, 8]. At CEUS abscesses present as rounded or geographical areas lacking of enhancement throughout the whole exam. Some present with rim enhancement or enhancing thick septa [11]. Moreover, US- and CT-guided percutaneous placement of drains helps most of the patients to improve clinical status and is sometimes a definitive procedure [8].

7.4 Chronic Infection

7.4.1 Chronic Pyelonephritis

Chronic pyelonephritis (CP) is a somewhat controversial disease that is debated on whether it reflects a long-standing infection, arises from multiple recurrent infections or represents the residuum of an old, inactive disease. In the past it was diagnosed when significant lymphocytic inflammation of the renal interstitium was noted. However, kidneys' scarring from non-infectious conditions is also accompanied by prominent, non-specific chronic inflammation [7]. Moreover, chronic inflammation in areas of tubulointerstitial scarring cannot fully support CP diagnosis [7]. CP is usually associated with multiple urinary infections, vesicoureteral reflux or a history of past or present urinary. However it can also occur in other clinical setting, such as calculi, urinary diversion and neurogenic bladder [8]. Scarring could determine renal failure, hypertension and complications during pregnancy [8]. At gross examination of the kidney, the capsular surface demonstrates broad "U-shaped" scars. A cortical and medullary thinning underlies these scarred areas [7]. Renal pelvis is normally dilated, blunted and deformed. At microscopic findings mononuclear inflammation involves the tubulointerstitial compartment of both the cortex and medulla, with severe tubular atrophy.

IVU was once considered the imaging modality of choice; however US and CT are more sensitive in the detection of CP. There are several typical imaging findings: renal scarring, atrophy and cortical thinning, hypertrophy of sparred renal parenchyma, thickening and dilatation of calyceal system and renal asymmetry. On US scars are linear hyperechoic areas perpendicular to kidney's surface [8]. Focal areas of fibrosis and cortical thinning may also be recognized as well as an increased echogenicity of renal pelvis due to an increased renal sinus fat [8]. Moreover a dilatation of calices and the entire collecting system may be seen due to parenchymal fibrosis [8].

7.4.2 Xanthogranulomatous Pyelonephritis

Xanthogranulomatous pyelonephritis (XGP) is a destructive, rare, chronic inflammatory process of the kidneys that was initially described by Schlagenhaufer in 1916. Middle-aged females (45–55 years) are more frequently affected than males in a ratio of 2:1 [15]. Even though almost all patients are symptomatic, symptoms are non-specific such as pain, fever, weight loss, lower urinary symptoms and malaise [3, 15], so XGP is commonly misdiagnosed because it mimics other pathologic conditions. Flank pain and haematuria may help in narrowing the differential diagnosis and direct imaging evaluation. The aetiology of XGP is not fully understood, but it is thought to derive from an atypical, incomplete immune response in association to a long-term UT obstruction and infection. Although calculi are not a prerequisite for the diagnosis of XGP, they are present in a wide percentage of cases; moreover staghorn type of calculi is frequent. The two most common pathogens associated with XGP are *Escherichia coli* and *Proteus mirabilis*. Three forms have been recognized: diffuse, segmental and focal. The long-lasting granulomatous immune response to recurrent infections led to a replacement of renal parenchyma with lipid-laden (foamy) macrophages [3, 15]. Loss of renal function is attributable to the severe renal inflammation rather than to UT obstruction [3]. At gross pathology affected kidneys are usually enlarged with single or multiple yellow to orange nodules, abscess, cortical scarring and atrophy and involvement of perinephric fat [15]. As detailed before in the microscopic evaluation, the inflammatory infiltrate mainly composed of xanthomatous cells, which have a foamy cytoplasm with an abundant clear to vacuolated cytoplasm and are consistent with histiocytes, is mixed with fibrosis and cholesterol clefts. The parenchyma nearby is characterized by calyceal mucosa ulceration, necrotic debris and tubular atrophy.

A large staghorn is commonly depicted in most, but not all, cases at abdominal radiographs even though it is a non-specific sign (Fig. 7.4). Renal contour enlargement and loss of the ipsilateral psoas margin are additional radiographic find-

ings [3]. IVU demonstrates a markedly decreased renal function with an extremely retarded or absent excretion of contrast medium even at delayed imaging. US findings in diffuse XGP demonstrate an enlarged kidney, with a loss of the typical architecture and a large amorphous central echogenicity that corresponds to the staghorn calculus which generally is associated with acoustic shadowing [3, 15]. Contrary there are no specific US imaging features in focal XGP; in fact it is impossible to differentiate it from a renal abscess.

7.4.3 Tubercular Infection

The genitourinary system involvement in patients with extrapulmonary tuberculosis is well known and accounts for 15–20% of patients. The cor-

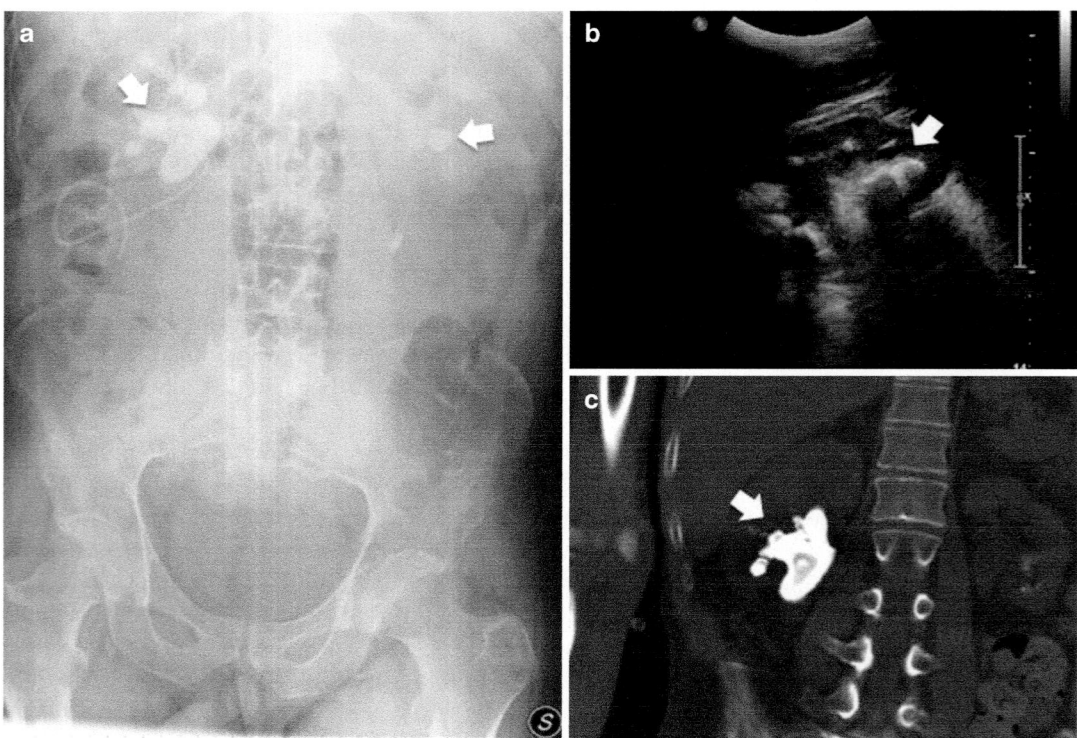

Fig. 7.4 Plain film (**a**), US (**b**) and CT (**c**) of a young man with fever and abdominal pain; he suffered of severe perinatal brain hypoxia. Large bilateral calculi (*arrows*) were identified at abdominal X-ray. The one on the right side had staghorn conformation. Abdominal US (**b**) examination performed to rule out presence of XGP confirmed the presence of a large, hyperechoic, staghorn calculus within the right collecting system, which produced acoustic shadowing underneath. A subsequent CT scan was acquired (**c**) which ruled out the presence of XGP, demonstrating acute cholecystitis (not shown), but better imaged the staghorn calculus

relation with pulmonary tuberculosis is debated in literature: some claim a relation between the two with a delay between pulmonary and genito-urinary disease that varies from 5 to 40 years [8, 16], while other suggests that less than 50% of patients with urinary tuberculosis actually have abnormal results from chest radiography [3]. Symptoms are non-specific and range from fever, weight loss and fatigue, which are less common to dysuria, increased frequency of micturition and microscopic or macroscopic haematuria associated with back, abdominal or flank pain. Also, purified protein derivative skin testing is inconclusive in 20% of patients, and cultures of urine from affected patients may be distorted or confounded by the simultaneous presence of more common urinary pathogens yielding to a difficult diagnosis.

Renal involvement is related to haematogenous spread of mycobacterium tuberculosis, and even though dissemination is possible bilaterally, clinical involvement is usually prominent on one side. The high oxygen tension and blood flow in glomeruli and peritubular capillary beds determine an excellent environment for bacteria development and proliferation [16]. Initially small cortical granulomas, nearby glomeruli, form when host immunity prevails and disease lasts dormant for decades [3, 8, 16]. The further compromission of immune system leads granulomas to enlarge and coalesce. With ruptured capillary bacteria gain access to proximal tubules and loops of Henle creating caseating granuloma and papillary necrosis [3, 16]. Further extension in the collecting system often occurs, which generates fibrosis [3]. Moreover, if left untreated, subsequent evolution of the disease determines a loss of renal function and may spread to retroperitoneal organs including the colon [3]. In fact, the involvement of the ureter and bladder is secondary to renal involvement. Granuloma formation within the transitional epithelium could lead to fibrosis, thus to ureteral strictures and ureteral shortening and calcification [8]. It is important to specify that there is no specific imaging clue for the diagnosis of urinary tuberculosis since similar imaging findings could be caused by several other pathogens; that is the reason why it is defined as the "great imitator". But nevertheless the presence of several abnormalities at the same time allows the correct diagnosis [4].

Several different types of calcifications may be seen at abdominal radiographs including amorphous, speckled or curvilinear patterns, "putty kidney" (calcified thick material filling a dilated collecting system) and calcium in parenchymal mass and lobar calcifications [8]. Calcifications are present in 24–44% of patients with UT tuberculosis [16]. Common findings on IVU include focal scars, dystrophic parenchymal calcifications, cavitary lesions and infundibular stenosis which lead to focal or generalized hydronephrosis [8]. Ureteral ulceration, wall thickening and focal dilatation determine a sawtooth- or corkscrew-like aspect of the ureter; the subsequent progressive fibrosis determines a straighter and more fixed appearance of the ureter, an aspect that is normally defined as "pipestem ureter" [8]. Even though US has limited use in the definition of urinary tuberculosis, two patterns have been described: an infiltrating one with higher echogenicity related to the presence of calcifications and an hydronephrotic or pyonephrotic one with dilated calices and a renal pelvis with reduced dimensions.

7.4.4 Human Immunodeficiency Virus Relate Infections and Nephropathy

Despite the prevention programme and their impact in controlling human immunodeficiency virus (HIV) spreading in population of some countries, the HIV-acquired immunodeficiency syndrome (AIDS) epidemic continues to grow, and by 2005 there were more than 40 million people infected worldwide [17]. Even though respiratory, neurologic and gastrointestinal involvement and imaging characteristics have been widely described, there is a lower definition of HIV renal and UT involvement and its imaging aspects. There are several different causes attributed to renal impairment in HIV patients: HIV acquired nephropathy, opportunistic infections, drug-related renal disease (especially in patients treated with HAART antiviral therapy), neoplasia and vascular causes [17]. The disease-related reduction in T-helper lymphocytes cells and the subsequent immunosuppression make AIDS patients highly susceptible of opportunistic fungal infections, such as *Pneumocystis jirovecii,* although *P. jirovecii* most frequently infects lung, haematogenous and lymphatic spread occur in 1% of patients [17]. Histological evaluation of kidneys infected with *P. jirovecii* demonstrated multiple calcific nodules particularly in renal cortex, representing areas of pathogen infiltration and consequent destruction of renal tubules [17].

Focal areas of increased echogenicity have been described in the renal cortex and medulla [18] but also in the liver, spleen, pancreas and adrenal gland. At CT evaluation calcification was described in the renal cortex [17]. However all these findings were non-specific for the diagnosis of *P. jirovecii* infection and in fact were subsequently described also in *Mycobacterium avium* infection and *Cytomegalovirus.*

Other fungal infections associated with AIDS are *Candida albicans* and *Aspergillus* infection. They can manifest as the presence of several focal microabscess in the kidney parenchyma and hydronephrosis. At histologic analysis, kidneys contain a combination of fungal spores, hyphae and pseudohyphae [17].

HIV-acquired nephropathy is a relatively new disease (the first published description was in 1984) recognized as a complication of HIV infections. HIV viruses directly infect renal epithelial cells and led to direct expression of HIV genes within those cells. It is characterized by progressive renal failure often associated with proteinuria and bland urinary sediment and has a mortality rate of 100% within 6 months from the onset of uraemia [8, 19]. HIV-related nephropathy is more frequent in patients with a CD4 cell count <200 cells/mm^3. On gross specimen evaluation at autopsy, the kidneys were pale, swollen and enlarged due to the presence of several tubular microcyst distending the parenchyma [19]. Even though imaging could help in the diagnostic workup of patients, an in vivo diagnosis is only achieved with renal biopsy. At microscopic evaluation in the acute setting a severe form of collapsing focal segmental glomeruloscle-rosis is seen. As the disease evolves, glomeruli evolve in a tight solidified ball crowded by overlying enlarged, vacuolated visceral epithelial cells [19]. In addition to glomeruli modifications also, tubular involvement is present with atrophy, interstitial fibrosis, oedema, inflammation and widespread tubular degenerative and regenerative changes which determine distended tubules containing loose proteinaceous casts to form tubular microcysts [19].

At US kidneys appear as normal size or enlarged. The initial enlargement is on axial dimension with kidneys losing their normal aspect and gaining a bulbous shape. A high echogenic parenchyma is the most characteristic feature, with a loss of differentiation between fat renal sinus and renal cortex which have to be related with parenchymal disease [17]. Moreover the reduction of renal sinus dimensions due to renal oedema has been described in up to 49% of patients. Also a thickening of pelvicalyceal system has also been described both at US and CT [17].

7.4.5 Malakoplakia

Malakoplakia is a rare granulomatous condition first reported by Michaelis and Gutmann in 1902, characterized histopathologically by von Hansemann histiocytes and Michaelis-Gutmann bodies. Von Hansemann cells are large ovoid eosinophilic macrophages with intracytoplasmic bodies, the Michaelis-Gutmann bodies [20]. The aetiology is unknown; it is believed to be associated with defective bacterial digestion due to impaired macrophage function [20]. It can present in several different ways; moreover since it can occur in almost any part of the body, symptoms depend on the organ involved, thus presenting a huge diagnostic challenge. Anyhow malakoplakia is most commonly found in the genitourinary tract [20]. The incidence rate is three to four times higher in middle-aged female who develop malakoplakia than their male counterparts. The most frequently recovered organism in urine culture and upon flexible cystoscopy is *Escherichia coli* [16]. Moreover malakoplakia is more frequent in immunosuppressed patients. It usually affects the bladder, prostate, ureters and kidneys. Advanced disease may lead to renal failure. Treatment of malakoplakia is not well established, usually medical with surgical intervention sometimes advocated.

Since it manifests as a mucosal mass of the bladder and ureters, renal findings are those of a lower urinary obstruction. When kidneys are directly involved, an infiltrative multifocal process is typically observed [16]. Kidney lesions range from a few millimetres up to 3–4 cm and tend to coalesce. At US lesions are poorly marginated, hypoechoic lesions in a markedly enlarged, deformed, renal parenchyma. There is scarce literature evidence in the usage of nuclear medicine; however an intense accumulation of fluorine 18 fluorodeoxyglucose was noted at positron emission tomography.

7.4.6 Fungal Infection

If yeast-like organisms, which are *Candida* species for the most of times, are discovered in the urine, it is important to decide whether or not this is the clue that outlines an infection or if it represents a colonization or a contamination. A new sample of urine helps in discriminating contamination from colonization and infection. Whether patients are symptomatic or not, candiduria in critically ill patients is very serious and should be considered as a potential marker of invasive candidiasis [13]. Systemic candidiasis is a well-known cause of morbidity and mortality in critically ill, hospitalized and immunocompromised patients such as patients with AIDS and hematologic malignancies or patients treated with immunosuppressive drugs after an organ transplant. In patients at risk, a prophylactic antifungal therapy is administered in order to reduce the prevalence of *Candida* infection [21]. *Candida* invades the intestinal mucosa and infects the liver through portal circulation. Acute infection is accompanied by generic symptoms such as non-specific gastrointestinal complaints, fever and hepatosplenomegaly. After this initial phase normally, there are three

different scenarios: patients die of overwhelming infection despite therapy, patients respond favourably to therapy or patients recover after candidiasis has become widespread and the resultant response to infection causes organ failure and death [21].

There is a paucity of descriptions on the aspects of US findings in renal candidiasis. The US manifestations are divided in two categories, which may coexist or may be consecutive to one another: parenchymal involvement and creation of a mycetoma (also known as fungus ball) in the collecting system [22]. In parenchymal involvement normally papillae become hyperechoic, a finding that is challenging to differentiate from nephrocalcinosis and transient hyperechogenicity of the pyramids in neonates. Moreover papillae may slough and a fungus ball, which appears as a non-shadowing hyperechoic focus, may develop in the collecting system [22]. IVU can reveal hydronephrosis, a focal mass in the collecting system or a non-functioning kidney.

7.4.7 Parasitic Infection

Several parasites (*Plasmodium malariae* and *falciparum*, *Leishmania donovani*, *Trypanosoma brucei*, *Filarioidea*, etc.) may cause renal damage and are associated with glomerular lesions [23]. Schistosomiasis or bilharzia is a tropical disease due to *Schistosoma* worms. The transmission involves the water where the larvae seek the skin of a suitable definitive hosts and migrate in the blood via the lungs to the liver and here transform into worms that gradually reach their perivesicular (*Schistosoma haematobium*) or mesenteric (other species) destination [24]. Females then produce hundreds to thousands of eggs that reach bladder or intestinal lumen and from there are eliminated in the environment. This complex life cycle determines a granulomatous inflammation, ulceration and pseudopolyposis of the bladder and ureteral walls [24]. Common signs are haematuria, dysuria, pollakiuria and proteinuria. Chronic lesions of the bladder and terminal part of ureters evolve to fibrosis or calcifications, subsequently resulting in hydroureter and hydronephrosis. Surprisingly renal function in early stages of the disease is preserved; contrary chronic compression is associated with parenchymal damage and renal failure [24].

Due to the specific involvement of the bladder, imaging findings mirror the pathologic course. Acute phase is characterized by nodular bladder wall thickening at IVU or CTU. End-stage schistosomiasis leads to bladder wall thickening, contraction and calcification; the latter is easily seen at plain radiograph. Calcifications are typically linear or curvilinear. Ureter involvement is rare and typically limited to the lower third. Findings in the affected part are the same described for the bladder walls. Fibrosis of the lower third ureters produces a partial urine obstruction. Upper parts of ureters initially compensate by dilatation hypertrophy that generates enough pressure to overcome distal obstruction. IVU and CTU may demonstrate ureteral calcifications and stenosis, ureterectasis and obstructive uropathy.

Hydatid disease is a zoonosis caused by *Echinococcus granulosus*' larvae. It is endemic in many regions of the world including the Mediterranean, Africa, South America, Australia, Middle East and New Zealand [25]. Sheep, cattle and camels are the common intermediate hosts for this worm. The worm's eggs are passed in stool and are transmitted to humans by dogs [23]. Larvae escape from eggs and penetrate the human body throughout the intestinal mucosa. From there they spread in the portal circulation. Even though the majority of larvae are filtered by the liver and the lungs, some of them reach the general circulation and involve other organs, such as the kidneys [23]. The undestroyed larvae form cysts. The wall of hydatid cyst is formed by three layers: the outermost (pericystic) is produced by modified host cell that forms in the presence of the parasite; the middle is a thin, easily ruptured, acellular, membrane that allows the passage of nutrients; and the inner is where the laminated membrane and scolices are produced [25]. Cyst fluid is a clear transudate that is antigenic if released into the host's body as a consequence of cyst rupture causing severe reactions and anaphylaxis. Of all human organs, renal involvement is rare (2–3% of cases) and patients are often asymptomatic for several years. Most common symptoms are flank mass, pain and dysuria [25]. Renal hydatid cysts are more frequently unilateral, solitary and localized in the cortex of the superior or inferior pole. A severe, but uncommon (18%), complication is the rupture of the cysts in the collecting system with resultant renal colic and hydatiduria [25].

Abdominal radiography images a soft tissue mass that corresponds to the cyst. In a minority of cases, curvilinear or ring-shaped calcifications may be seen. IVU demonstrates infundibular and calyceal distortion [25]. US appearance of renal hydatid cysts may vary between a unilocular simple renal cyst and multiseptated daughter cysts. Three signs raise suspicion on a cyst: a thick, bilayered wall, the "falling snowflake" which is the presence of multiple echogenic foci produced by hydatid sand that modify their locations as the patients change position and a "floating membrane" that represents the detachment of the endocyst from the pericyst [25].

References

1. Hooton T (2012) Uncomplicated urinary tract infection. N Engl J Med 366:1028–1037
2. Solomon CG, Schaeffer AJ, Nicolle LE (2016) Urinary tract infections in older men. N Engl J Med 374(6):562–571. https://doi.org/10.1056/NEJMcp1503950
3. Craig WD, Wagner BJ, Travis MD (2008) From the archives of the AFIP: pyelonephritis: radiologic-pathologic review. Radiographics 28:255–276
4. Quaia E (2014) In: Quaia E (ed) Radiological imaging of he kidney, 2nd edn. Springer, Heidelberg
5. Stacul F, Rossi A, Cova MA (2008) CT urography: the end of IVU? Radiol Med 113(5):658–669
6. Feldman MK (2009) US artifacts 1. Radiographics 29(4):1179–1189
7. Hou J, Herlitz LC (2014) Renal infections. Surg Pathol Clin 7(3):389–408
8. Browne RFJ, Zwirewich C, Torreggiani WC (2004) Imaging of urinary tract infection in the adult. Eur Radiol Suppl 14(3):168–183
9. Mitterberger M, Pinggera GM, Colleselli D et al (2008) Acute pyelonephritis: comparison of diagnosis with computed tomography and contrast-enhanced ultrasonography. BJU Int 101(3):341–344
10. Roy C, Pfleger DD, Tuchmann CM, Lang HH, Saussine CC, Jacqmin D (2001) Emphysematous pyelitis: findings in five patients. Radiology 218:647–650

11. Fontanilla T, Minaya J, Corteás C et al (2012) Acute complicated pyelonephritis: contrast-enhanced ultrasound. Abdom Imaging 37(4):639–646
12. Rossleigh MA (2001) Renal cortical scintigraphy and diuresis renography in infants and children. J Nucl Med 42(1):91–95
13. Kauffman CA, Fisher JF, Sobel JD, Newman CA (2011) Candida urinary tract infections - diagnosis. Clin Infect Dis 52(SUPPL. 6):S452–S456
14. Laway BA, Bhat MA, Bashir MI, Ganie MA, Mir SA, Daga RA (2012) Conservative management of emphysematous pyelonephritis. Indian J Endocrinol Metab 16(2):303–305
15. Li L, Parwani AV (2011) Xanthogranulomatous pyelonephritis. Arch Pathol Lab Med 135(5):671–674
16. Wong A, Dhingra S, Surabhi VR (2012) AIRP best cases in radiologic- pathologic correlation genitourinary tuberculosis. Radiographics 32(3):839–844
17. Symeonidou C, Standish R, Sahdev A, Katz RD, Morlese J, Malhotra A (2008) Imaging and Histopathologic features of HIV-related renal disease. Radiographics 28(5):1339–1354
18. Kay CJ (1992) Renal diseases in patients with AIDS: sonographic findings. AJR Am J Roentgenol 159(3):551–554
19. Wyatt CM, Klotman PE, D'Agati VD (2009) HIV-associated nephropathy: clinical presentation, pathology, and epidemiology in the era of antiretroviral therapy. Semin. Nephrol. 28(6):513–522
20. Dong H, Dawes S, Philip J, Chaudhri S, Subramonian K (2015) Malakoplakia of the urogenital tract. Urol Case Reports 3(1):6–8
21. Moore NJE, Leef JL, Pang Y (2003) Systemic candidiasis. Radiographics 23(5):1287–1290
22. Daneman A, Navarro OM, Somers GR, Mohanta A, Jarrín JR, Traubici J (2010) Renal pyramids: focused sonography of normal and pathologic processes. Radiographics 30(5):1287–1307
23. Van Velthuysen MLF, Florquin S (2000) Glomerulopathy associated with parasitic infections. Clin Microbiol Rev 13(1):55–66
24. Gryseels B, Polman K, Clerinx JKL (2006) Human schistosomiasis. Lancet 368(9541):1106–1118
25. Ishimitsu DN, Saouaf R, Kallman C, Balzer BL (2010) Best cases from the AFIP: renal hydatid disease. Radiographics 30(2):334–337

Cross-Sectional Imaging of Acute Pyeloureteritis and Pyonephrosis

8

Massimo Tonolini

8.1 Computed Tomography (CT) Role and Techniques in Acute Urinary Infections

Albeit with disadvantages of radiation exposure, superior cost compared to ultrasound, and the use of iodinated contrast medium, multidetector computed tomography (CT) currently represents the "workhorse" modality to investigate emergency patients with acute abdominal complaints, fever or elevated acute-phase reactants of unclear source [1–4].

Furthermore, CT is arguably the preferred technique to comprehensively investigate most urologic disorders. Unless contraindicated by history of allergy or renal impairment, contrast medium (CM) administration is recommended to comprehensively assess the renal parenchyma structure, perfusion and function as well as the walls of the collecting systems, ureters and bladder. As most European radiologists do, we suggest to refer to the guidelines from the European Society of Urogenital radiology (ESUR) to prevent CM-induced nephrotoxicity in patients with risk factors. Alternatively, the latest American College of Radiologists (ACR) Manual on contrast media may be used [5, 6].

Nowadays, the widely available fast multidetector scanners allow to image the abdominal organs in well-defined dynamic phases of enhancement. In the setting of suspected urinary infection or abdominal sepsis, the nephrographic phase which acquired 75–100 s after intravenous CM injection provides the maximum detection and visualization of both infectious and solid renal changes and is therefore warranted as the only indispensable acquisition. A preliminary unenhanced phase may allow to detect unilateral renal enlargement, perinephric fat stranding and thickening of Gerota's fascia, coexisting urolithiasis or the presence of blood. However, precontrast phase may be obviated, particularly in younger patients, in order to limit the CT radiation dose administered. Unless characterization of a suspected solid or complex renal mass is required, the corticomedullary phase scan (25–45 s after CM injection) is generally unnecessary, as characteristic imaging appearances of acute pyelonephritis are barely or not perceptible. Additional excretory-phase imaging obtained 8–10 min after CM may be acquired at the discretion of the attending radiologist, is recommended in cases of obstructive uropathy and may be useful to improve characterization in cases of delayed nephrogram, renal hypoattenuating changes or filling defects in the urinary tract. Multidetector CT studies tailored to the urinary tract should be routinely reviewed along both axial

M. Tonolini, M.D.
Radiology Department, "Luigi Sacco" University
Hospital, Via G.B. Grassi 74, Milan 20157, Italy
e-mail: mtonolini@sirm.org

© Springer International Publishing AG 2018
M. Tonolini (ed.), *Imaging and Intervention in Urinary Tract Infections and Urosepsis*,
https://doi.org/10.1007/978-3-319-68276-1_8

and coronal planes: the latter provide a panoramic representation the renal and excretory structures and easily allow assessment of renal length, contours and parenchymal enhancement. Image reading using narrow CT window settings may allow an improved identification of perinephric fat changes and of subtle renal hypoenhancing regions [7–13].

8.2   Acute Pyeloureteritis

Due to the widespread use of multidetector CT, acute pyeloureteritis (APU) currently represents a not uncommon finding in cross-sectional studies performed to investigate haematuria, flank pain or suspected urinary tract infection (UTI). Moreover, its characteristic imaging signs are sometimes incidentally encountered in patients with unrelated clinical features: in this situation, the aware radiologist provides the first indication of the presence of an active UTI. APU may be observed in the context of acute pyelonephritis (APN) or cystitis; alternatively, it may represent the only feature suggesting an ongoing ascending UTI, before characteristic renal changes of APN appear. Therefore early CT diagnosis allows preventing further disease progression [8, 12, 14–16].

AT CT, infectious APU is heralded by diffuse, mild or moderate circumferential pelvicalyceal and/or ureteral mural thickening (≥2 mm) with uniform, more or less prominent contrast enhancement corresponding to urothelial inflammation; inflammatory stranding of the peripelvic and periureteral fat is commonly associated (Figs. 8.1, 8.2, 8.3, and 8.4). These

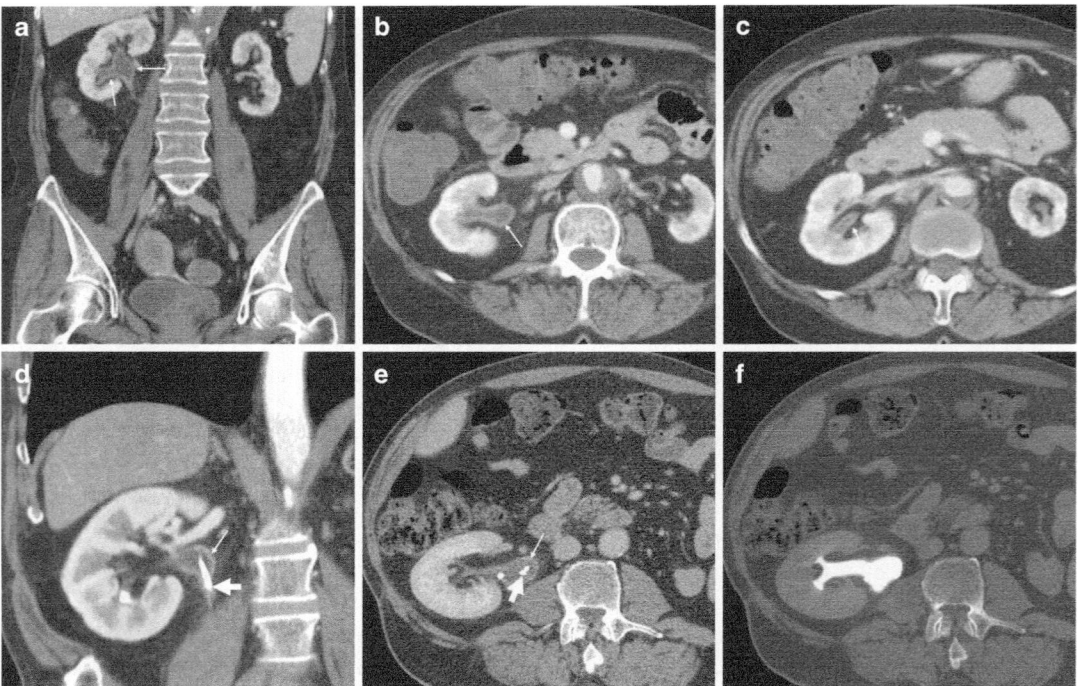

Fig. 8.1 A 59-year-old female with chronic HIV and hepatitis C virus coinfection was hospitalized because of low-grade fever, lumbar pain, dysuria and urinary incontinence. Multiplanar images from contrast-enhanced CT (**a–c**) showed mild, uniform, diffusely enhancing pelvicalyceal mural thickening (thin arrows) as the only sign of active urinary tract infection (UTI) from multiresistant *Escherichia coli*; the same finding was absent on the contralateral collecting system. A 69-year-old male with solitary right kidney and urolithiasis was investigated with multidetector CT (**d–f**) after retrograde ureteroscopy and stent (thick arrows) positioning. The thin, hyperenhancing mural thickening (thin arrows) was best perceptible in corticomedullary (**d**) and nephrographic (**e**) phase images and obscured in the delayed excretory phase (**f**). Note normal renal parenchymal enhancement and function, calyceal stone at lower renal pole in (**d**)

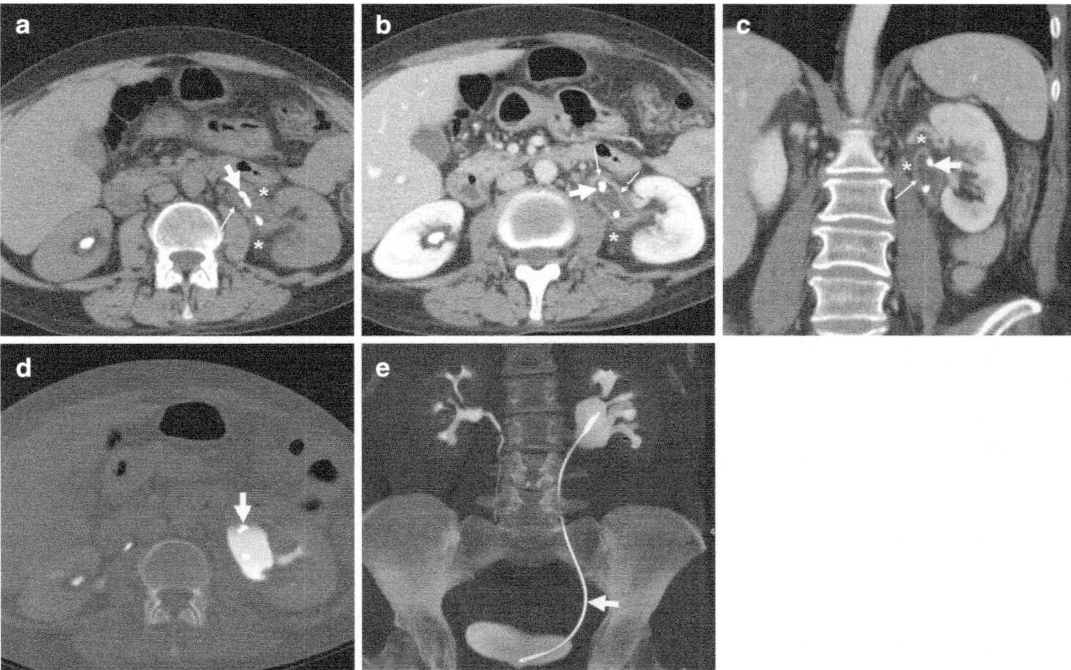

Fig. 8.2 A 59-year-old female suffered from postprocedural fever after left-sided ureteral stenting (thick arrows) to relieve pyeloureteral junction syndrome and underwent CT including unenhanced (**a**), nephrographic (**b**, **c**) and delayed excretory (**d**, **e** with maximum intensity projection reconstruction) acquisition phases. With normal renal function on both sides, the left renal pelvis showed mild-enhancing mural thickening (thin arrows) and subtle inflammatory stranding of the peripelvic fat (*)

CT appearances are often relatively subtle, best perceptible in comparison with the unaffected contralateral side, by far most conspicuous in the nephrographic phase of enhancement, and potentially reversible with successful treatment of UTI (Fig. 8.3). Occasionally, the presence of air within the collecting system or ureter (Fig. 8.5) without previous instrumentation or surgery indicates UTI by gas-forming bacteria [8, 12, 14–16].

Conversely, CT signs consistent with APU are often obscured in the excretory phase because of the decreased mural enhancement and the adjacent high-attenuation-enhanced urine. This is true not only for the usual multiphasic CT studies including preliminary unenhanced, corticomedullary, nephrographic and delayed phases but also for the modern dual or triple split-bolus CT

urography techniques which provide combined nephrographic and excretory imaging in a single acquisition [15, 17, 18].

The CT differential diagnosis of APU encompasses tuberculosis, primary urothelial malignancies, ureteral metastases and other uncommon conditions such as ureteritis cystica, amyloidosis and periureteral haematoma (Fig. 8.6). The key consideration is that APU does not narrow nor obstruct the renal pelvis and ureter. Conversely, the identification of focal, asymmetric or mass-forming mural thickening and of filling defects protruding in the renal pelvis or ureteral lumen suggests an underlying malignant process, most usually transitional cell carcinoma (Fig. 8.7). As discussed in the dedicated chapter of this book, urinary tuberculosis results from haematogenous spread and often involves the ureters with

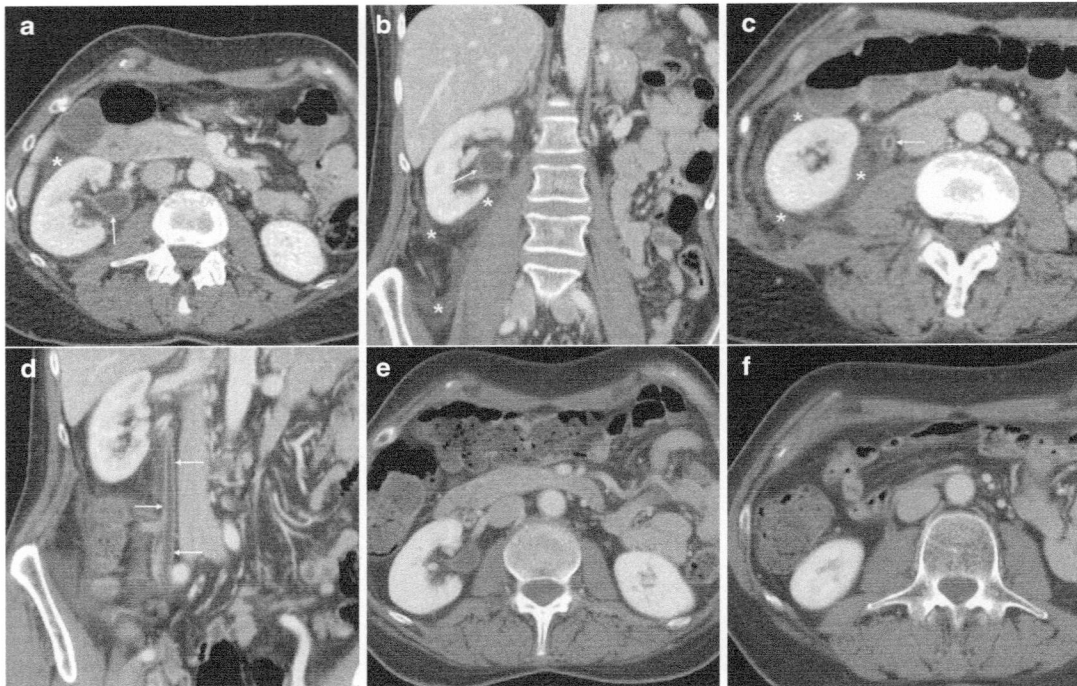

Fig. 8.3 A 49-year-old woman with demyelinating disease suffered from diffuse abdominal pain, emesis and irritative voiding symptoms, without fever. Contrast-enhanced multidetector CT (**a–d**) showed normal, symmetric size, parenchymal thickness and enhancement of both kidneys. On the right side, some perinephric and pararenal fluid (*) was present. The ipsilateral renal pelvis showed mild, circumferential mural thickening with urothelial hyperenhancement (thin arrows) compared to the contralateral side, which extended along the ureter and was consistent with an acute ascending UTI without signs of pyelonephritis. Urine cultures disclosed infection from multiple Gram-negative bacteria. After prompt clinical and laboratory improvement on antibiotic therapy, repeated CT (Fig. **e**, **f**) depicted regression of perinephric changes and of pyeloureteritis (Adapted with permission from Ref.no. [21])

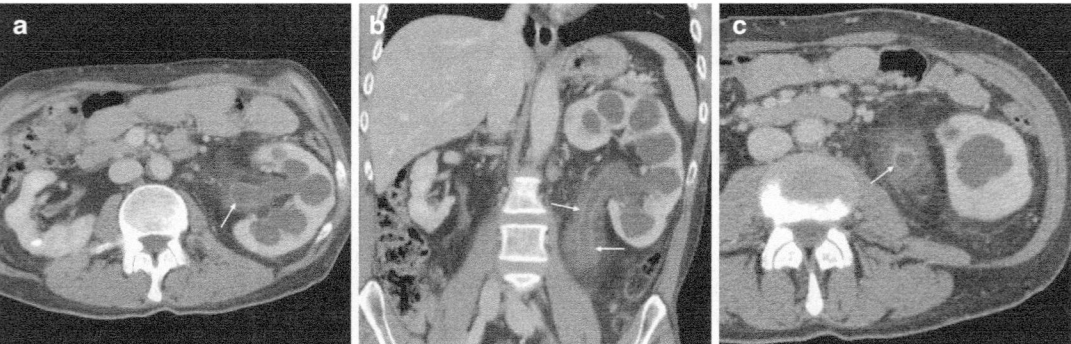

Fig. 8.4 A 44-year-old male had history long-standing HIV infection on antiretroviral treatment, known left-sided hydronephrosis and previously resected nephrogenic adenoma of the urinary bladder. Currently suffering from fever and macroscopic haematuria, he underwent contrast-enhanced CT (**a–c**) which showed worsening hydronephrosis compared to previous studies (not shown) with parenchymal thinning and appearance of urothelial enhancement (thin arrows) and of marked periureteral stranding. The patient's clinical conditions and laboratory changes improved after ureteral stenting

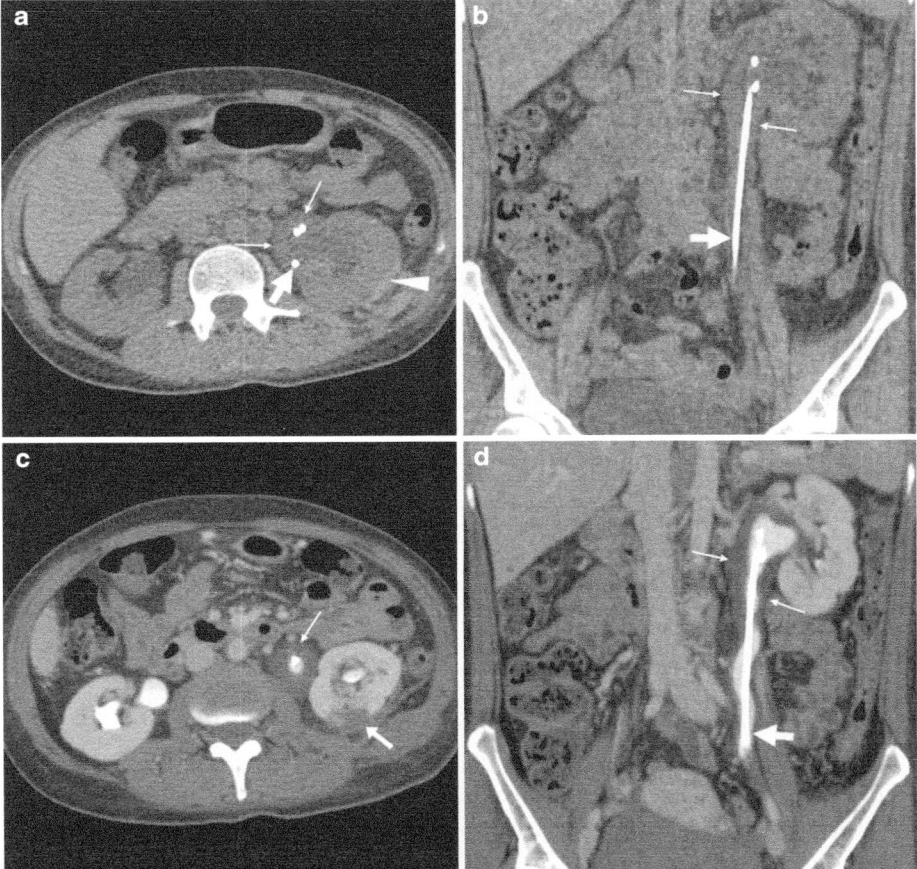

Fig. 8.5 A 34-year-old female suffered from recurrent UTIs after caesarean section a few months earlier. After inconclusive sonography and without previous instrumentation, contrast-enhanced CT showed some air (thin arrows in **a**, **b**) in the right ureter, with minimally thickened walls and inhomogeneous perfusion at the upper third of the contralateral kidney (**c**)

Fig. 8.6 Following percutaneous nephrolithotomy (PCNL) treatment performed to treat a 2-cm left renal pelvis stone, a 46-year-old woman was not discharged because of progressive, asymptomatic haemoglobin drop (nadir 8.4 g/dL). Four days later, unenhanced CT showed ureteral stent (thick arrows) in place, hyperattenuating (50 HU) circumferential mural thickening of the renal pelvis and proximal ureter (thin arrows in **a**, **b**) consistent with suburothelial haemorrhage and minimal blood in the ipsilateral perirenal and posterior pararenal spaces (arrowhead in **a**). CT urography (**c**, **d**) showed functioning left kidney with a 2-cm devascularized injury (arrow in **c**) at the dorsal middle third and hypodense suburothelial haemorrhage (thin arrows) compared to the well-opacified pyeloureteral lumen. Conservative management including blood transfusions allowed hospital discharge in a few days, normalization of clinical, biochemistry and imaging abnormalities within a month (Reproduced from Open Access Ref. no. [22])

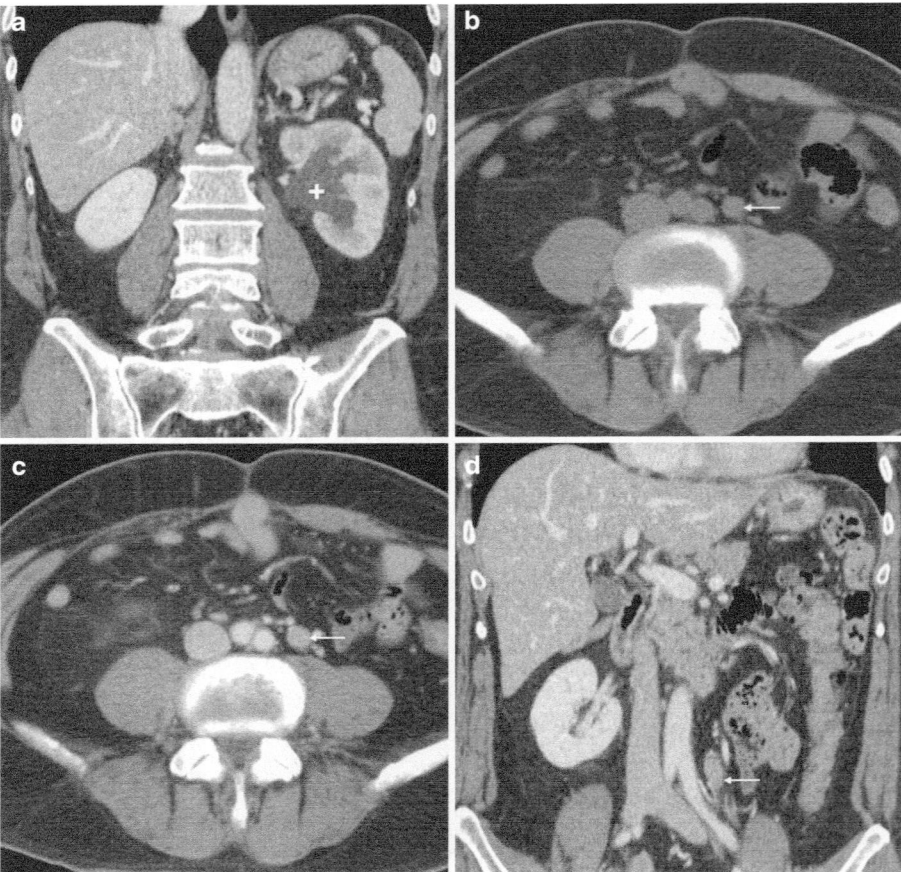

Fig. 8.7 In a 60-year-old male undergoing follow-up for resected colon cancer, multidetector CT (**a–d**) showed first-degree hydronephrosis (+) with delayed nephrogram on the left side (**a**). The ipsilateral lumbar ureter (thin arrows) showed higher-than-water precontrast attenuation (**b**) with homogeneous mural enhancement and strictured lumen, corresponding to metachronous transitional cell carcinoma

"ragged" irregular mural thickening, ureteral filling defects, calcification and strictures [14, 15].

8.3 Pyonephrosis

In the context of UTI, hydronephrosis represents a key finding, which requires early diagnosis and immediate treatment. Pyonephrosis, defined by an infected and obstructed collecting system, represents a true urological emergency: if left untreated, it is associated with impending risk of sepsis and rapid and permanent loss of renal function. In the adult population, pyonephrosis may result from either acute or chronic obstruction from lithiasis, tumours, strictures or congenital anomalies with superimposed infection. Clinically, patients with pyonephrosis generally present with the usual signs and symptoms of UTI, but more subtle manifestations such as low-grade fever, malaise, weight loss and dull pain are not uncommon: it has been reported that as many as 15% of patients are afebrile. Practically, pyonephrosis should be suspected in any patient with urinary tract obstruction and accompanying fever and flank pain. As discussed in the interventional radiology chapters of this book, prompt decompression of pyonephrosis should be performed by means of percutaneous nephrostomy or ureteral stenting, to relieve obstruction and also to confirm the diagnosis [8, 12, 19].

Radiologists should maintain a high level of suspicion, since imaging differentiation of pyonephrosis from noninfected dilatation is challenging. Although it readily detects pelvicalyceal dilatation, ultrasound has limited sensitivity for pyonephrosis, which may be confidently diagnosed only when mobile echogenic intraluminal debris or a urine-debris level are visualized within the distended renal collecting system. Pyonephrosis is difficult to distinguish from uninfected hydronephrosis also at CT. Its most specific findings are rarely observed and include:

(a) Gas bubbles within hydronephrosis without history of previous instrumentation
(b) Higher-than-water (10–50 HU) attenuation of the dilated collecting system corresponding to purulent fluid
(c) Contrast layering with opacified urine above dependent purulent urine in excretory-phase acquisition

However, distinguishing simple hydronephrosis on the basis of fluid attenuation measurements is unreliable. As with APU, the key finding which should be always sought for is pelvic mural thickening which has a reported sensitivity of 76% for pyonephrosis (Figs. 8.8 and 8.9). Other useful but nonspecific accessory findings suggesting infection include perinephric fat stranding, thickening of the bridging septa and Gerota's fascia (Figs. 8.8 and 8.9), variable degrees of renal oedematous enlargement with poor nephrographic enhancement or the characteristic "striated nephrogram" of APN.

The key differential diagnosis is acute obstructive uropathy without infection, which is commonly associated with perinephric stranding (Fig. 8.10) and decreased or delayed parenchymal enhancement (Fig. 8.11). However, noninfected acute obstruction generally lacks the characteristic hyperenhancing pyeloureteral thickening and has a detectable obstructing

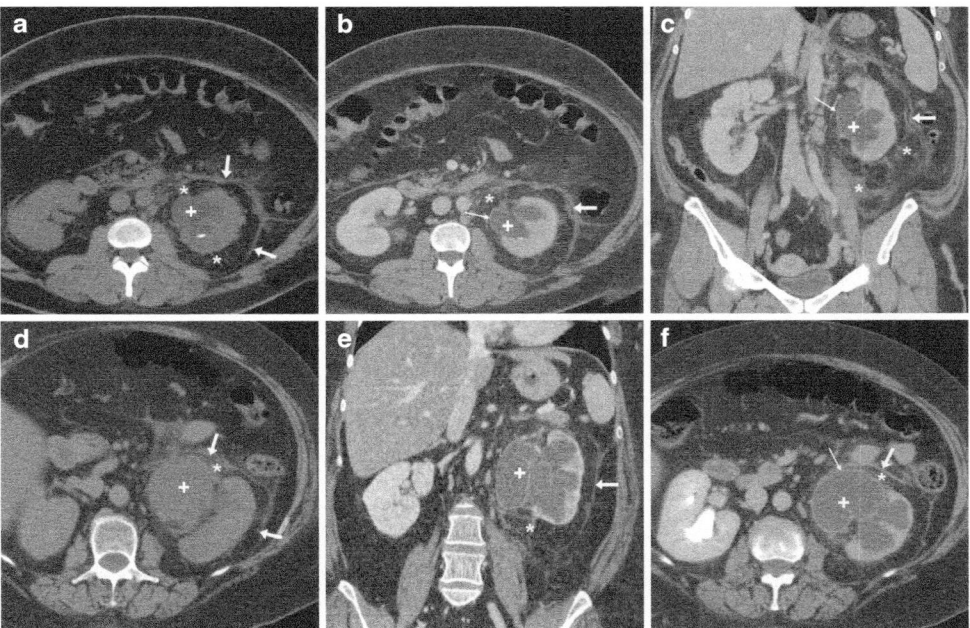

Fig. 8.8 A 40-year-old female experienced septic fever 3 days after a PCNL treatment. Unenhanced (**a**) and contrast-enhanced (**b, c**) images showed left-sided pelvicalyceal dilatation with inflammatory-type stranding of the surrounding fat (*), mild-enhancing urothelial thickening (thin arrow in **b**), ipsilateral fascial effusion (arrows) and decreased nephrographic parenchymal enhancement compared to the contralateral kidney. Hydronephrosis was due to small residual stone fragments in the lumbar ureter

(not shown). Clinical and imaging suspicion of pyonephrosis was confirmed and relieved by positioning of ureteral stent plus intensive antibiotic therapy (Adapted from Open Access Ref. no. [22]). Analogous pre- (**d**) and post-contrast (**e, f**) CT signs were present in a 53-year-old female with history of psychiatric disease and acute lumbar pain, consistent with superimposed UTI on pre-existent pyeloureteral junction stricture, which was relieved by long-term ureteral stenting

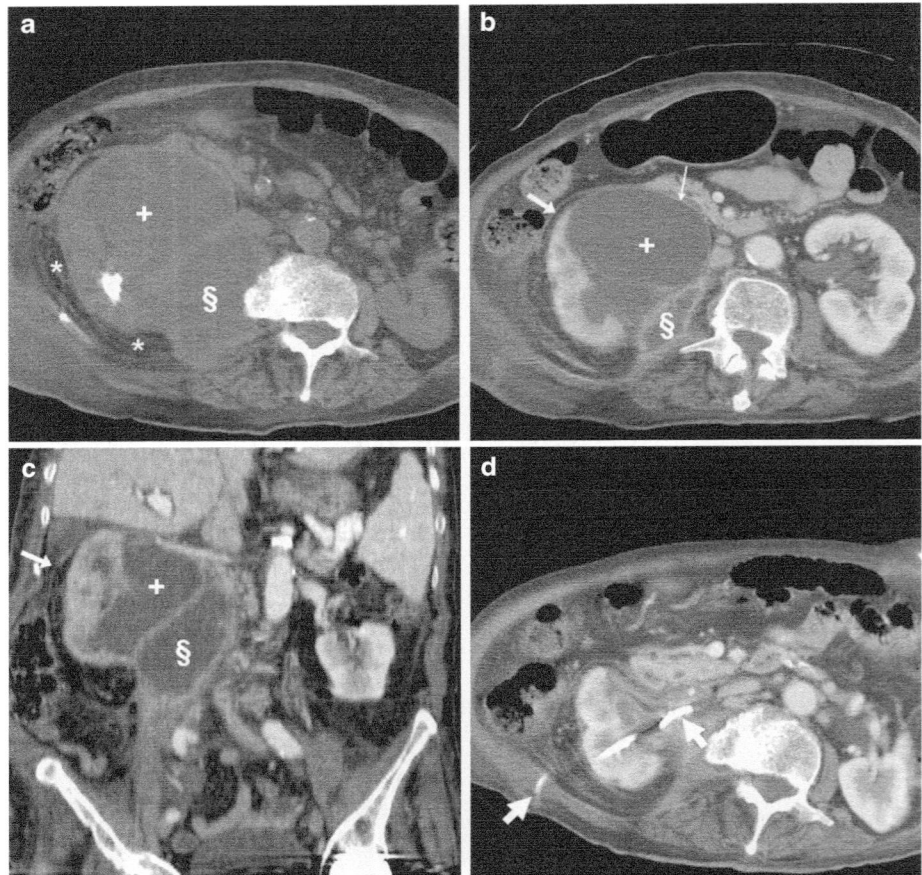

Fig. 8.9 An elderly female with septic fever and abdominal pain had CT diagnosis of severe right-sided hydronephrosis (+) with associated perinephric fat stranding (on unenhanced image **a**), hyperenhancing pyelic wall (thin arrow), fascial effusion (arrows) and psoas muscle abscess (§) in post-contrast images (**b** and **c**). Note calcific calyceal lithiasis in **a**. The picture resolved after percutaneous drainage of psoas abscess and nephrostomy (thick arrow in follow-up CT **d**)

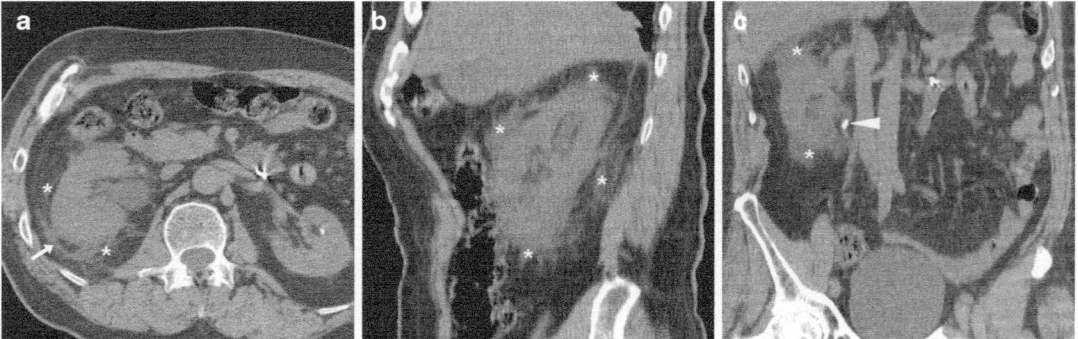

Fig. 8.10 A 78-year-old overweight male suffered from acute right flank pain. Unenhanced CT (urolithiasis protocol, **a**–**c**) showed mild thickening of the renal parenchyma, marked perinephric fat stranding (*) and fascial fluid (arrows) and first-degree hydronephrosis caused by a 6-mm stone (arrowhead in **c**) of the pyeloureteral junction

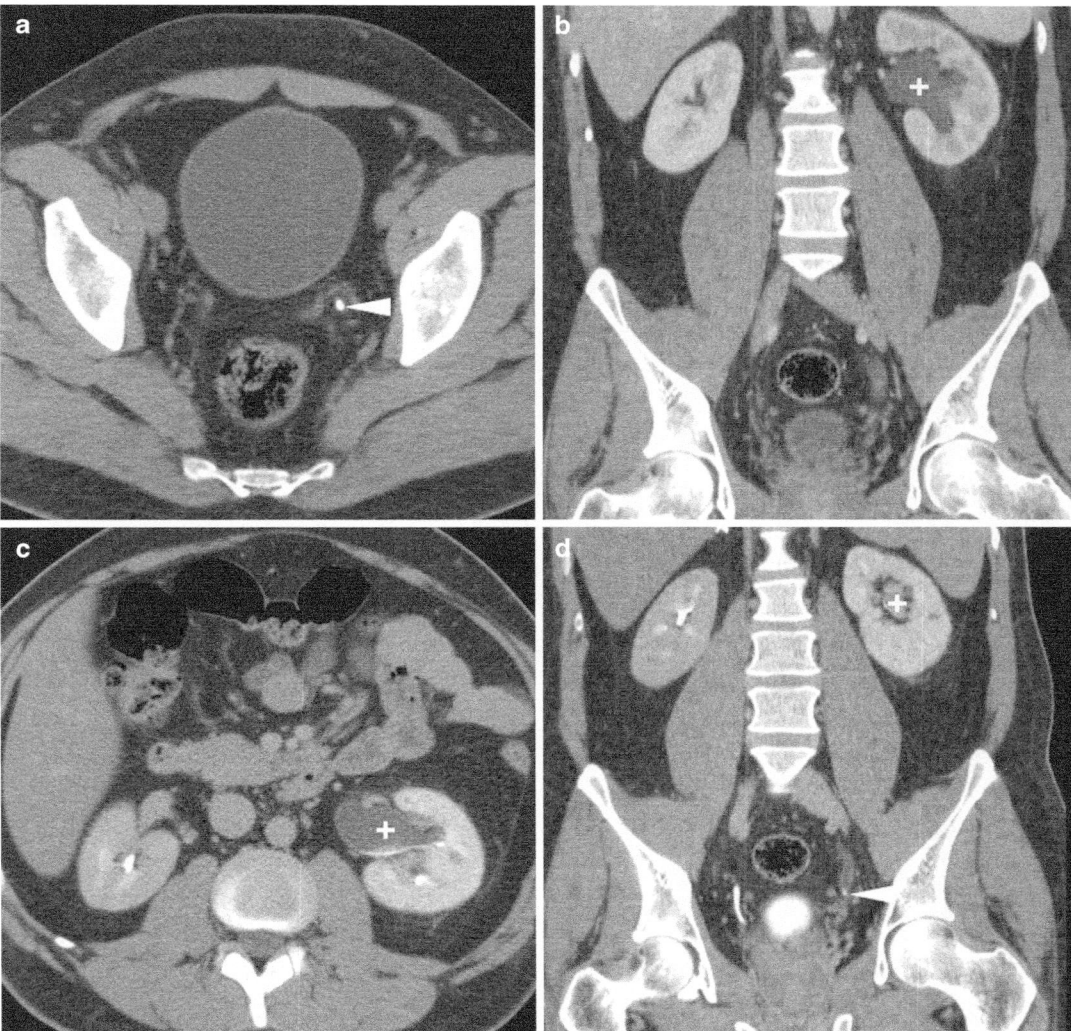

Fig. 8.11 In a 49-year-old male suffering from acute left renal colic, urgent unenhanced CT (**a**) detected a small-sized calculus (arrowhead) of the distal ureter. The attending urologist requested study completion with intravenous contrast (**b–d**), which confirmed ipsilateral first-degree hydronephrosis (+) with associated delayed nephrogram (**b**) compared to the contralateral kidney, preserved contrast excretion (**c**, **d**) and persistent ureteral calculus (arrowhead in **d**), without signs of UTI

cause, most commonly a ureteral stone (Figs. 8.10 and 8.11) [8, 11–13, 19].

Although seldom used, MRI consistently depicts the urine-filled collecting system by the use of static-fluid MR urography techniques. In pyonephrosis, dependent debris and fluid-fluid levels may be seen within the dilated urine-filled cavities. Furthermore, increasing reports describe that the use of diffusion-weighted MRI with calculation of apparent diffusion coefficients (ADC) is highly reliable in the differentiation between hydronephroses from pyonephrosis (Fig. 8.12): the infected pelvicalyceal system appears markedly hyperintense on high b-value DWI images, with corresponding very low $(0.64 \pm 0.35 \times 10^{-3}$ mm^2/s) ADC values compared to $2.98 \pm 0.65 \times 10^{-3}$ mm^2/s of noninfected urine [19, 20].

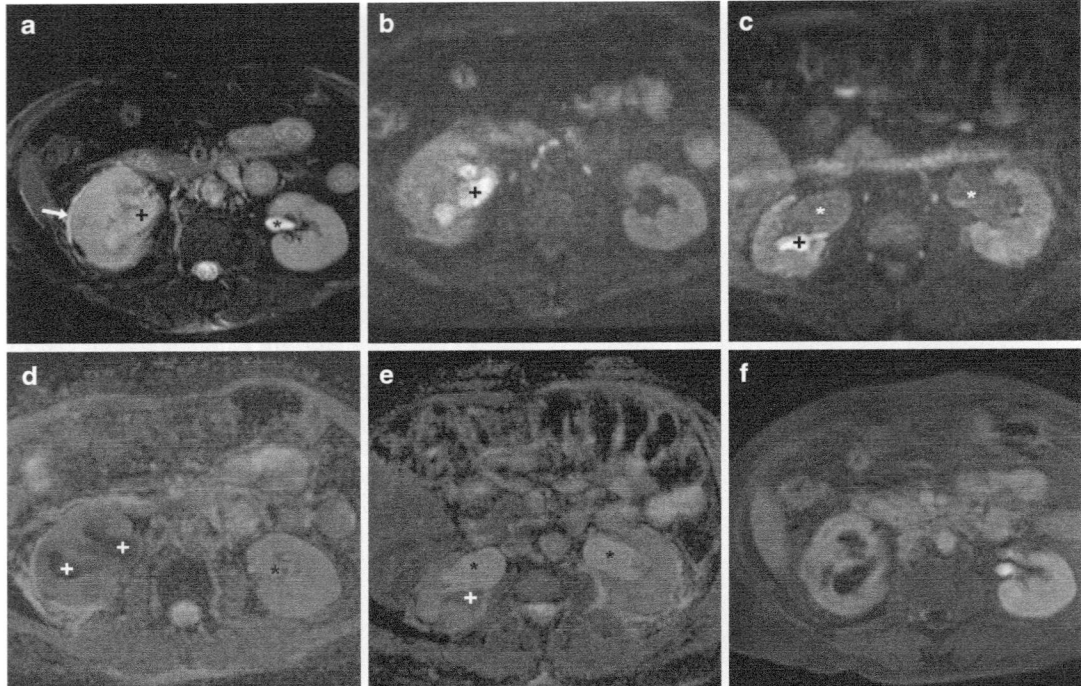

Fig. 8.12 In a 68-year-old male with previous radical cystectomy with ileal conduit (Bricker's technique), fat-suppressed T2-weighted MR image (**a**) showed enlarged right kidney with perinephric fluid (arrows) and hydronephrosis (+) characterized by different signal intensity of urine compared to the contralateral renal pelvis (*). Diffusion-weighted images (**b** value 700) showed visually high signal (+) of urine in the dilated right collecting system consistent with pyonephrosis, forming a fluid-fluid level (in **c**) with the nondependent, noninfected urine with normal low signal (*). Corresponding apparent diffusion coefficient (ADC) maps (**d, e**) showed hypointensity from low ADC values in infected (+) compared to noninfected urine (*). Excretory-phase T1-weighted acquisition after intravenous gadolinium contrast (**f**) showed lack of urinary opacification in the right-sided dilated urinary cavities. Pyonephrosis ultimately resolved after 2 months of intensive antibiotic therapy (Courtesy of dr. D.Gned, Hospital "San Luigi Gonzaga", Orbassano—Italy)

References

1. Sartelli M, Viale P, Catena F et al (2013) 2013 WSES guidelines for management of intra-abdominal infections. World J Emerg Surg 8:3
2. Chin JY, Goldstraw E, Lunniss PJ et al (2012) Evaluation of the utility of abdominal CT scans in the diagnosis, management, outcome and information given at discharge of patients with non-traumatic acute abdominal pain. BJR 85:e596–e602
3. Raja AS, Mortele KJ, Hanson R et al (2011) Abdominal imaging utilization in the emergency department: trends over two decades. Int J Emerg Med 4:19
4. Rosen MP, Siewert B, Sands DZ et al (2003) Value of abdominal CT in the emergency department for patients with abdominal pain. Eur Radiol 13:418–424
5. European Society of Urogenital Radiology (2016) ESUR guidelines on contrast media 9.0. Available at: "www.esur.org/guidelines". Accessed 25 March 2017
6. American College of Radiologists (2015) ACR manual on contrast media. Version 10.2. Available at: "https://www.acr.org/Quality-Safety/Resources/Contrast-Manual". Accessed 25 March 2017
7. Coppenrath EM, Mueller-Lisse UG (2006) Multidetector CT of the kidney. Eur Radiol 16:2603–2611
8. Craig WD, Wagner BJ, Travis MD (2008) Pyelonephritis: radiologic-pathologic review. Radiographics 28:255–277. quiz 327-258
9. Ifergan J, Pommier R, Brion MC et al (2012) Imaging in upper urinary tract infections. Diagn Interv Imaging 93:509–519
10. Yu M, Robinson K, Siegel C et al (2016) Complicated genitourinary tract infections and mimics. Curr Probl Diagn Radiol 46(1):74–83. https://doi.org/10.1067/j.cpradiol.2016.1002.1004
11. Browne RF, Zwirewich C, Torreggiani WC (2004) Imaging of urinary tract infection in the adult. Eur Radiol 14(Suppl 3):E168–E183

12. Stunell H, Buckley O, Feeney J et al (2007) Imaging of acute pyelonephritis in the adult. Eur Radiol 17:1820–1828
13. Demertzis J, Menias CO (2007) State of the art: imaging of renal infections. Emerg Radiol 14:13–22
14. Wasnik AP, Elsayes KM, Kaza RK et al (2011) Multimodality imaging in ureteric and periureteric pathologic abnormalities. AJR Am J Roentgenol 197:W1083–W1092
15. Potenta SE, D'Agostino R, Sternberg K et al (2015) CT urography for evaluation of the ureter. Radiographics 35:709–726
16. Uyeda JW, Gans BS, Sodickson A (2015) Imaging of acute and emergent genitourinary conditions: what the radiologist needs to know. AJR Am J Roentgenol 204:W631–W639
17. Kekelidze M, Dwarkasing RS, Dijkshoorn ML et al (2010) Kidney and urinary tract imaging: triple-bolus multidetector CT urography as a one-stop shop--protocol design, opacification, and image quality analysis. Radiology 255:508–516
18. Van Der Molen AJ, Cowan NC, Mueller-Lisse UG et al (2008) CT urography: definition, indications and techniques. A guideline for clinical practice. Eur Radiol 18:4–17
19. Das CJ, Ahmad Z, Sharma S et al (2014) Multimodality imaging of renal inflammatory lesions. World J Radiol 6:865–873
20. Chan JH, Tsui EY, Luk SH et al (2001) MR diffusion-weighted imaging of kidney: differentiation between hydronephrosis and pyonephrosis. Clin Imaging 25:110–113
21. Tonolini M (2013) Acute pyelo-ureteritis: MDCT diagnosis and follow-up {Online}. EuroRAD URL: http://www.eurorad.org/case.php?id=10764
22. Tonolini M, Villa F, Ippolito S et al (2014) Cross-sectional imaging of iatrogenic complications after extracorporeal and endourological treatment of urolithiasis. Insights Imaging 5:677–689

CT Imaging and Differential Diagnosis of Acute Pyelonephritis

Adriana Vella and Massimo Tonolini

Albeit with disadvantages of radiation exposure, cost and the use of iodinated contrast medium, multidetector computed tomography (CT) currently represents the "workhorse" modality in emergency departments and the preferred technique to comprehensively investigate abdominal sepsis and most urologic disorders [1–3].

As discussed in the introductory clinical chapters of this book, CT consistently detects and stages acute pyelonephritis (APN), identifies both early subtle and full-blown changes and evaluates the perinephric structures and entire urinary tract [4–10].

Based upon our experience at a tertiary care hospital devoted to diagnosis and treatment of infectious illnesses, this chapter reviews with imaging examples of the CT imaging appearances of uncomplicated bacterial APN including typical and unusual renal changes, accessory signs, intrarenal abscesses and long-term sequelae. Afterwards, the differential diagnosis of APN from other entities which can show similar imaging changes is presented.

9.1 Multidetector CT of Acute Pyelonephritis

9.1.1 Technique and Typical Renal Findings

In the vast majority of situations, imaging evaluation of patients with suspected acute urinary tract infection (UTI) or sepsis requires a single CT acquisition encompassing the abdomen and pelvis in the nephrographic phase (75–100 s) after intravenous administration of iodinated contrast medium (CM), which provides the maximum detection and visualization of both infectious and solid renal changes. Unless contraindicated by history of allergy or renal impairment, CM administration is warranted to comprehensively assess the renal parenchyma structure, perfusion and function as well as the walls of the collecting systems, ureters and bladder. We recommend to follow the guidelines from the European Society of Urogenital Radiology (ESUR) to prevent CM-induced nephrotoxicity in patients with risk factors. Alternatively, the latest American College of Radiologists (ACR) Manual on contrast media may be used [11, 12].

Albeit it may be useful to detect asymmetric renal enlargement, urolithiasis, perinephric fat stranding and thickening of Gerota's fascia, a preliminary unenhanced phase is generally obviated, particularly in younger patients, in order to limit the CT radiation dose administered. With

A. Vella, M.D. • M. Tonolini, M.D. (✉)
Radiology Department, "Luigi Sacco" University Hospital, Via G.B. Grassi 74, Milan 20157, Italy
e-mail: adriana.vella1984@gmail.com; mtonolini@sirm.org

© Springer International Publishing AG 2018
M. Tonolini (ed.), *Imaging and Intervention in Urinary Tract Infections and Urosepsis*,
https://doi.org/10.1007/978-3-319-68276-1_9

current multidetector CT scanners, standard acquisition parameters and the use of automated tube current modulation, the radiation dose erogated by a single-pass CT study of the abdomen and pelvis is approximately 10–12 mSv [1, 2].

The cross-sectional imaging findings of uncomplicated APN reflect the presence of zones of hypoperfused, poor or non-functioning renal parenchyma secondary to vasospasm, tubular obstruction and/or interstitial oedema. The earliest but characteristic CT appearance is the "striated nephrogram" sign, which corresponds to discrete linear streaks of alternating hypo- and hyperattenuation, orthogonal to and reaching the cortex, corresponding to obstructed tubules with intervening functioning parenchyma (Fig. 9.1).

In our experience, APN from ascending UTI is most commonly unilateral rather than bilateral. The most characteristic CT appearance is represented by more or less well-defined regions of decreased enhancement within the renal parenchyma, typically radiating from the papilla towards and oriented perpendicularly to the cortex (Figs. 9.2 and 9.3). Practically, with consistent clinical and laboratory findings, all hypoenhancing intraparenchymal regions

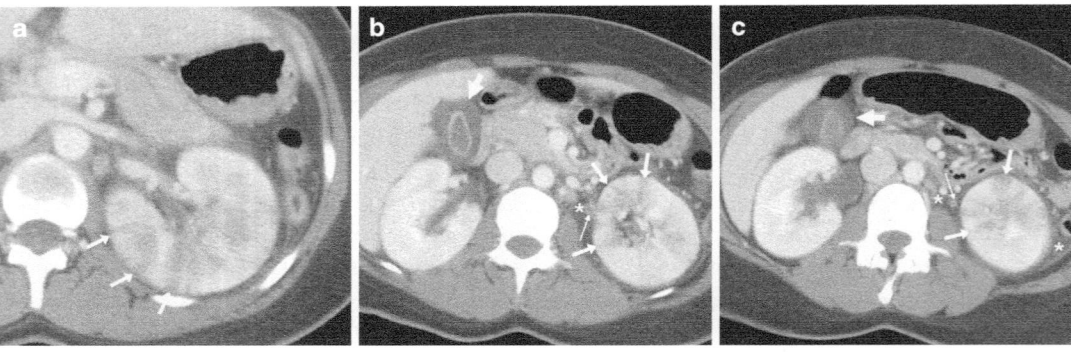

Fig. 9.1 Early acute pyelonephritis (APN) with "striated nephrogram" appearance and common accessory signs in a 32-year-old female suffering from acute abdominal pain with clinical and laboratory signs of sepsis. Nephrographic phase images from contrast-enhanced CT show left kidney with upper normal limit size and parenchymal thickness, mildly inhomogeneous perfusion with thin hypoattenuating "streaks" (arrows) oriented perpendicularly to the cortex, best visualized in detail image (**a**). Accessory signs consistent with APN included mild hyperenhancing pyeloureteral thickening (thin arrows), ipsilateral perinephric fat stranding (*) and pronounced gallbladder mural oedema (thick arrows in **b**, **c**)

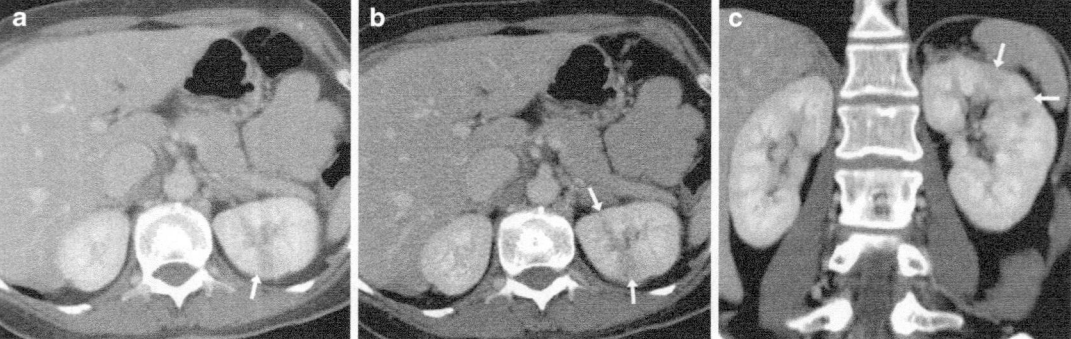

Fig. 9.2 Unilateral APN in a 49-year-old female with characteristic clinical manifestations and laboratory signs consistent with urinary tract infection (UTI). Nephrographic phase CT viewed at standard abdominal window settings (**a**) showed a circumscribed hypoenhancing intraparenchymal focus (arrow) at the upper third of the left kidney. The presence and extent of focal APN is best assessed using modified CT window settings (**b**) and coronal image review (**c**). Infection was confirmed by associated CT finding of ipsilateral pyelitis (not shown)

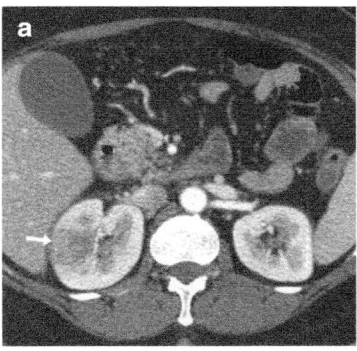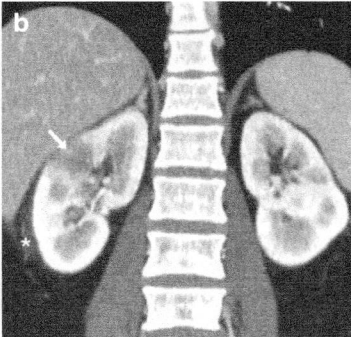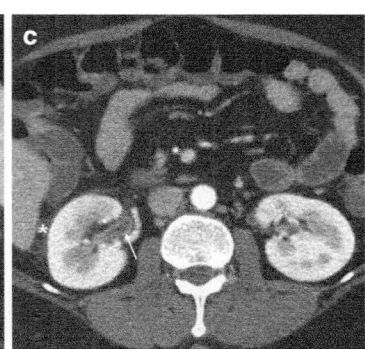

Fig. 9.3 Unilateral APN in a 50-year-old HIV-positive female with fever, flank pain and increased acute phase reactants. Unfortunately acquired in a corticomedullary phase, contrast-enhanced images detected an ill-defined intraparenchymal focus of inhomogeneous perfusion (arrows in **a**, **b**) measuring approximately 2.5 cm in maximum diameter at the upper third of right kidney. Infection was confirmed by associated CT finding of ipsilateral pyelitis (thin arrow in **c**)

should be attributed to APN, particularly if band-like or wedge-shaped widest at the cortical surface and tapering towards the papillae. Subtle APN changes are best appreciated by reviewing the study at non-standard window settings (Fig. 9.2) such as window width (WW)/window level (WL) 470/130 Hounsfield units rather than at the usual abdominal WW/WL 350/50 settings [4, 5, 7–10, 13].

Early APN changes including the "striated nephrogram" are barely perceptible on corticomedullary phase scans (Fig. 9.3) obtained 25–45 s after CM injection, which are not recommended in this clinical setting, unless characterization of a sonographically suspected solid or complex renal mass is required. Furthermore, APN changes are relatively inconspicuous on both additional excretory phase acquisitions (obtained 8–10 min after CM injection) and CT urography studies (Fig. 9.4) [4, 5, 7–10, 13].

We recommend routine CT review along both axial and coronal planes, since the latter provide a panoramic representation of the urinary tract and allow an easy comparative assessment of renal size, contours and parenchymal enhancement (Figs. 9.2, 9.3, 9.4, and 9.5). Coronal CT reconstructions generally allow in identifying the typical wedge-shaped configuration of APN regions and the common "patchy" multifocal distribution of APN with intervening spared parenchyma (Figs. 9.6, 9.7, 9.8, and 9.9).

When reporting CT studies in patients with UTI, we suggest to categorize APN as uni- or bilateral (Figs. 9.7 and 9.8), focal or diffuse, causing none, focal or global renal enlargement. Currently very uncommon because of timely diagnosis, the diffuse APN appears as global oedematous renal enlargement, with delayed nephrogram and poor or absent contrast excretion [4, 5, 7–10, 13].

Findings which suggest APN originating from haematogenous dissemination (Fig. 9.9) over the more common ascending UTI include:

(a) Bilaterality
(b) Multifocal, peripherally distributed changes
(c) Small-sized, round-shaped changes
(d) Changes located at or immediately below the cortex at a distance from the collecting system [4, 5, 7–10, 13]

9.1.2 Accessory CT Signs of Acute Pyelonephritis

Ancillary signs which may be present in patients with APN include, in descending order of specificity:

(a) Ipsilateral pyeloureteritis represented by mild or moderate pelvicalyceal and/or ureteral thickening with increased urothelial enhance-

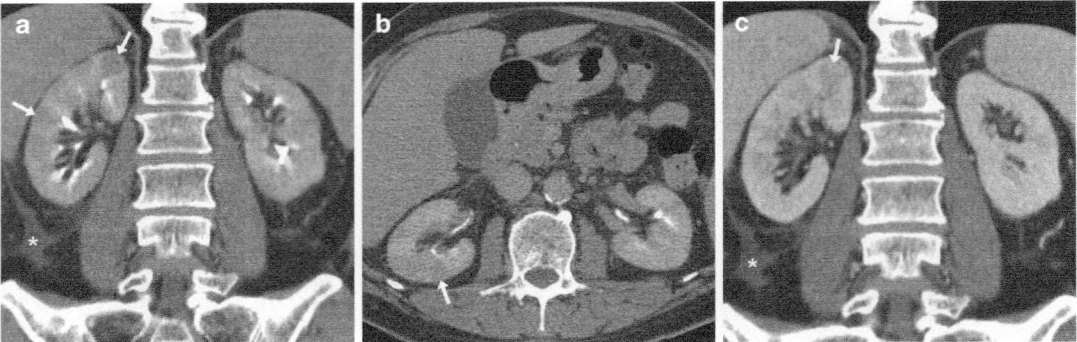

Fig. 9.4 A 70-year-old male experienced septic fever 3 months after radical cystectomy with orthotopic neobladder reconstruction (not shown). Multidetector CT urography (**a**, **b**) detected at least two faintly hypoenhancing intraparenchymal foci (arrows) in the right kidney consistent with clinical diagnosis of acute UTI. Repeated nephrographic phase CT (**c**) during antibiotic therapy showed persistence of an APN focus at the upper pole (arrow), which ultimately regressed at further follow-up (not shown)

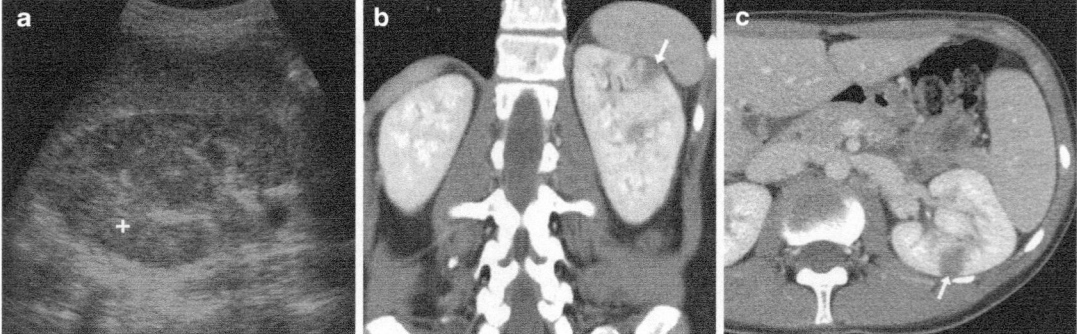

Fig. 9.5 Unilateral APN in a young 20-year-old female with fever and flank pain. Initially, ultrasound (**a**) detected a focal area of increased parenchymal echogenicity at the upper third of right kidney (+). Nephrographic phase post-contrast CT (**b**, **c**) confirmed a solitary hypoenhancing renal focus (arrows) without abscessualization and perinephric extension, thus allowing appropriate treatment choice

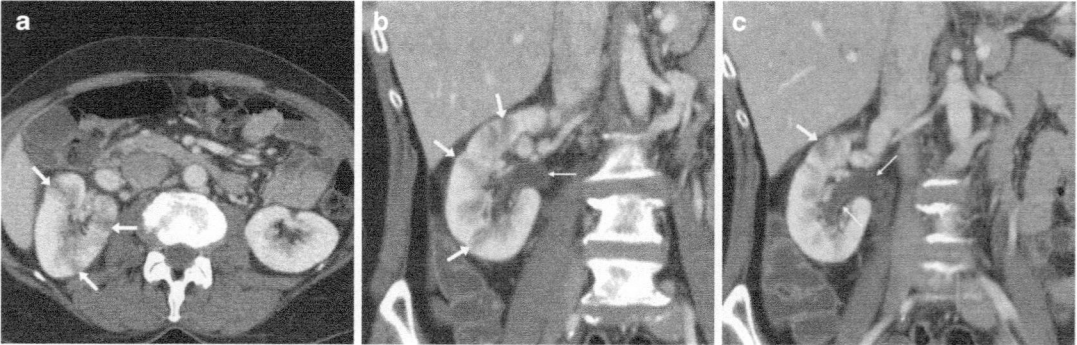

Fig. 9.6 Characteristic appearance of multifocal unilateral APN in a 53-year-old female with fever and lower right quadrant pain. CT was requested to differentiate acute appendicitis from APN. Nephrographic phase CT images (**a–c**) showed multiple hypoenhancing bands orthogonal to the renal cortex (arrows) throughout the normal-sized right kidney, with associated ipsilateral mild hyperenhancing pyeloureteral thickening (thin arrows in **b**, **c**)

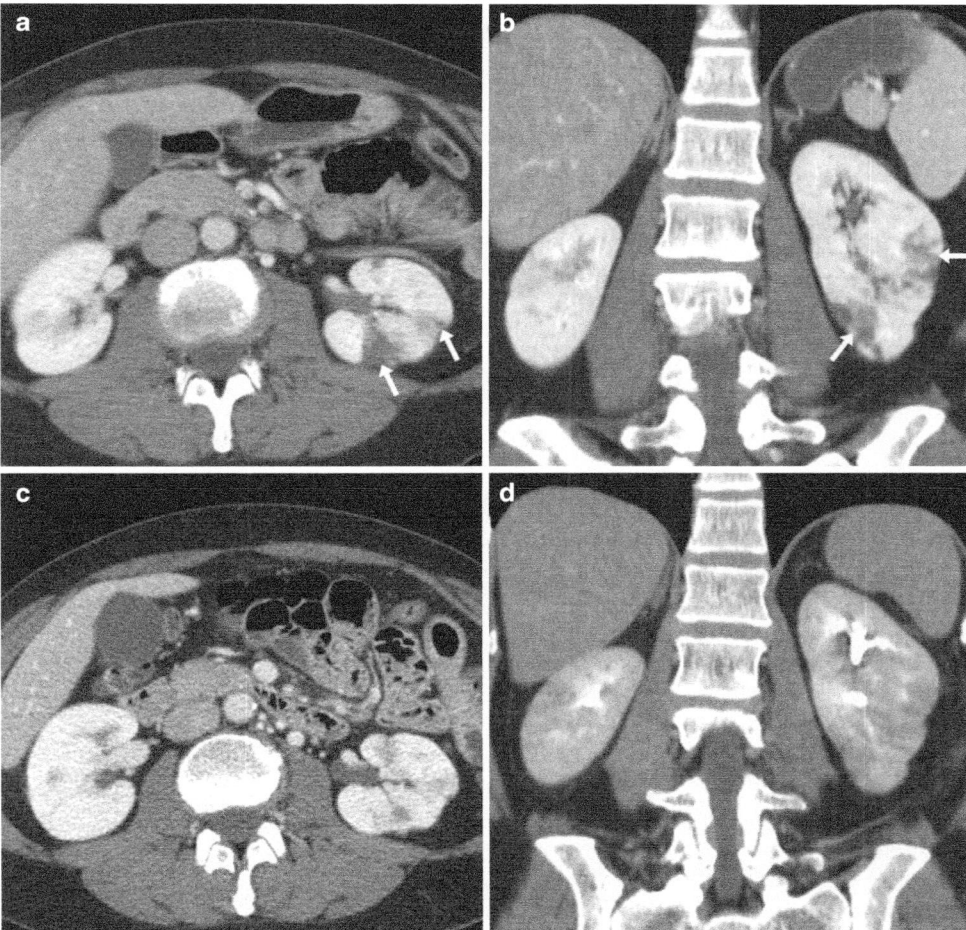

Fig. 9.7 Usual appearance of multifocal unilateral APN in a 51-year-old female with abdominal pain and hyperleukocytosis. Initial CT (**a**, **b**) showed at least four wedge-shaped hypoenhancing parenchymal regions in the left kidney (arrows) plus minimal thickening of ipsilateral fascia. Ten weeks later, repeated CT (**c**, **d**) after antibiotic treatment showed regression of APN changes, with development of multiple contour changes and cortical irregularities consistent with early scarring

ment (Figs. 9.1, 9.3, and 9.6) as extensively described in the previous chapter.

(b) Ipsilateral perinephric fat stranding and/or thickening of Gerota's fascia (Figs. 9.1, 9.3, 9.4, 9.7, 9.8, and 9.9), which may be also present in acute obstruction, urinoma or other inflammatory conditions such as acute pancreatitis [14].

(c) Periportal fluid "tracking" and gallbladder oedema (Fig. 9.1) which should not be confused with cholecystitis.

(d) Hepatic "mosaic" reticular enhancement pattern in the arterial-dominant or portal venous phases, with complete homogenization on delayed phase: this appearance has been recently described in patients with acute extrahepatic infectious or inflammatory disorders including APN, reflects sepsis-associated liver dysfunction and corresponds histologically to liver sinusoidal dilatation and is reversible in 82% of cases at follow-up after resolution of the underlying disorders [15, 16].

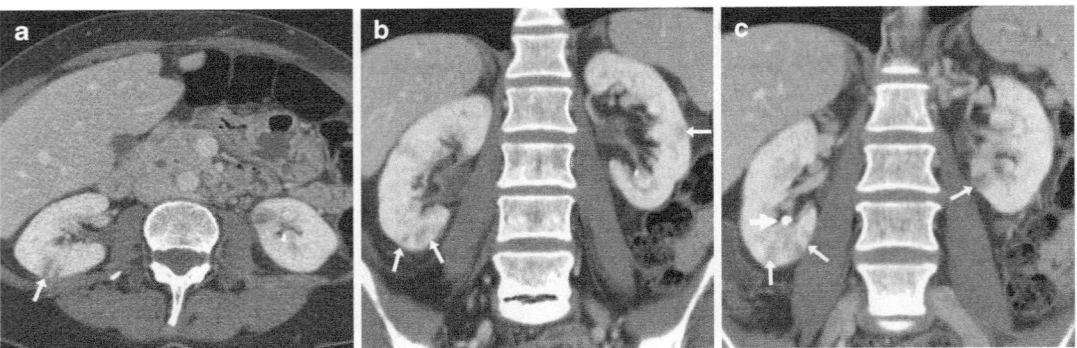

Fig. 9.8 Mild, bilateral APN in a 54-year-old female with history of urolithiasis, suffering from culture-proven UTI. At CT (**a–c**) both kidneys showed small-sized hypoenhancing bands (arrows). Note lower pole calculus (thick arrow in **c**)

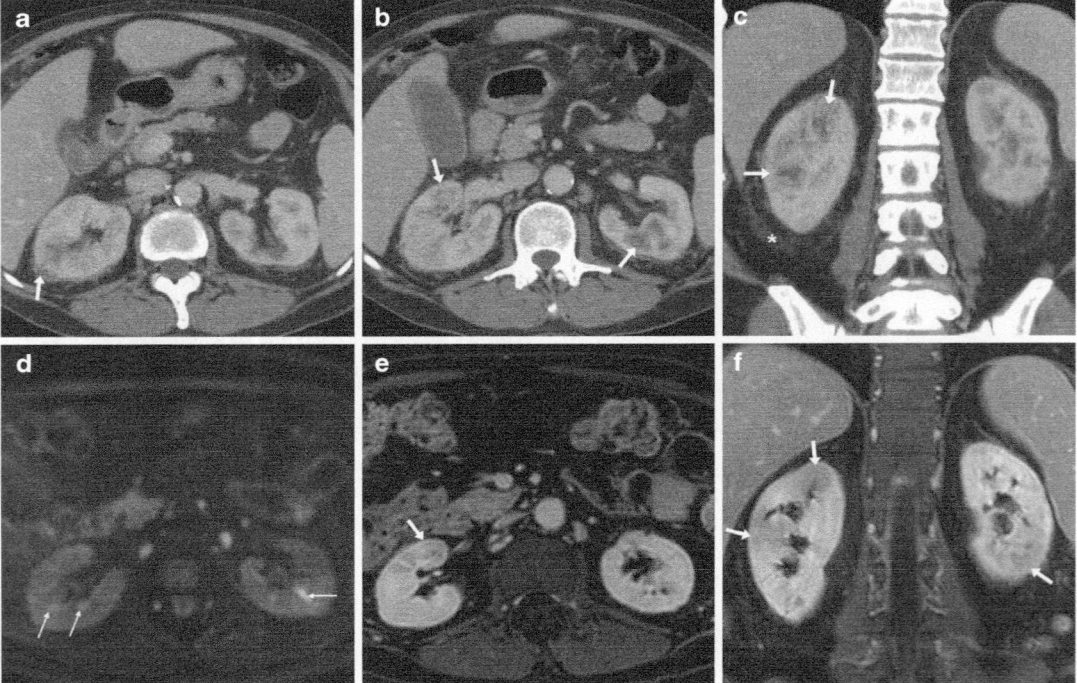

Fig. 9.9 Urinary sepsis from *Escherichia coli* APN in a 49-year-old male. Initial CT (**a–c**) showed multiple ill-defined cortical hypoenhancing foci (arrows) in both kidneys, consistent with haematogenous dissemination of infection. After prompt improvement on intravenous anti-biotics, a week later MRI showed tiny bilateral foci of restricted diffusion (thin arrows in **b** 800 diffusion-weighted image **d**) and subtle hypoenhancing parenchymal regions (arrows in post-gadolinium T1-weighted images **e** and **f**)

(e) Lung base effusions, particularly if ipsilateral [4, 5, 7–10, 13].

9.1.3 Abscess-forming Pyelonephritis and Prediction of Severity

If undiagnosed, APN may progress to form intrarenal abscesses, which appear as peripheral round small- (Figs. 9.10 and 9.11) or moderate-sized (Fig. 9.12) nonenhancing fluidlike collections demarcated by a thin rim-like enhancing capsule and surrounded by hypoenhancing oedematous parenchyma [4, 5, 7–10, 13].

Albeit non-validated, an APN severity score has been proposed to identify those patients at high risk for deterioration and includes clinical features such as diabetes, tachycardia, hypotension, persistent fever and pyuria along with imaging signs including global renal enlargement, pelvicalyceal air, infected hydronephrosis, effacement of renal sinus and poor contrast excretion [17].

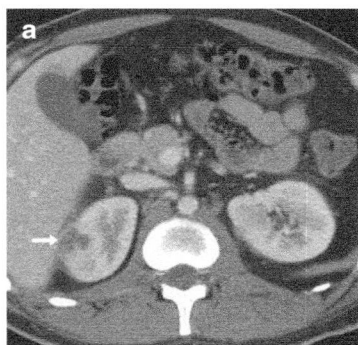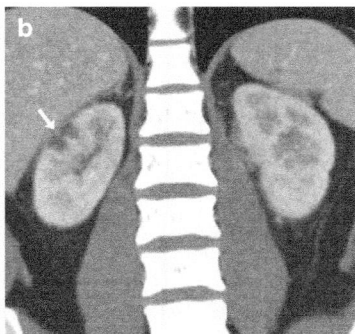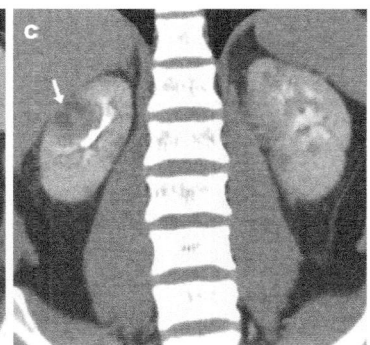

Fig. 9.10 Focal APN with tiny abscess formation at the upper third of the right kidney in a 34-year-old immunosuppressed male. Nephrographic phase CT (**a**, **b**) showed two centimetric nonenhancing fluidlike cortical areas (arrows), which on delayed excretory phase (arrow in **c**) appeared to be surrounded by hypoenhancing oedematous parenchyma

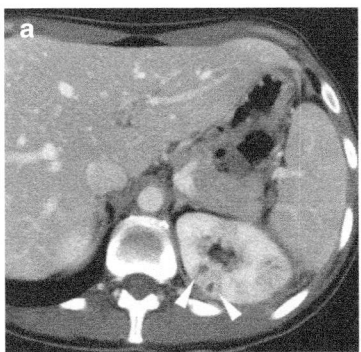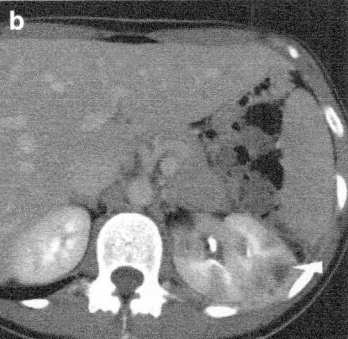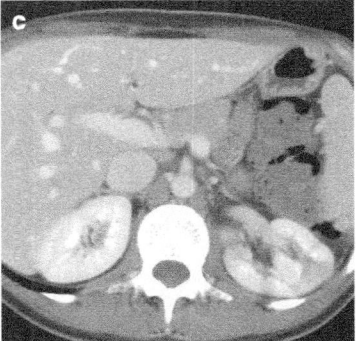

Fig. 9.11 Bacterial APN in a 30-year-old female. Nephrographic (**a**) and excretory (**b**) phase CT acquisitions showed minimally enlarged left kidney with multiple centimetric fluidlike abscess cavities (arrowheads) surrounded by thin rim-like enhancement and by hypoenhancing oedematous parenchyma. Follow-up CT (**c**) after antibiotic therapy showed near-complete normalization of APN changes

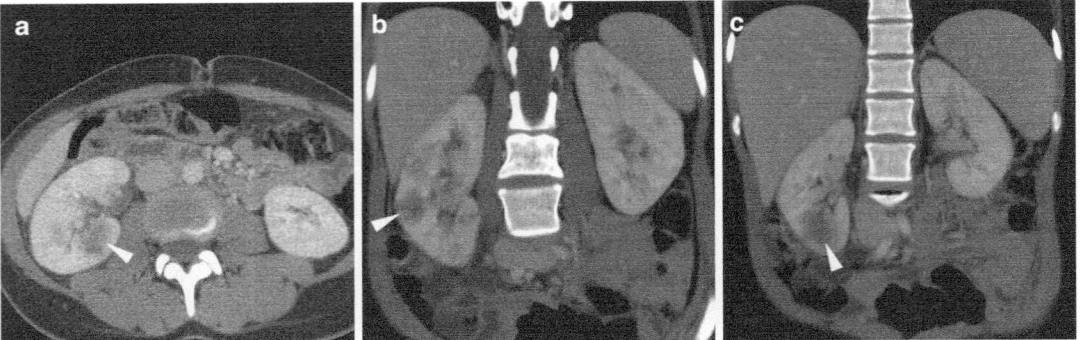

Fig. 9.12 Abscess-forming APN in a 30-year-old female with fever, hypotension, abdominal pain and vaginal discharge shortly after removal of intrauterine contraceptive device. Nephrographic phase CT (**a–c**) showed three intraparenchymal abscesses (arrowheads) of the right kidney, measuring up to 3 cm in size, with central fluidlike content and irregular peripheral enhancement

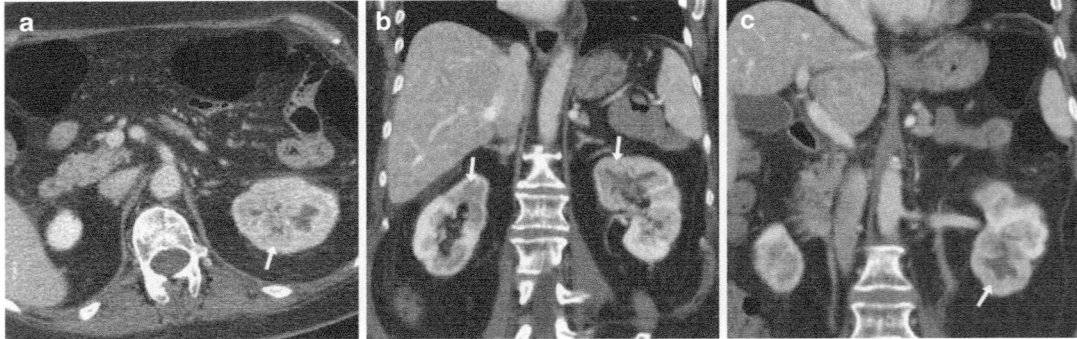

Fig. 9.13 Bilateral long-standing APN in a 70-year-old female with malaise, weakness and weight loss after improperly treated, recurrent UTIs. At contrast-enhanced CT (**a–c**), both kidneys showed polar regions (arrows) with poor medullary enhancement and calyceal deformities

9.1.4 Long-Term Sequelae of Acute Pyelonephritis

In our experience CT represents the most reliable modality to perform follow-up of APN (Figs. 9.4, 9.7, and 9.11). Unfortunately, despite clinical and laboratory improvement, imaging appearances of APN may persist for weeks or months during or after therapy, and CT follow-up may thus prove confusing for the clinician. As discussed in the Introduction, currently there is convincing evidence on the potential detrimental effect of APN on renal function. Anatomically, the long-term anatomic sequelae of APN consist in irreversible parenchymal destruction. Corresponding CT findings consistent with chronic pyelonephritis include renal "scarring" seen as focal or lobar cortical thinning with underlying calyceal distortion from retraction of papillae (Fig. 9.13). Ultimately long-standing or recurrent UTI may cause segmental atrophy of the affected kidney or diffuse reduction of renal size and parenchymal thickness [4, 5, 7–10, 13].

9.2 Differential Diagnosis of Acute Pyelonephritis

The main differential diagnosis of focal APN is represented by renal infarction (RI), which most commonly occurs secondary to atrial fibrillation, systemic infections such as endocarditis and sometimes coagulopathies or antiblastic thera-

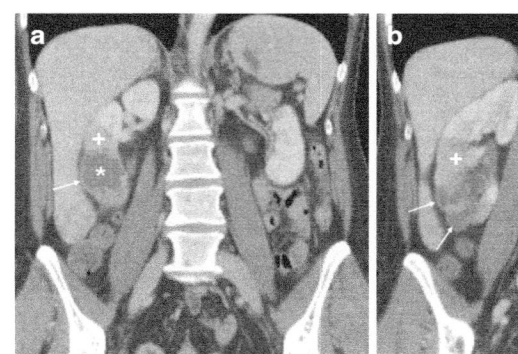
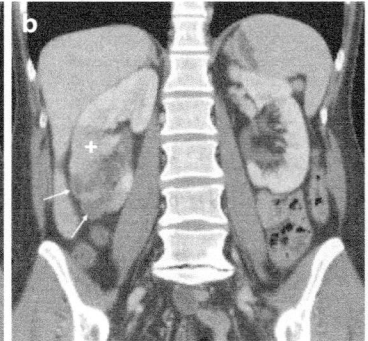
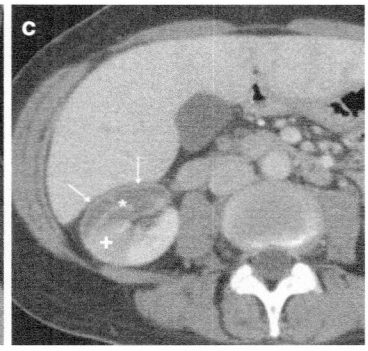

Fig. 9.14 Ventral infarct of the lower third of right kidney mimicking renal abscess: at CT (**a–c**) the nonenhancing parenchymal region (*) causes minimal bulging of the renal contour without formation of a round-shaped cavity shows preserved capsular "brim" enhancement (thin arrows) characteristic of renal infarctions. Note adjacent region of hypoenhancing ischaemic—oedematous parenchyma (+). Consistent clinical history and lack of acute phase reactants confirmed diagnosis over infection

pies. Albeit the clinical context is generally different, patients may present with similar symptoms and leukocytosis may be present [18]. At CT imaging, the infarcted renal parenchyma is differentiated from APN by the presence of the "cortical brim" sign, which is a thin layer of capsular enhancement representing preserved flow to the capsule through collateral vessels, overlying the nonperfused RI (Fig. 9.14).

A universal and highly specific indicator of renovascular compromise, the "cortical brim" sign may be also observed in renal venous thrombosis along with "striated nephrogram". Multifocal reversible changes closely resembling RIs (Fig. 9.15) are the hallmark of a characteristic yet uncommon syndrome, namely, acute renal failure (ARF) with loin pain (LP) and patchy renal vasoconstriction (PRV) which generally develops after anaerobic exercise, sometimes with other precipitating factors such as heavy alcohol ingestion, upper respiratory infections and medication (analgesics and diuretics) use. Luckily, ARF-LP-PRV has a relatively good prognosis since symptoms and renal impairment are transient, and renal scarring does not occur [19, 20].

Sometimes, unifocal APN may raise concern for the presence of a neoplastic lesion: useful considerations to differentiate APN from tumour include:

(a) Clinical manifestations and laboratory data
(b) Associated inflammatory-type perinephric fat stranding and fascial thickening
(c) Poorly defined interface between the affected area and surrounding parenchyma
(d) Presence of microabscesses (Fig. 9.16)
(e) Regression at follow-up imaging [4, 5, 7–10, 13]

Furthermore, diffuse changes which may be confused with APN may be observed in the setting of non-infected acute urinary obstruction (Fig. 9.17), including perinephric fat stranding and delayed and attenuated nephrogram; however in these occurrences, hydronephrosis with a detectable cause is generally observed.

Finally bilateral renal changes are commonly observed after chemotherapy, which may correspond to either acute interstitial nephritis (AIN) or acute tubular necrosis (ATN): the former mostly occurs after ipilimumab and sorafenib treatment and unspecifically appears as oedematous renal enlargement; conversely ATN results from toxic damage to the tubular epithelial cells. In both entities, "streaky" parenchymal hypoattenuation zones similar to multifocal APN may be observed; analogously to RI, the preserved "cortical brim" sign may be useful to distinguish ATN from APN [21].

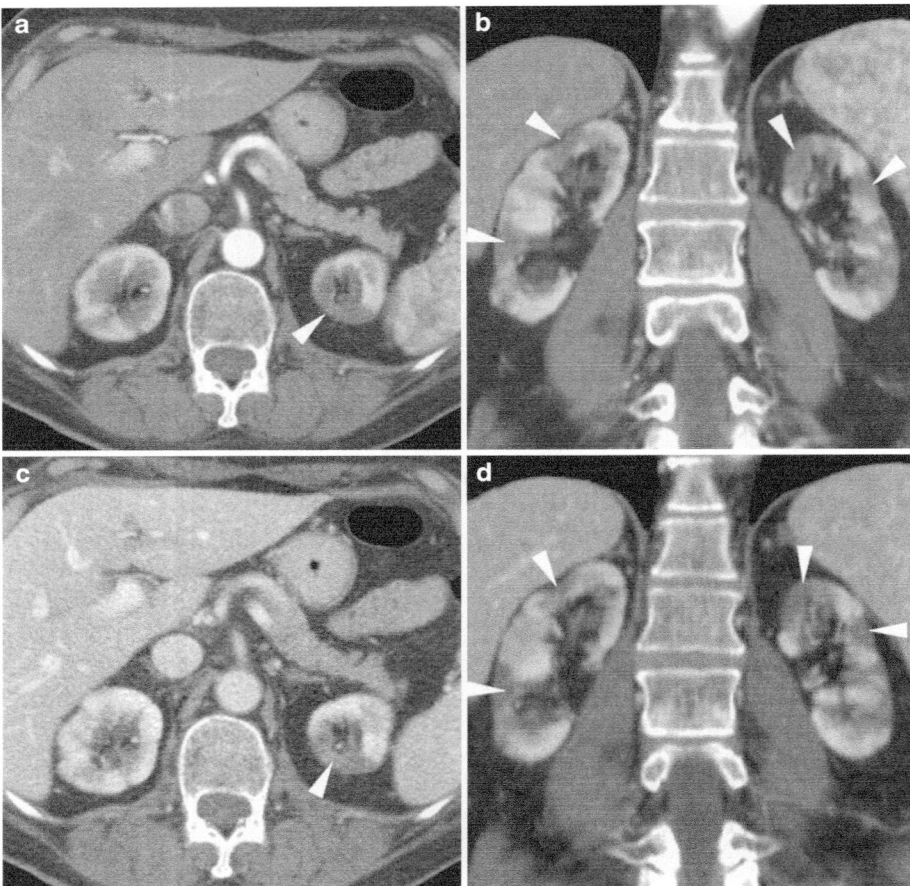

Fig. 9.15 Characteristic CT appearance of acute renal failure with loin pain and patchy renal vasoconstriction syndrome in a 58-year-old female: corticomedullary (**a**, **b**) and corresponding nephrographic (**c**, **d**) phase images showed normal-sized kidneys with scattered infarct-like wedge-shaped nonenhancing parenchymal regions (arrowheads), resulting from temporary vasoconstriction of renal vessels, without function impairment and scarring at follow-up imaging (not shown) (Adapted from Open access ref. no. [19])

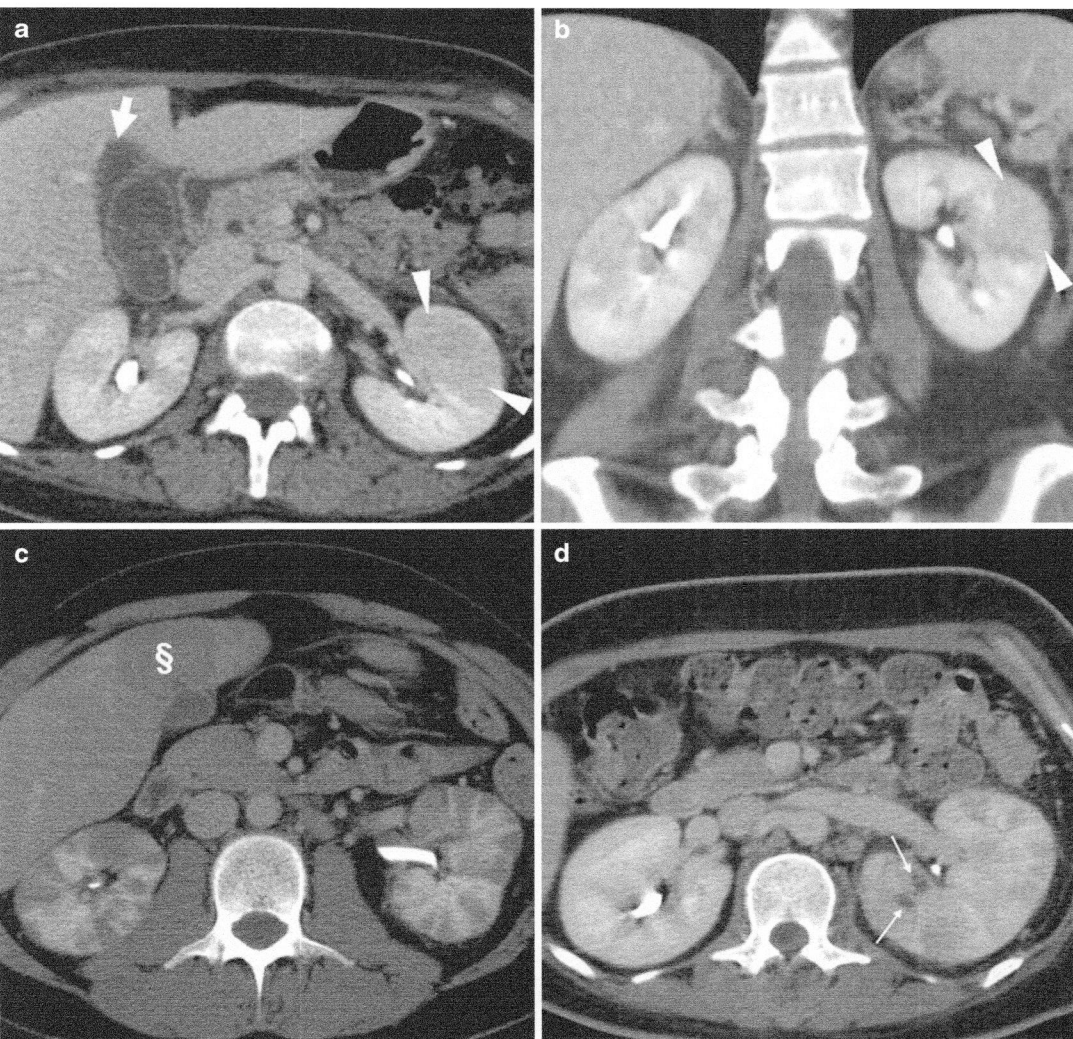

Fig. 9.16 Atypical mass-forming APN in a 44-year-old female with abdominal pain and fever. Combined nephrographic-excretory CT urography showed moderately swollen, hypoenhancing ventral aspect at middle third of the right kidney (arrowheads) without liquefaction. The wedge-shaped appearance on coronal image (**b**) and gallbladder oedema (thick arrow in **a**) favoured infection over tumour, which was confirmed by clinical and laboratory findings. Bilateral multifocal non-Hodgkin lymphomatous infiltration in a 35-year-old male presenting with testicular mass: CT (**c**) showed several small-sized hypovascular foci in both kidneys and intrahepatic masses (§); the latter appearance is closely similar to a unilateral APN (**d**) which shows enlarged left kidney with intraparenchymal hypoattenuating bands, plus microabscesses (thin arrows)

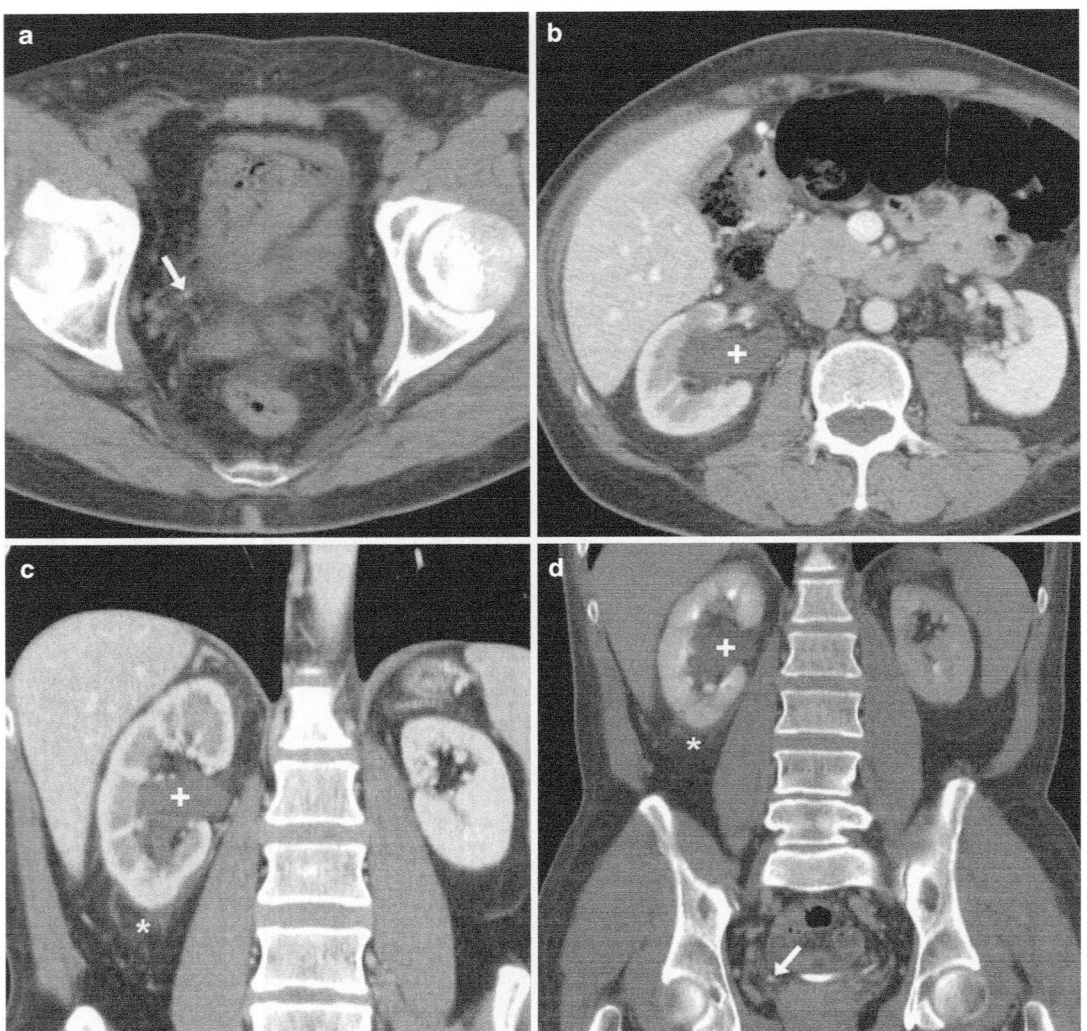

Fig. 9.17 Acute urinary obstruction without infection in a 55-year-old male with tiny stone at the distal right ureter (arrows in **a**, **d**). Note upstream hydronephrosis (+), delayed and attenuated nephrogram (**b–d**) compared to contralateral kidney, mild fluid stranding of ipsilateral perinephric fat (* in **c**, **d**)

References

1. Stoker J, van Randen A, Lameris W et al (2009) Imaging patients with acute abdominal pain. Radiology 253:31–46
2. Rosen MP, Siewert B, Sands DZ et al (2003) Value of abdominal CT in the emergency department for patients with abdominal pain. Eur Radiol 13:418–424
3. Sartelli M, Viale P, Catena F et al (2013) 2013 WSES guidelines for management of intra-abdominal infections. World J Emerg Surg 8:3
4. Browne RF, Zwirewich C, Torreggiani WC (2004) Imaging of urinary tract infection in the adult. Eur Radiol 14(Suppl 3):E168–E183
5. Craig WD, Wagner BJ, Travis MD (2008) Pyelonephritis: radiologic-pathologic review. Radiographics 28:255–277. quiz 327-258
6. Das CJ, Ahmad Z, Sharma S et al (2014) Multimodality imaging of renal inflammatory lesions. World J Radiol 6:865–873
7. Demertzis J, Menias CO (2007) State of the art: imaging of renal infections. Emerg Radiol 14:13–22
8. Ifergan J, Pommier R, Brion MC et al (2012) Imaging in upper urinary tract infections. Diagn Interv Imaging 93:509–519
9. Stunell H, Buckley O, Feeney J et al (2007) Imaging of acute pyelonephritis in the adult. Eur Radiol 17:1820–1828
10. Yu M, Robinson K, Siegel C, et al (2016) Complicated genitourinary tract infections and mimics. Curr Probl Diagn Radiol doi: https://doi.org/10.1067/j.cpradiol.2016.1002.1004
11. European Society of Urogenital Radiology (2016) ESUR guidelines on contrast media 9.0. Available at: www.esur.org/guidelines. Accessed 31 Jan 2017
12. American College of Radiologists (2015) ACR manual on contrast media. American College of Radiologists (ACR) Version 10.2. Available at: https://www.acr.org/Quality-Safety/Resources/Contrast-Manual. Accessed 20 Mar 2017
13. Coppenrath EM, Mueller-Lisse UG (2006) Multidetector CT of the kidney. Eur Radiol 16:2603–2611
14. Heller MT, Haarer KA, Thomas E et al (2012) Acute conditions affecting the perinephric space: imaging anatomy, pathways of disease spread, and differential diagnosis. Emerg Radiol 19:245–254
15. Ronot M, Kerbaol A, Rautou PE et al (2016) Acute extrahepatic infectious or inflammatory diseases are a cause of transient mosaic pattern on CT and MR imaging related to sinusoidal dilatation of the liver. Eur Radiol 26(9):3094–3101
16. Han GJ, Lee NK, Kim S et al (2013) Septic liver: clinical relevance of early inhomogeneous enhancement of the liver in patients with acute pyelonephritis. Acta Radiol 54:975–980
17. Kim SH, Kim YW, Lee HJ (2012) Serious acute pyelonephritis: a predictive score for evaluation of deterioration of treatment based on clinical and radiologic findings using CT. Acta Radiol 53:233–238
18. Antopolsky M, Simanovsky N, Stalnikowicz R et al (2012) Renal infarction in the ED: 10-year experience and review of the literature. Am J Emerg Med 30:1055–1060
19. Tonolini M (2017) Acute renal failure with loin pain and patchy renal vasoconstriction [Online]. EuroRAD URL: http://www.eurorad.org/case.php?id=14370
20. Ishikawa I (2002) Acute renal failure with severe loin pain and patchy renal ischemia after anaerobic exercise in patients with or without renal hypouricemia. Nephron 91:559–570
21. Jia JB, Lall C, Tirkes T et al (2015) Chemotherapy-related complications in the kidneys and collecting system: an imaging perspective. Insights Imaging 6:479–487

Imaging of Extrarenal Spread, Fistulising and Atypical Pyelonephritis

10

Massimo Tonolini

10.1 Emphysematous Pyelonephritis

As mentioned in the introductory chapter of this book, diabetes mellitus (DM) is a common predisposing factor in patients with complicated urinary tract infections (UTI). Compared to the general population, diabetics and particularly those with uncontrolled DM frequently experience more severe pyelonephritis with a similar mortality rate but poorer treatment outcome, common worsening of renal function and greater need for nephrectomy [1, 2].

A rare yet characteristic form of complicated UTI, emphysematous pyelonephritis (EPN) affects diabetics in the vast majority (90%) of cases with a 3:1 female predominance; the rare nondiabetic occurrences are related to either immunosuppression or urinary tract obstruction. EPN is a severe necrotizing renal infection with a complex pathogenesis involving a combination of factors, namely, gas-forming bacteria, high tissue glucose level, impaired tissue perfusion and defective immune response. The commonest pathogens isolated from pus cultures include *Escherichia coli* (49–71% of cases), *Klebsiella pneumoniae* (19%) and *Proteus mirabilis* (17%) in descending order of frequency, with frequent antibiotic resistance [3–6].

The clinical presentation is similar to that of severe forms of bacterial acute pyelonephritis (APN) and mostly includes fever, chills, flank pain, dysuria and pyuria. The usual laboratory abnormalities include leukocytosis, thrombocytopenia and altered renal function. Timely diagnosis is crucial, since untreated EPN generally progresses to sepsis and is potentially lethal [3–8].

The diagnostic hallmark of EPN is represented by abnormal gas collections within the renal parenchyma and sometimes also perinephric space. Traditionally, the usual radiographic appearance included 'mottled' gas over the affected kidney or crescent-shaped air collections within Gerota's fascia corresponding to perinephric extension; however plain abdominal radiographs have moderate (70%) sensitivity for retroperitoneal air, which is commonly misinterpreted as bowel gaseous content. Ultrasound (Fig. 10.1a) may detect renal enlargement with nondependent hyperechoic foci corresponding to gas causing 'dirty' reverberation artefacts. Despite use of ionizing radiation, multidetector CT is by far the preferred imaging technique to diagnose EPN. Unenhanced CT images readily detect the presence, extent and position of renal gas, which may show several different patterns

M. Tonolini, M.D.
Radiology Department, "Luigi Sacco" University Hospital, Via G.B. Grassi 74, Milan 20157, Italy
e-mail: mtonolini@sirm.org

© Springer International Publishing AG 2018
M. Tonolini (ed.), *Imaging and Intervention in Urinary Tract Infections and Urosepsis*,
https://doi.org/10.1007/978-3-319-68276-1_10

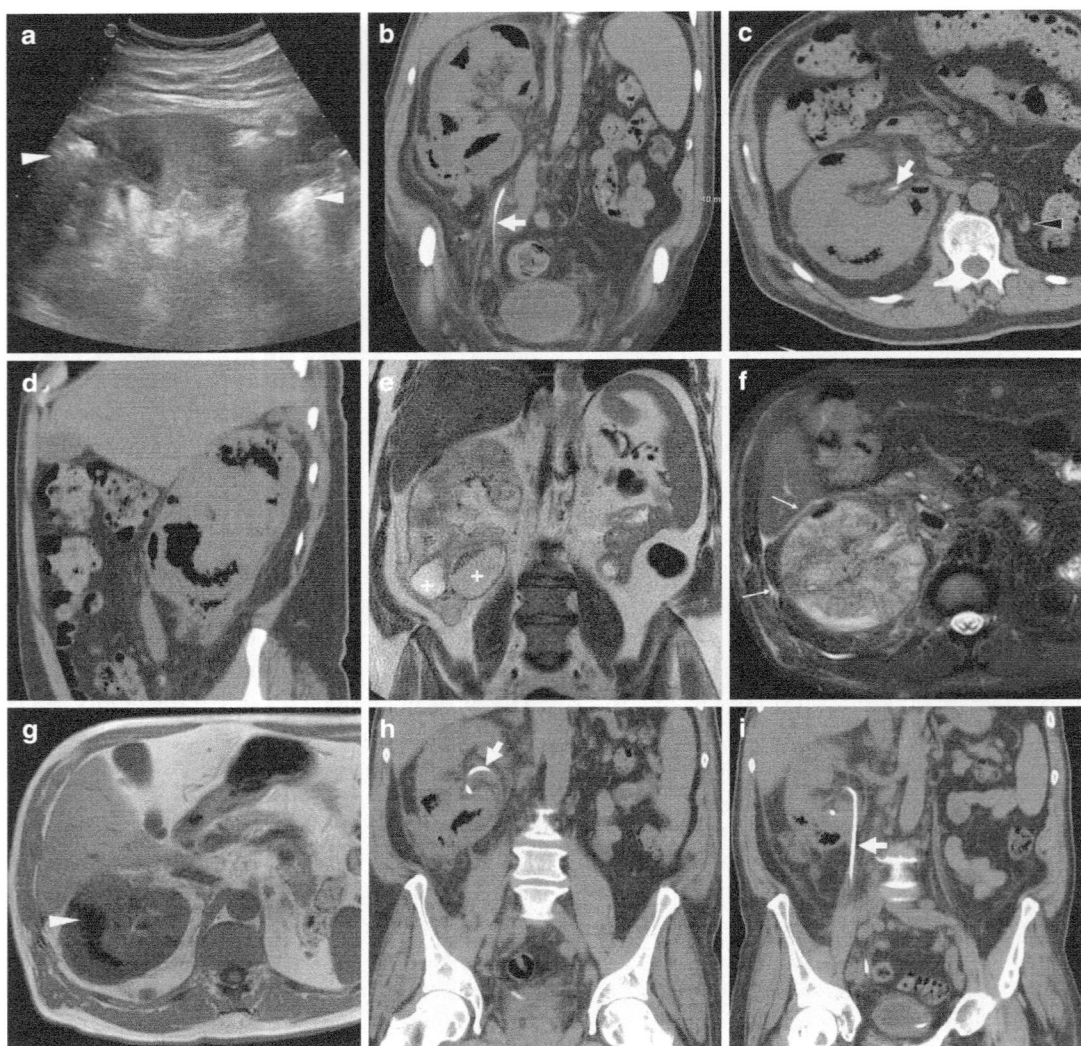

Fig. 10.1 A 63-year-old male admitted to emergency department because of high fever, dysuria and distended tender abdomen was diagnosed with decompensated diabetes mellitus, severe renal impairment (7.5 mg/dl serum creatinine), markedly increased C-reactive protein and metabolic acidosis. Initial ultrasound (**a**) showed enlargement of the right kidney, with parenchymal hyperechoic bands (arrowheads), posterior acoustic shadowing and previously unknown congenital left renal aplasia. After ureteral stenting (thick arrows), multiplanar unenhanced CT images (**a–d**) confirmed enlarged solitary right kidney with strongly hypoattenuating gaseous components, consistent with emphysematous pyelonephritis. MRI follow-up (**e–g**) better showed parenchymal oedema of the right kidney, intraparenchymal fluid collections (plus in T2-weighted image (**f**)) and ipsilateral fascial thickening (thin arrows in (**g**) with fat saturation); conversely gas was less perceptible (arrowhead in T1-weighted image (**e**)). The patient's clinical conditions and laboratory changes slowly improved during conservative treatment including haemodialysis, repeated unenhanced CT studies (**h, i**) showed progressive decrease of renal emphysematous changes and the patient ultimately obviated the need for nephrectomy (Adapted from Open Access Ref. no [16])

such as bubbly, linear, streaky or crescent-shaped. The use of intravenous contrast is reserved for those patients with preserved renal function. The nephrographic enhancement is diffusely altered with or without focal tissue necrosis, fluid-containing abscesses and delayed excretion (Fig. 10.1). Other CT findings include variable degrees of parenchymal enlargement and destruction and possible associated conditions such as urolithiasis and obstruction. Compared to CT, MRI (Fig. 10.1) is more sensitive for the presence of parenchymal oedema and fluid collections but is limited in the assessment of gas which has very low signal intensity [9–16].

In the past, Wan et al. differentiated type-1 EPN characterised by renal necrosis with parenchymal destruction and gas but no fluid collection, from the less aggressive type-2 EPN lacking renal or perirenal fluid collections, respectively, with 69 and 18% mortality rates. Nowadays, EPN should be more comprehensively staged according to classification proposed by Huang and Tseng (Table 10.1). Included in the staging system as grade I EPN, emphysematous pyelitis corresponds to intraluminal gas in the collecting system only and represents a milder form with better prognosis [9–16].

Alternatively, gas may be detected in the urinary tract after surgery, instrumentation or catheterisation, occasionally when fistulisation with the gastrointestinal tract occurs and exceptionally from penetrating trauma [13, 14, 16].

Nowadays, with a timely CT diagnosis, conservative management of EPN is increasingly feasible and effective, particularly in classes I and II, resulting in decreased mortality, currently below 25%. The aggressive treatment includes resuscitation, intravenous fluids and antibiotics, glycaemic control, dialysis and drainage of obstruction as needed. The risk factors for unfavourable outcome include higher CT grade, shock, emergency haemodialysis, altered sensorium and thrombocytopenia. However, conservative treatment fails in almost one-third of cases. Nephrectomy is not associated with improved survival and should be reserved for EPN classes III and IV with adverse prognostic factors or failed conservative treatment [3–5, 7, 16–19].

10.2   Extrarenal Spread of Acute Pyelonephritis

As discussed in the previous chapter of this book, acute pyelonephritis (APN) may worsen as tiny suppurative foci coalesce leading to the formation of variable-sized round or geographic collections: these abscesses are progressively demarcated by a more or less thick and irregular inflammatory wall. Albeit sonography may identify abscesses as hypo-anechoic cavities without internal colour flow signals, multidetector CT is by far superior in the assessment of APN complications such as abscesses (Fig. 10.2) [10–12, 20–22].

When APN is not timely recognized and treated, intrarenal abscesses may cross or rupture through the renal capsule and extend into the perirenal space and sometimes even progress to involve other retroperitoneal compartments. Perinephric abscesses (PNAs) represent organized collections of purulent material which may either result from a urinary tract infection, from superinfection of a pre-existing haematoma or urinoma or form separately from the kidney such as in haematogenous dissemination. Cross-sectional CT imaging consistently and comprehensively depicts PNAs extending from or abutting the adjacent kidney. The characteristic imaging appearance includes a central near-water hypoattenuation which occasionally contains gas bubbles, corresponding to pus and liquefaction, surrounded by a peripheral enhancing wall and by regions of decreased parenchymal enhancement reflecting non-necrotic infected kidney. Representing the hallmark of the mature abscess, the 'rim' enhancement may be more or less (typically several millimetres) thick, intense and often irregular (Figs. 10.2, 10.3 and 10.4). In the proper clinical setting, the CT diagnosis of PNA is relatively straightforward and dictates appropriate

Table 10.1 Classification of emphysematous pyelonephritis proposed by Huang and Tseng (Adapted from Open Access Ref. no [16])

Class	Description
I	Emphysematous pyelitis—gas in collecting system only
II	Intraparenchymal gas only (no extrarenal involvement)
IIIA	Gas extending into the perinephric space
IIIB	Extension of gas into the pararenal spaces
IV	Emphysematous pyelonephritis in solitary kidney or bilateral involvement

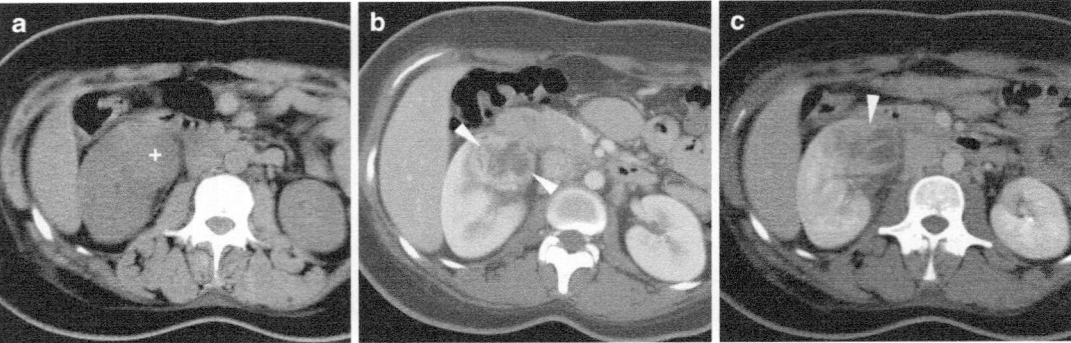

Fig. 10.2 An 18-year-old female with clinical and laboratory signs of acute urinary infection and inconclusive ultrasound findings underwent unenhanced (**a**) and post-contrast (**b**) multidetector CT. The anterior labrum of the right kidney showed mixed attenuation enlargement (plus) with nonenhancing centre and thin, irregular peripheral enhancement (arrowheads) consistent with an abscess, which measured approximately 4 × 3 cm and protruded ventromedially into the perinephric space. Repeated contrast-enhanced CT (**c**) showed decreased size and purulent content of the abscess after antibiotic therapy

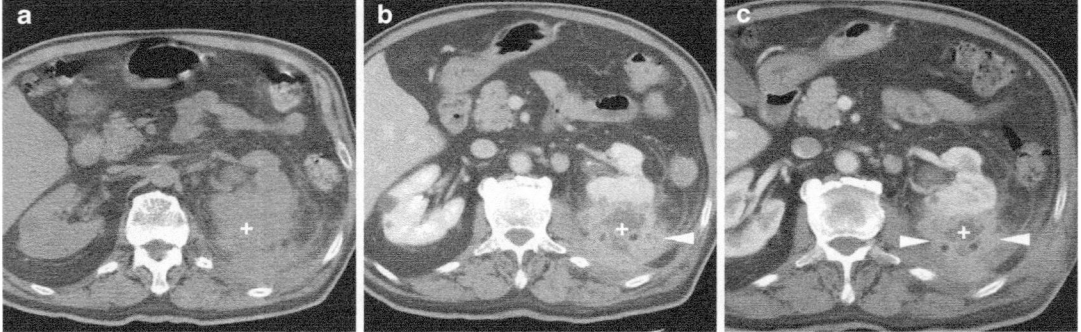

Fig. 10.3 In a 72-year-old male with history of urolithiasis and recurrent urinary infections, unenhanced (**a**) and post-contrast (**b**) CT acquisitions showed extensive inhomogeneous abnormality of the posterior aspect of the left kidney (plus) which largely occupied the dorsal perinephric and posterior pararenal spaces, thus displacing ventrally the kidney. The very thick, irregular peripheral enhancement (arrowheads) and fluidlike content were consistent with an abscess. Despite mild size decrease at follow-up CT (**c**) after 3 weeks of in-hospital treatment, nephrectomy was ultimately performed to relieve the infection

treatment with image-guided percutaneous drainage plus antibiotics [10–12, 20–22].

As discussed in the appropriate chapter of this book, although hampered by longer examination time and need for cooperation, MRI is an increasingly attractive option to comprehensively image renal infections without the use of ionizing radiation. At MRI, the mature renal abscess appears as a fluid collection with fluidlike high T2-weighted signal and internal restricted diffusion, surrounded by a variably thick capsule with relatively lower signal intensity which enhances strongly after gadolinium contrast (Fig. 10.5) [21, 23].

The most important differential diagnoses of a PNA include:

(a) Haematomas
(b) Urinomas (Fig. 10.6)
(c) Complex cystic masses (Fig. 10.7a–c)
(d) Necrotic renal tumours (Fig. 10.7d–f)

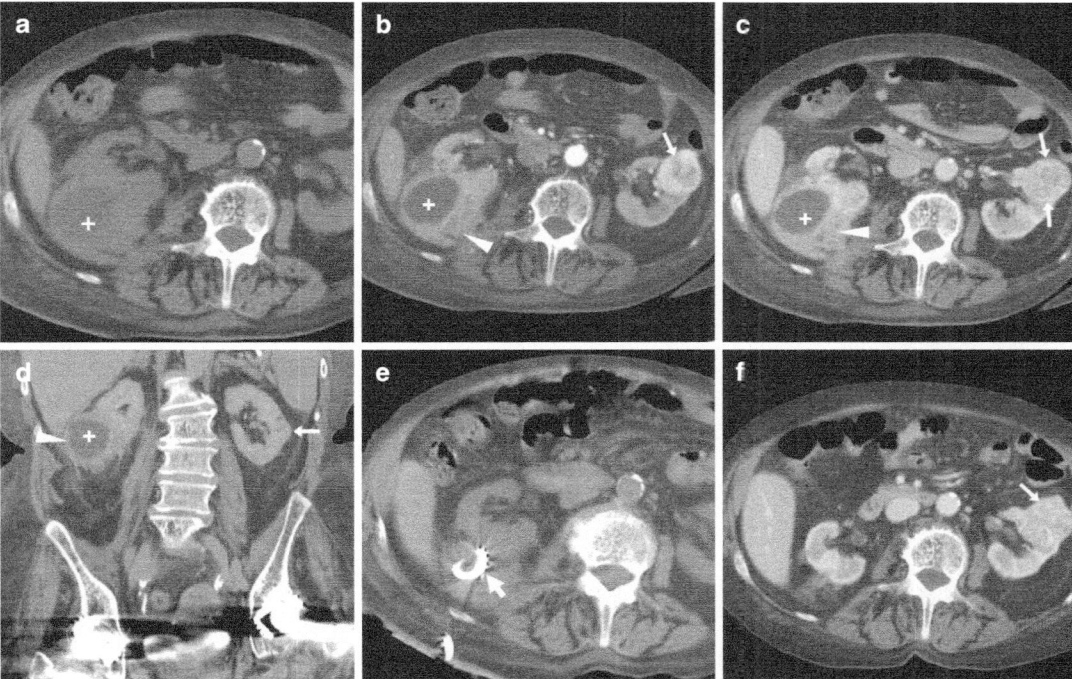

Fig. 10.4 In a 73-year-old diabetic woman hospitalized because of malaise and weight loss, unenhanced (**a**) and post-contrast (**b–d**) multidetector CT showed anterior displacement of the right kidney by a 7-cm hypoattenuating mass (plus) with nonenhancing fluid content (plus) and uneven peripheral enhancement (arrowheads), consistent with perinephric abscess. The abscess was treated by percutaneous drainage (thick arrow in (**e**)) and ultimately resolved (**f**). The incidentally detected 3-cm left renal mass with strong, early enhancement (arrows) consistent with renal cell carcinoma was subsequently treated by nephrectomy

Apart from the trauma setting, a perinephric haematoma may result from ruptured neoplasms (particularly angiomyolipoma), vascular lesions (such as aneurysms, arteriovenous malformations or vasculitides), bleeding diathesis or excessive anticoagulation: the diagnosis is suggested by acute clinical manifestations, dropping haematocrit and by the fact that thickened perirenal septa and acute haematoma have higher unenhanced attenuation than the renal parenchyma [24–27].

Urinomas may develop after iatrogenic injury or trauma or result from increased intraluminal pressure secondary to acute or chronic obstructive uropathy. The extravasated urine shows near-water CT attenuation and MRI signal intensity, but chronic urinomas may appear as complex fluid collections with enhancing rim and septa from chronic inflammation; the diagnostic hallmark of a urinoma is its opacification on delayed excretory-phase CT acquisition (Fig. 10.6) [28, 29].

Finally, rim-enhancing abscess lesions with internal inhomogeneity and thick, enhancing septa commonly raise a concern for a cystic or necrotic neoplasm which may suggest the need for biopsy or close follow-up (Fig. 10.7). The differential diagnosis of a complex cystic renal lesion requires careful assessment of presence and features of calcifications, quantification of internal attenuation and post-contrast enhancement, multiloculation, number and thickness of septa, mural thickness, nodularity and enhancement. An infectious process is suggested by the consistent clinical features and

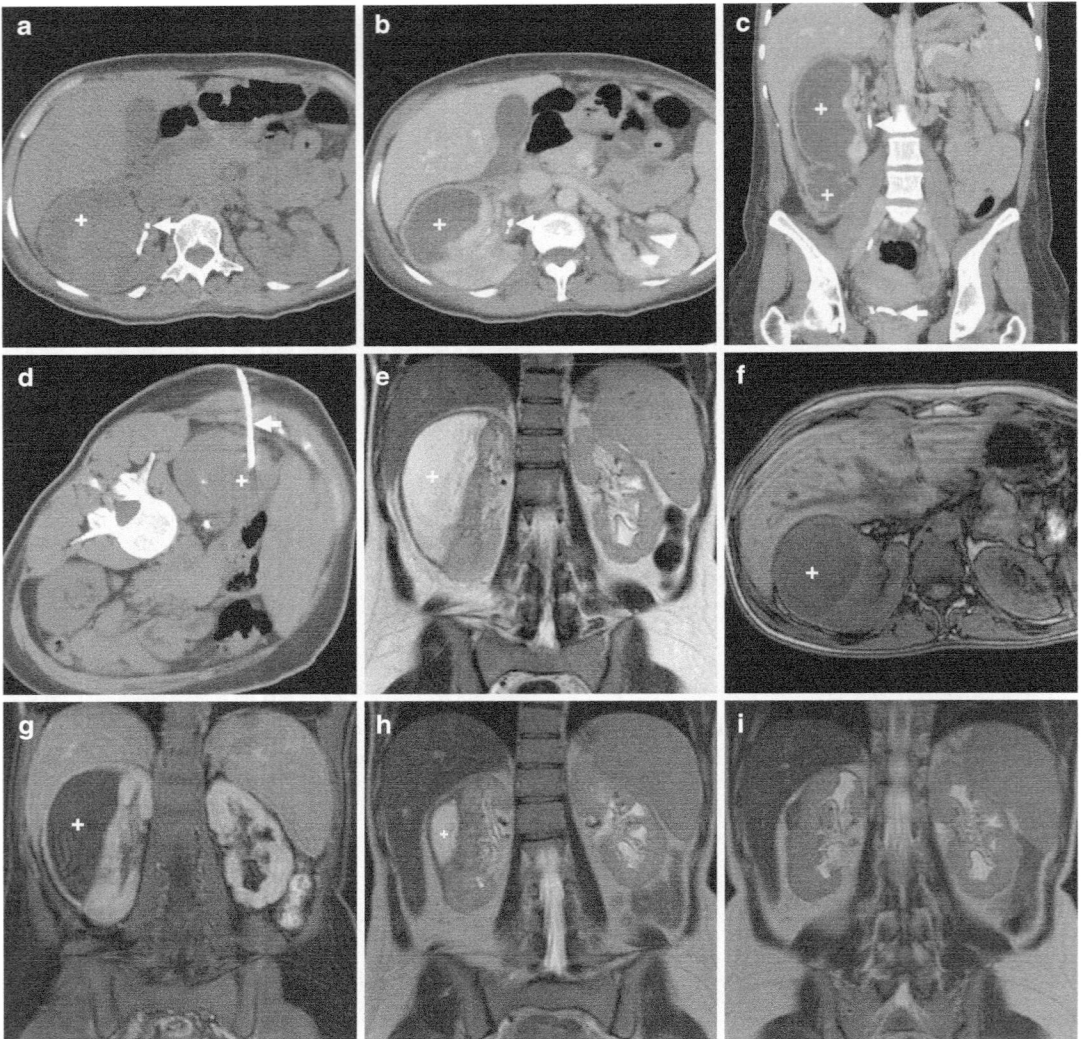

Fig. 10.5 A 37-year-old female had persistent fever and pain following right-sided lithotripsy and ureteral stenting (thick arrows) because of lithiasis and urinary infection. Unenhanced (**a**) and post-contrast (**b, c**) multidetector CT images showed severe compression of right kidney by hypoattenuating subcapsular collection (plus) with thin peripheral enhancement consistent with abscess, which extended distally to the lower renal pole into the inferior perinephric space (**c**). After percutaneous CT-guided drainage (thick arrow in (**d**)) yielded pus, MRI showed persistence of subcapsular abscess (plus) with inhomogeneous, non-haemorrhagic content (**e–g**) and thin peripheral enhancement (**h**). MRI follow-up showed progressive decrease (plus in (**h**) at 8 weeks) and ultimate resolution ((**i**) after 4 months) of the abscess

laboratory abnormalities and by imaging detection of perinephric fat infiltration and thickening of the retroperitoneal fasciae; however, the latter findings are non-specific as they may be also seen in other conditions such as acute pancreatitis [30, 31].

10.3 Xanthogranulomatous Pyelonephritis

Xanthogranulomatous pyelonephritis (XGPN) is a rare, chronic granulomatous infection which begins in the renal pelvis and then diffuses to

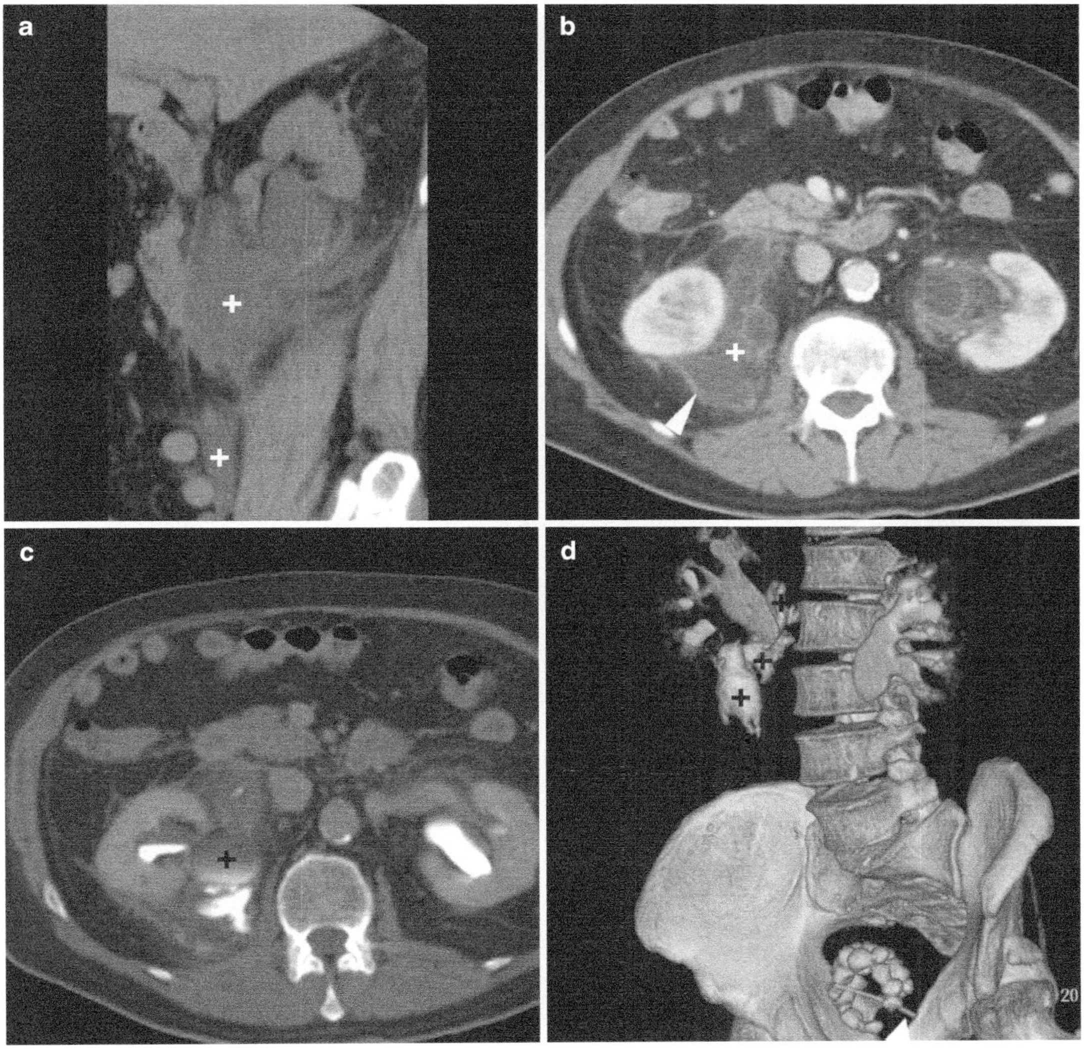

Fig. 10.6 A 70-year-old male patient with benign prostatic hyperplasia suffered from acute right flank pain. Performed to investigate suspected ureteral colic, unenhanced CT (**a**) showed moderate right-sided hydronephrosis plus a sizeable fluidlike collection (plus) which surrounded the renal pelvis and proximal ureter, extending into the medial perinephric space. The collection showed thin peripheral enhancement (arrowhead in (**b**)) after intravenous contrast which was initially interpreted as suggestive of infection. The nephrographic phase and urinary excretion were normal. Delayed phase acquisition (**c**) revealed strong hyperattenuation of the perinephric and pararenal collection (plus) corresponding to extravasated urine from forniceal rupture. The urinoma (plus) was clearly depicted by three-dimensional volume rendering images (**d**) in its size and spatial relationship to the kidney, pelvis and proximal ureter. Note Foley catheter (thick arrow in (**d**)) in the bladder, filled by calculi from chronic urinary retention. The urinoma ultimately resolved on conservative treatment. (Adapted with permission from Ref. no. [53])

the medulla and cortex, leading to a progressive parenchymal destruction of the kidney which is characteristically replaced by lipid-laden 'foamy' macrophages (xanthoma cells). Further extension of XGPN to the perinephric space is commonly encountered in approximately two-thirds of cases. The poorly understood pathogenesis involves an incomplete immune response to a subacute bacterial infection superimposed on long-standing urinary obstruction. Almost invariably unilateral,

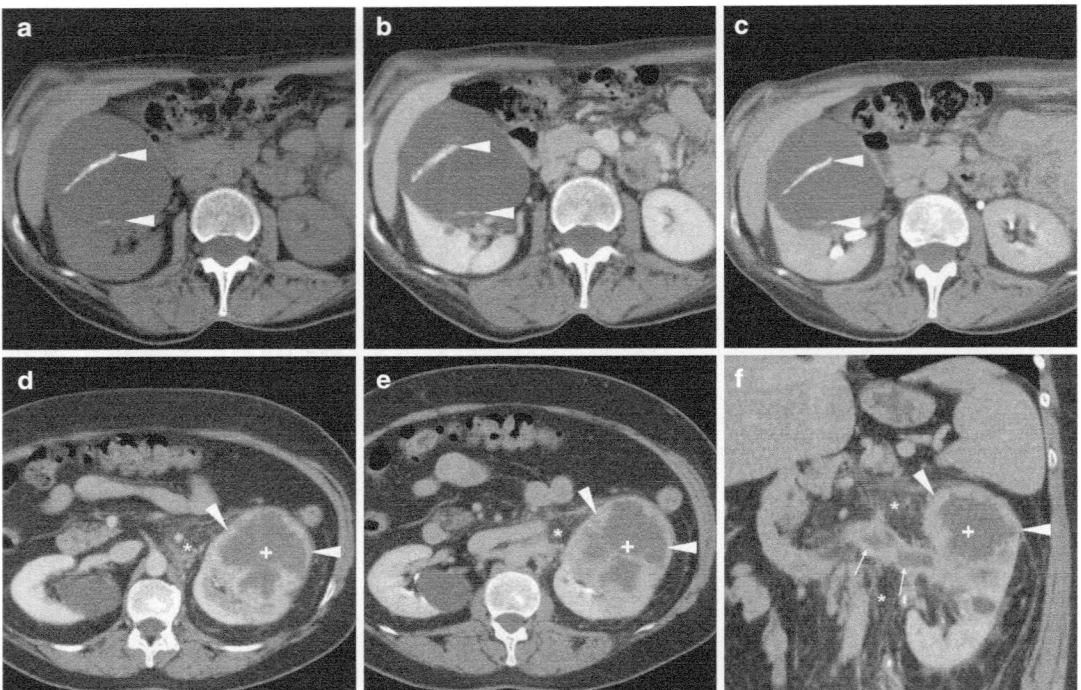

Fig. 10.7 A 62-year-old diabetic female with recurrent urinary infection was requested CT (**a–c**) on the basis of sonographic suspicion of renal abscess. The large right-sided renal lesion showed water-like attenuation on unenhanced scans (**a**), peripheral and septal calcifications (arrowheads) and absent enhancement on both nephrographic (**b**) and excretory phases (**c**), thereby excluding an infectious nature. A 58-year-old female with left-sided abdominal pain and low-grade fever underwent CT (**d–f**) to investigate suspected renal colic and/or pyelonephritis. The left kidney showed a 7-cm centrally nonenhancing mass (plus) with irregular peripheral enhancement (arrowheads). Despite perinephric fat stranding (asterisk) and mild fascial thickening, the presence of ipsilateral renal vein thrombosis (thin arrows) favoured necrotic renal cell carcinoma over abscess, as confirmed at surgery and pathology

XGPN mostly occurs in middle age, with a predilection for perimenopausal women with history of urolithiasis and long-standing urinary infection or obstruction. Compared to EPN, XGPN affects diabetic patients in 10% of cases only. The clinical manifestations are non-specific, often insidious compared to the severity of the imaging abnormalities. Symptoms include low-grade fever, flank pain and tenderness, malaise, weight loss, lethargy, leukocytosis and pyuria. Sometimes a palpable mass is clinically appreciated. *E. coli* and *P. mirabilis* are the commonest identifiable microorganisms [32, 33].

In XGPN, the initial sonographic evaluation shows extensive replacement of the normal renal architecture by hypo-anechoic masses corresponding to dilated calyces and abscesses filled with pus and debris (Fig. 10.11a) and amorphous central hyperechoic structures with acoustic shadowing representing 'staghorn' lithiasis; however these complex ultrasound findings invariably require multidetector CT for a correct characterisation, including intravenous contrast medium unless contraindicated by renal impairment. Cross-sectional imaging findings include an enlarged, non-functioning kidney with poor and heterogeneous contrast enhancement. The majority (75–90%) of cases have obstructing pelvis or ureteral lithiasis, often in a central 'staghorn' configuration. The destroyed parenchyma is replaced by multiple rounded hypodense cavities representing dilated, pus-filled calyces (Fig. 10.8): recognising

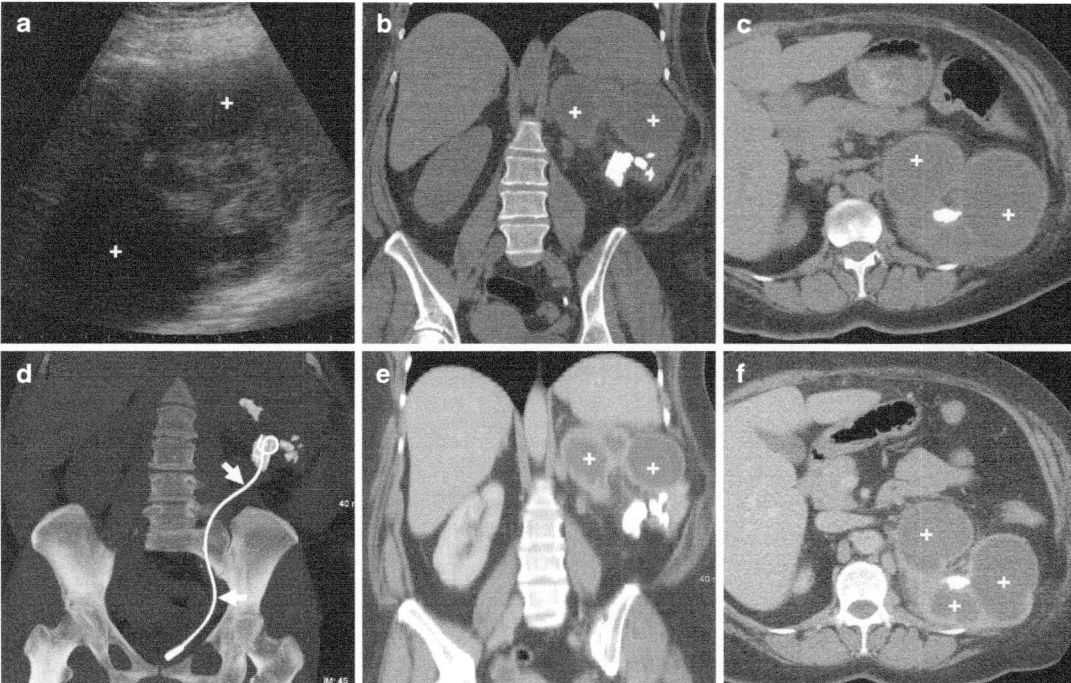

Fig. 10.8 A 48-year-old obese female with history of left-sided pyelolithotomy 15 years earlier was hospitalized with presumptive diagnosis of acute pyelonephritis. Ultrasound (**a**) showed extensive left renal replacement by large hypo-anechoic regions (plus) with poorly perceptible residual parenchyma. Unenhanced (**b**, **c**) CT images confirmed renal parenchymal thinning with sizeable, confluent water-attenuation cavities (plus) and 'staghorn' calcific lithiasis of the renal pelvis and upper and lower calyces. Ureteral stenting (thick arrows in (**d**)) was per- formed to relieve pyonephrosis (as seen in maximum intensity projection (MIP) reconstruction). Six weeks later, after stent removal, contrast-enhanced CT (**e**, **f**) con- firmed poorly enhancing renal parenchyma and uneven calyceal dilatation; the enlarged left kidney occupied and compressed the ipsilateral perirenal and pararenal spaces. After prolonged antibiotics, laparoscopic nephrectomy was performed. Histopathology diagnosed xanthogranu- lomatous pyelonephritis. (Adapted from Open Access ref.no [37])

the hydronephrotic pattern of the fluidlike cavities is crucial for a correct diagnosis. The highly spe- cific fatty xanthomatous deposits with negative CT attenuation are detected in approximately 30% of cases. Contrast excretion into urine is rarely seen at diagnosis. Furthermore, CT readily detects extrarenal extension of XGPN into the perinephric space and other adjacent structures such as the posterior pararenal space and psoas muscles. Although less used in this setting, MRI may depict similar changes, with a lower sensitivity for neph- rolithiasis. The pus-filled cavities show fluidlike very high T2-weighted signal intensity and vari- ably hypointense T1 signal depending on the pro- tein concentration; conversely the solid parts may be T1 isointense or hyperintense from adipose

component and iso- to slightly T2 hypointense [10, 11, 21, 32–38].

The combination of characteristic CT fea- tures, particularly:

(a) Non-functioning kidney
(b) Central lithiasis
(c) Calyceal dilatation
(d) Perinephric involvement

is strongly suggestive of XGPN, a diagnosis which is generally confirmed by histopathology on the nephrectomy specimen. The imaging diag- nosis is challenging in atypical cases, such as in absence of calculi (10% of cases) and the rare (below 10% of cases) focal XGPN which appears as a minimally enhancing renal mass and is commonly misinterpreted as bacterial abscess or tumour [10, 11, 21, 32–37].

10.4 Fistulising Renal Infections

Unrecognised acute or chronic pyelonephritis may further breach through the anterior or posterior renal fasciae and involve other retroperitoneal compartments, most often the posterior pararenal spaces, the iliopsoas and quadratus lumborum muscles (Fig. 10.9) and occasionally to the abdominal wall (Fig. 10.10) giving rise to more or less extensive abscess collections. Urinary tract fistulisation represents an abnormal communication between the renal parenchyma (nephro-) or the pelvis (pyelo-) and other structures: nowadays, the vast majority of urinary fistulas are iatrogenic in origin, secondary to surgical interventions or percutaneous procedures such as nephrostomy, nephrolithotomy or extracorporeal shock wave lithotripsy. Nowadays, cases of renal fistulas from penetrating trauma, tumours or infections are occasionally encountered [39, 40].

Multidetector CT represents the mainstay imaging modality to image fistulising complications, as it promptly provides a comprehensive diagnosis of retroperitoneal infectious involvement even in acutely ill patients and in nonfunctioning kidneys and represents a consistent basis to choose between conservative, percutaneous or surgical treatment [41].

Muscular abscesses such as those involving the psoas present on cross-sectional imaging with variable enlargement of the muscle belly compared to the contralateral one. CT generally shows a hypoattenuating, sometimes multiloculated, lesion with peripheral 'rim' enhancement. Similarly, at MRI muscle abscesses appear as fluidlike cavities with low T1-weighted, high T2 signal intensity and strong 'rim' enhancement. Additional findings suggesting infection over haemorrhage or tumour include indistinct margins, obliteration of the surrounding fat planes and occasionally air-fluid levels; although uncommon, the presence of gas bubbles is considered specific [41–44].

Nowadays, psoas abscesses are most commonly secondary to direct infectious spread from adjacent organs such as the kidneys and urinary tract, the bowel, the lumbar spine or the aorta. When faced with a retroperitoneal abscess, the radiologist should suggest the likely cause between complicated urinary infection, gastrointestinal lesions, musculoskeletal and exceptionally aortic infections (Table 10.2). Generally encountered in association with HIV infection, intravenous drug abuse, immunosuppression or

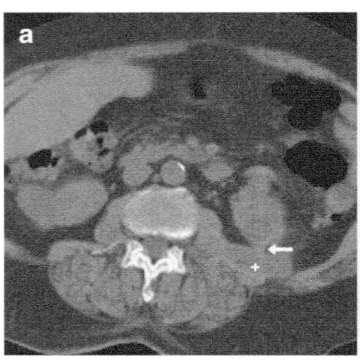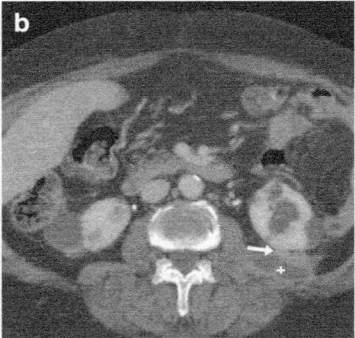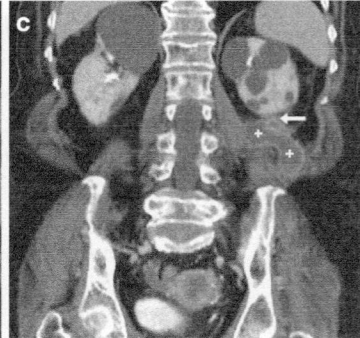

Fig. 10.9 A 78-year-old female with urinary infection and previously unknown multicystic chronic kidney disease underwent unenhanced (**a**) and post-contrast (**b**, **c**) multidetector CT. The posterior aspect of the left kidney was seen adherent and communicating (arrows) with an enlarged quadratus lumborum muscle (plus), character-ised by fluidlike content and peripheral 'rim' enhancement consistent with muscle abscess from renal fistulisation. The patient did well with conservative treatment; the abscess was unchanged and anechoic at ultrasound follow-up (not shown)

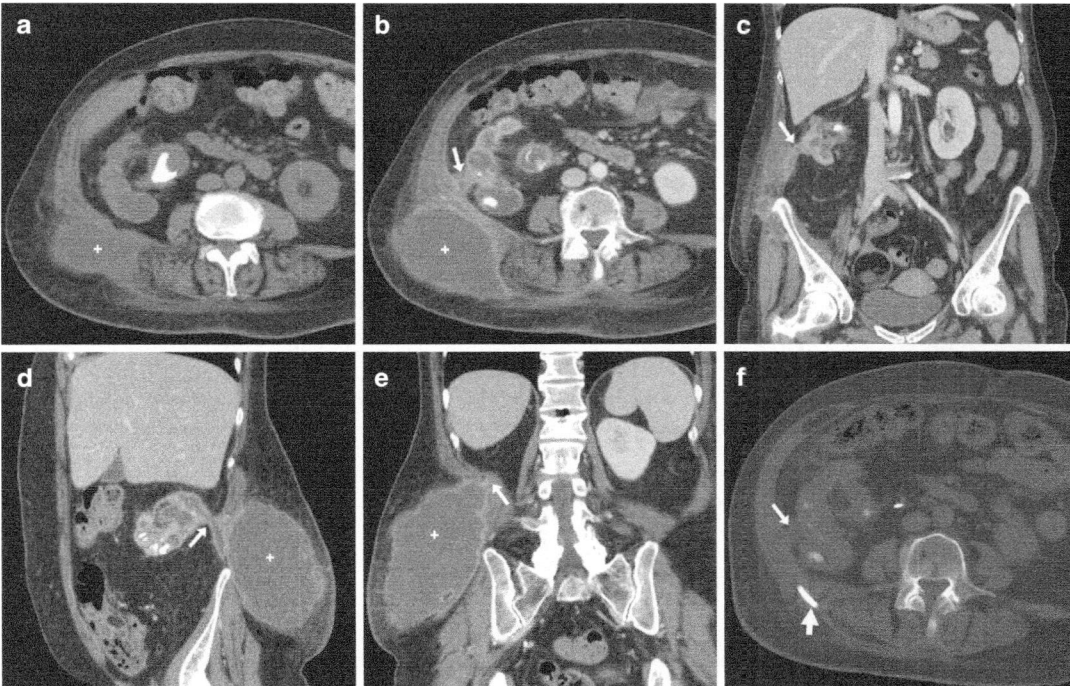

Fig. 10.10 A 64-year-old female presented to emergency department with low-grade fever and painful erythematous swelling in her right lumbar region, without any previous surgical or interventional procedures. Urgent unenhanced (**a**) and post-contrast (**b–e**) CT images showed right kidney with reduced, poorly functioning parenchyma, calcific pelvicalyceal stones. A fluid-containing track with enhancing walls (arrows) consistent with spontaneous fistulisation was seen crossing through the perinephric, posterior pararenal spaces and abdominal wall muscles, to form a large abscess (plus) that displaced the superficial fascia. Percutaneous drainage (thick arrow in (**f**)) yielded 500 ml of pus from *P. mirabilis* infection. Follow-up unenhanced CT (**f**) confirmed disappearance of the abscess. Later on, laparoscopic nephroureterectomy was performed, and surgical pathology confirmed extensive renal infection breaching through the renal capsule

Table 10.2 Causes of psoas muscle abscesses

Source	Main underlying conditions
Urinary	Acute pyelonephritis
	Renal abscess
	Pyonephrosis
	Xanthogranulomatous pyelonephritis
Digestive tract	Fistulising Crohn's disease
	Colonic diverticulitis
	Complicated acute appendicitis
	Perforated colorectal cancer
Musculoskeletal	Pyogenic spondylodiskitis
	Spinal tuberculosis
	Infectious sacroiliitis
Vascular	Infected aortic aneurysms
	Prosthetic vascular infection
Haematogenous	Primary psoas abscess

DM, the rare primary iliopsoas abscesses originate from haematogenous spread and are diagnosed when no obvious local cause can be identified [44–46].

In current urological practice, spontaneous nephrocutaneous fistulas (NCFs) without history of surgery or other instrumentation are exceptionally encountered, invariably associated with long-standing nephrolithiasis and chronic UTI. A NCF involves the development of an abnormal communication between the kidney and the skin, classically crossing through the retroperitoneum and abdominal wall structures following the lowest resistance points such as Petit's triangle and the Grynfeld quadrilateral. Most reported cases are associated with 'staghorn' calculi and poorly functioning kidneys and attributed to XGPN,

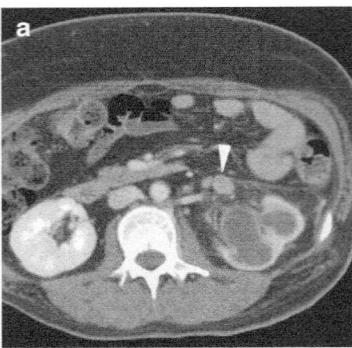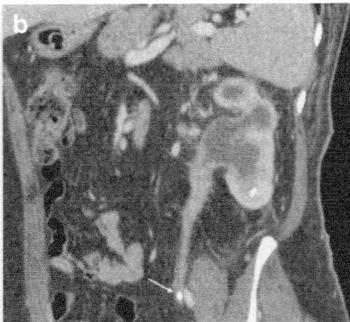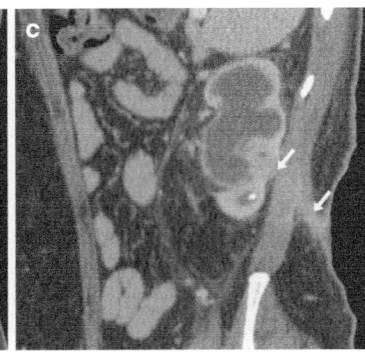

Fig. 10.11 Four months after lithotripsy, a 45-year-old female with diabetes, HIV infection and 'staghorn' nephrolithiasis experienced a painful lumbar swelling. Careful inspection revealed a cutaneous ulcer on her left flank draining smelly greenish fluid. Compared to previous studies (not shown), contrast-enhanced multidetector CT (**a**–**c**) showed appearance of hydronephrosis with enhancing inflammatory urothelial thickening along the pelvis and proximal and mid-ureter, a residual stone fragment (thin arrow in (**b**)) and ipsilateral adenopathies (arrowhead in (**a**)). Furthermore, a thin fluidlike track with enhancing wall (arrows in (**c**)) consistent with nephrocutaneous fistulisation was recognised, directed posteroinferiorly through the posterior pararenal space and abdominal wall to reach the skin orifice (Partially reproduced from Open Access Ref.no [39])

pyogenic infections such as renal abscesses or pyelocalyceal diverticula, tuberculosis, renal trauma or malignancies. The characteristic clinical manifestation is flank or lumbar tenderness and swelling with a cutaneous orifice draining urine or pus [47–52].

In the past, most patients were investigated with fluoroscopic retrograde pyelogram and or fistulography: the injected contrast medium directly opacified the abnormal tract and urinary collecting system, without providing any cross-sectional information on the involved renal and perirenal anatomical structures [40, 47, 51]. Conversely, CT comprehensively and noninvasively depicts the fistulous track even in poorly or non-functioning kidneys (Fig. 10.11). When contrast excretion is preserved, the NCF may be seen opacified on delayed excretory CT acquisitions obtained 20–120 min after intravenous injection. In the setting of urinary fistulisation, CT reliably provides:

(a) Key information about size, parenchymal thickness and function of the involved kidney

(b) Comprehensive characterisation and extent assessment of the underlying infectious or neoplastic disease

(c) A surgical road map for nephrectomy and fistula debridement

(d) Identification of abscesses amenable to drainage [40, 52]

Particularly in patients with non-functioning kidneys and complex lithiasis, nephrectomy plus fistulectomy is the standard surgical treatment which prevents sepsis, that should be planned after interventional treatment of pyonephrosis and abscesses with stenting or percutaneous drainage.

Conservative treatment with antibiotics is reserved for debilitated patients [47, 51].

References

1. Kumar S, Ramachandran R, Mete U et al (2014) Acute pyelonephritis in diabetes mellitus: single center experience. Indian J Nephrol 24:367–371
2. Garg V, Bose A, Jindal J et al (2015) Comparison of clinical presentation and risk factors in diabetic and non-diabetic females with urinary tract infection assessed as per the european association of urology classification. J Clin Diagn Res 9:PC12–PC14
3. Aboumarzouk OM, Hughes O, Narahari K et al (2014) Emphysematous pyelonephritis: time for a management plan with an evidence-based approach. Arab J Urol 12:106–115

4. Behera V, Vasantha Kumar RS, Mendonca S et al (2014) Emphysematous infections of the kidney and urinary tract: a single-center experience. Saudi J Kidney Dis Transpl 25:823–829

5. Dhabalia JV, Neligvi GG, Kumar V et al (2010) Emphysematous pyelonephritis: tertiary care center experience in management and review of the literature. Urol Int 85:304–308

6. Sharma PK, Sharma R, Vijay MK et al (2013) Emphysematous pyelonephritis: our experience with conservative management in 14 cases. Urol Ann 5:157–162

7. Fatima R, Jha R, Muthukrishnan J et al (2013) Emphysematous pyelonephritis: a single center study. Indian J Nephrol 23:119–124

8. Lu YC, Hong JH, Chiang BJ et al (2016) Recommended initial antimicrobial therapy for emphysematous pyelonephritis: 51 cases and 14-year-experience of a tertiary referral center. Medicine (Baltimore) 95:e3573

9. Tasleem AM, Murray P, Anjum F et al (2014) CT imaging is invaluable in diagnosing emphysematous pyelonephritis (EPN): a rare urological emergency. BMJ Case Rep 2014: bcr2014204040–bbcr201420404

10. Demertzis J, Menias CO (2007) State of the art: imaging of renal infections. Emerg Radiol 14:13–22

11. Craig WD, Wagner BJ, Travis MD (2008) Pyelonephritis: radiologic-pathologic review. Radiographics 28:255–277. quiz 327-258

12. Stunell H, Buckley O, Feeney J et al (2007) Imaging of acute pyelonephritis in the adult. Eur Radiol 17:1820–1828

13. Portnoy O, Apter S, Koukoui O et al (2007) Gas in the kidney: CT findings. Emerg Radiol 14:83–87

14. Tsitouridis I, Michaelides M, Sidiropoulos D et al (2010) Renal emphysema in diabetic patients: CT evaluation. Diagn Interv Radiol 16:221–226

15. Huang JJ, Tseng CC (2000) Emphysematous pyelonephritis: clinicoradiological classification, management, prognosis, and pathogenesis. Arch Intern Med 160:797–805

16. Tonolini M, Vella A, Romanò AL, et al (2016) Emphysematous pyelonephritis in a solitary kidney. EuroRAD URL: http://www.eurorad.org/case.php?id=13869

17. Alsharif M, Mohammedkhalil A, Alsaywid B et al (2015) Emphysematous pyelonephritis: is nephrectomy warranted? Urol Ann 7:494–498

18. Kangjam SM, Irom KS, Khumallambam IS et al (2015) Role of conservative management in emphysematous pyelonephritis - a retrospective study. J Clin Diagn Res 9:PC09–PC11

19. Lu YC, Chiang BJ, Pong YH et al (2014) Predictors of failure of conservative treatment among patients with emphysematous pyelonephritis. BMC Infect Dis 14:418

20. Browne RF, Zwirewich C, Torreggiani WC (2004) Imaging of urinary tract infection in the adult. Eur Radiol 14(Suppl 3):E168–E183

21. Das CJ, Ahmad Z, Sharma S et al (2014) Multimodality imaging of renal inflammatory lesions. World J Radiol 6 865–873

22. Ifergan J, Pommier R, Brion MC et al (2012) Imaging in upper urinary tract infections. Diagn Interv Imaging 93:509–519

23. Dunn DP, Kelsey NR, Lee KS et al (2015) Non-oncologic applications of diffusion-weighted imaging (DWI) in the genitourinary system. Abdom Imaging 40:1645–1654

24. Tonolini M, Ierardi AM, Carrafiello G (2015) Letter to the editor: spontaneous renal haemorrhage in end-stage renal disease. Insights Imaging 6:693–695

25. Diaz JR, Agriantonis DJ, Aguila J et al (2011) Spontaneous perirenal hemorrhage: what radiologists need to know. Emerg Radiol 18:329–334

26. Daskalopoulos G, Karyotis I, Heretis I et al (2004) Spontaneous perirenal hemorrhage: a 10-year experience at our institution. Int Urol Nephrol 36:15–19

27. Zhang JQ, Fielding JR, Zou KH (2002) Etiology of spontaneous perirenal hemorrhage: a meta-analysis. J Urol 167:1593–1596

28. Titton RL, Gervais DA, Hahn PF et al (2003) Urine leaks and urinomas: diagnosis and imaging-guided intervention. Radiographics 23:1133–1147

29. Gayer G, Zissin R, Apter S et al (2002) Urinomas caused by ureteral injuries: CT appearance. Abdom Imaging 27:88–92

30. Heller MT, Haarer KA, Thomas E et al (2012) Acute conditions affecting the perinephric space: imaging anatomy, pathways of disease spread, and differential diagnosis. Emerg Radiol 19:245–254

31. Hartman DS, Choyke PL, Hartman MS (2004) From the RSNA refresher courses: a practical approach to the cystic renal mass. Radiographics 24(Suppl 1):S101–S115

32. Loffroy R, Guiu B, Watfa J et al (2007) Xanthogranulomatous pyelonephritis in adults: clinical and radiological findings in diffuse and focal forms. Clin Radiol 62:884–890

33. Zorzos I, Moutzouris V, Korakianitis G et al (2003) Analysis of 39 cases of xanthogranulomatous pyelonephritis with emphasis on CT findings. Scand J Urol Nephrol 37:342–347

34. Rajesh A, Jakanani G, Mayer N et al (2011) Computed tomography findings in xanthogranulomatous pyelonephritis. J Clin Imaging Sci 1:45

35. Kim JC (2001) US and CT findings of xanthogranulomatous pyelonephritis. Clin Imaging 25:118–121

36. Yu M, Robinson K, Siegel C et al (2016) Complicated genitourinary tract infections and mimics. Curr Probl Diagn Radiol 45(1):74–83. https://doi.org/10.1067/j.cpradiol.2016.1002.1004

37. Tonolini M, Bonzini M (2016) Xanthogranulomatous pyelonephritis: when CT findings suggest the diagnosis. EuroRAD URL: http://www.eurorad.org/case.php?id=14129

38. Nikken JJ, Krestin GP (2007) MRI of the kidney-state of the art. Eur Radiol 17:2780–2793

39. Tonolini M, Vila F, Ippolito S et al (2014) Cross-sectional imaging of iatrogenic complications after

extracorporeal and endourological treatment of uro-lithiasis. Insights Imaging 5:677–689

40. Yu NC, Raman SS, Patel M et al (2004) Fistulas of the genitourinary tract: a radiologic review. Radiographics 24:1331–1352
41. Tonolini M, Campari A, Bianco R (2012) Common and unusual diseases involving the iliopsoas muscle compartment: spectrum of cross-sectional imaging findings. Abdom Imaging 37:118–139
42. Zissin R, Gayer G, Kots E et al (2001) Iliopsoas abscess: a report of 24 patients diagnosed by CT. Abdom Imaging 26:533–539
43. Muttarak M, Peh WC (2000) CT of unusual iliopsoas compartment lesions. Radiographics 20(Suppl 1):S53–S66
44. Cronin CG, Lohan DG, Meehan CP et al (2008) Anatomy, pathology, imaging and intervention of the iliopsoas muscle revisited. Emerg Radiol 15:295–310
45. van den Berge M, de Marie S, Kuipers T et al (2005) Psoas abscess: report of a series and review of the literature. Neth J Med 63:413–416
46. Mallick IH, Thoufeeq MH, Rajendran TP (2004) Iliopsoas abscesses. Postgrad Med J 80:459–462
47. Antunes AA, Calado AA, Falcao E (2004) Spontaneous nephrocutaneous fistula. Int Braz J Urol 30:316–318
48. Ansari MS, Singh I, Dogra PN (2004) Spontaneous nephrocutaneous fistula--2 unusual case reports with review of literature. Int Urol Nephrol 36:239–243
49. Singer AJ (2002) Spontaneous nephrocutaneous fistula. Urology 60:1109–1110
50. Qureshi MA (2007) Spontaneous nephrocutaneous fistula in tuberculous pyelonephritis. J Coll Physicians Surg Pak 17:367–368
51. Charles JC (1990) Nephrocutaneous fistula. J Natl Med Assoc 82:589–590
52. Cooper SG, Richman AH, Tager MG (1989) Nephrocutaneous fistula diagnosed by computed tomography. Urol Radiol 11:33–36
53. Tonolini M (2011) Spontaneous perinephric urinoma complicating obstructive uropathy {Online}. EuroRAD URL: http://www.eurorad.org/case.php?id=9710

MRI and DW-MRI of Acute Pyelonephritis (APN)

11

Andrea Veltri, Agostino De Pascale,
and Dario Gned

11.1 Background

Acute pyelonephritis (APN) is a non-specific suppurative inflammatory process due to hematogenous bacterial diffusion or secondary to ascending
infection from the urinary bladder [1]. In fact, it is
frequently associated with lower urinary tract
infections (UTI) and involves all kidney structures,
with *E. coli* as the most commonly found organism. UTI is more commonly seen in women [2].

Urinary tract infections accounted for two
million emergency department visits in the USA
in 2007 [3–6]. In that country acute pyelonephritis (APN) has an incidence as high as 250,000
cases per year, mostly in young women, and
necessitates 200,000 hospitalizations every year
[7–9]. There are very few data on the overall incidence of APN in Europe, being influenced by the
type of sanitary system and the hospitalization
policy; however, based on a previous surveillance
on the referral area to our University Hospital,
the gross incidence of hospitalized APN cases
can be estimated as about 26.5 new cases per year
per 100,000 inhabitants [10].

According to the British Medical Research
Council Bacteriuria Committee [7], the definition
of APN is clinical, based on a classic tetrad of
high fever, costovertebral angle tenderness, signs
or symptoms of lower UTI (leukocytosis, pyuria),
and positive urinary cultures. As this definition
does not discriminate between upper UTI with
and without renal parenchymal involvement,
other authors follow a "pathological" criterion,
based upon the demonstration of kidney involvement by imaging techniques [8].

A general consensus is reached for the definition
of "complicated" versus "noncomplicated" APN
[9–12]. "Complicated" refers to the presence of systemic (any factor affecting the immune response,
including diabetes, collagen disease, neoplasia, chemotherapy, HIV positivity, neuromuscular disease,
hemoglobinopathies) or anatomical (any factor
causing obstruction, including active stone disease,
prostatic hypertrophy, kidney malformations, reflux
nephropathy, polycystic kidney disease, and
indwelling catheters) predisposing factors.
"Noncomplicated" refers to their absence [10].

11.2 MRI and DW-MRI in the Workup of APN

In view of its low sensitivity for the presence of
parenchymal lesions [13] but high sensitivity for
obstructive lesions, conventional ultrasound (US) is
used to identify the presence of anatomical or other
predisposing factors for complicated APN, and further investigation is adopted based on US findings.
In cases with a clinical suspicion of APN in which
no predisposing condition is found at US, noncom-

A. Veltri (✉) • A. De Pascale • D. Gned
Radiology Department, "San Luigi Gonzaga"
University Hospital, Regione Gonzole, 10,
Orbassano, TO 10043, Italy
e-mail: andrea.veltri@unito.it; ago.depascale@libero.it

© Springer International Publishing AG 2018
M. Tonolini (ed.), *Imaging and Intervention in Urinary Tract Infections and Urosepsis*,
https://doi.org/10.1007/978-3-319-68276-1_11

113

plicated APN should be suspected, and a second-line imaging test has to be performed as well. Computed tomography (CT) or magnetic resonance imaging (MRI) examination allows precise definition of the inflammatory areas and evidence of abscesses [1, 14–15]. As patients with noncomplicated APN are mostly women of childbearing age, MR might be chosen as the preferred imaging technique, and CT should be performed only in the case of contraindications or logistical problems (i.e., long wait before the availability of an MRI) [16].

MRI, using a parallel imaging technique acquisition, is able to perform dynamic enhanced studies, with diagnostic accuracy comparable to CT [17]. It does not use ionizing radiation, and it is equipped with considerable contrast resolution. Between sequences performed in a basal setting, diffusion-weighted magnetic resonance imaging (DW-MRI) has recently gained particular interest [18]. It is realizable by analyzing the spin dephasing and signal loss caused by random motion along magnetic field gradients. The apparent diffusion coefficient (ADC), as a quantitative parameter calculated from the DW-MRI acquisition, combines the effects of capillary perfusion and water diffusion in the intracellular extravascular space.

The development of echo-planar imaging (EPI), high-gradient amplitudes, multichannel coils, and parallel imaging has been helpful in increasing the applications of DW sequences. In particular, the introduction of parallel imaging, such as sensitivity encoding (SENSE), which allowed reduction in the echo-train length (TE) and the K-space filling time, led to considerably less motion artifacts at image acquisition, thus enabling high-quality DW images of the body to be acquired. Hence, DWI might be useful in differentiating APN, with the advantage of lower costs and execution times than gadolinium-enhanced MRI (GE-MRI). The following protocol is used at our institution.

11.3 MRI and DW-MRI Diagnosis of APN

Our study protocol is presented in Table 11.1. As summarized in Table 11.2, the MRI findings consistent with APN include:

At basal MRI:

- Changes in renal volume (kidney enlargement, presumably due to edema from active infection) often associated with perinephric inflammatory fluid and stranding of the perinephric fat (Fig. 11.1a, b, c)

Table 11.1 Pre- and post-contrast MRI acquisition protocol

Basal MRI study
• Survey BFFE (balanced fast field echo) sequences along the three orthogonal axes (x, y, and z)
• Axial TSE SENSE (turbo spin echo SSH T2-weighted) sequences (TR = 375 ms; double TE = 100 ms, Sp 7.0/1.0, turbo factor 47; EPI factor 1, NSA 1, SENSE torso XLcoil)
• Axial TSE SENSE (turbo spin echo sSSH T2-weighted) sequences (TR = 375 ms; double TE = 100 ms, Sp 7.0/1.0, turbo factor 47; EPI factor 1, NSA 1, SENSE torso XLcoil)
• Axial SPAIR SENSE Sat-SPIR (spectral attenuation inversion recovery) sequences (TR = 418 ms; TE = 80 ms, Sp 7.0/1.0, turbo factor 47; EPI factor 1, NSA 1, SENSE torso Xlcoil)
• Axial DWI—SENSE Sat-SPIR sequences (TR = 1275–2572 ms; TE = d0.0 62–65 ms, Sp 7.0/1.0 mm, turbo factor 62–65; EPI factor 62–65, NSA 4, matrix 190/256; SENSE torso XLcoil; b 0 and b 600 with breath-hold and imaging time 20–25 s)
• Axial basal T1 3D FFE DIXON sequence (TR = 5,88 ms; TE = 1,80 ms, Sp 4/0, breath-hold SENSE torso XLcoil)
GE-MRI study: after bolus intravenous administration of contrast agent (gadobutrol, 1 mmol/kg), 2 mL/s
• Coronal 2D bolus-track sequences (TR = 4.0 ms, TE = 0.9 ms, Sp 80/0.0 mm, turbo factor 1; EPI factor 1, NSA 1, matrix 128/224; SENSE body coil) in the course of administration of contrast medium by an injector to determine dynamic sequences (care bolus)
• Coronal Angio-RM 3D RES sequences (TR = 5.1 ms, TE = 1.5 ms, Sp 3.0/−1.5 mm, turbo factor 1; EPI factor 1; SENSE body coil), after about 20–30 s (cortical-arterial phase). The beginning of MR data acquisition is determined by the vision of the initial opacification of the abdominal aorta using a care bolus
• Axial dynamic T1 3D FFE DIXON sequences—(TR = 5,88 ms; TE = 1,80 ms, Sp 4/0, breath-hold SENSE torso XLcoil). In the course of administration of contrast medium at 60–80 s (nephrographic phase) and 100–120 s (nephrographic/early excretory phase)

Table 11.2 Multiparametric MRI diagnosis of acute pyelonephritis

Findings of APN at basal MRI

• Partial or entire kidney enlargement, perinephric inflammatory fluid, and stranding of the fat

• Reduced or cancelled corticomedullary delineation

• Focal or diffuse parenchymal signal alteration on T2-weighted images, with slight hyperintensity in mild inflammatory tissue alterations and heavy hyperintensity in abscesses

Findings of APN at DWI sequences

• Hyperintensity, with high b value and hypointensity in the same area on ADC maps, correlating with focal reduction of enhancement at T1-weighted sequences in the contrast-enhanced study

Findings of APN at GE-MRI

• Reduction of parenchymal enhancement in the affected area. Multiple areas quickly affected, with lesions mostly well-defined, wedge-shaped with their bases at the periphery and apexes toward the renal sinus, and parenchyma sometimes demonstrating a striated appearance, due to hypoperfusion secondary to arteriolar vasoconstriction and inflammatory response

• Abscessed areas, as fluid lesions delineated by a peripheral halo dilation of the collecting system

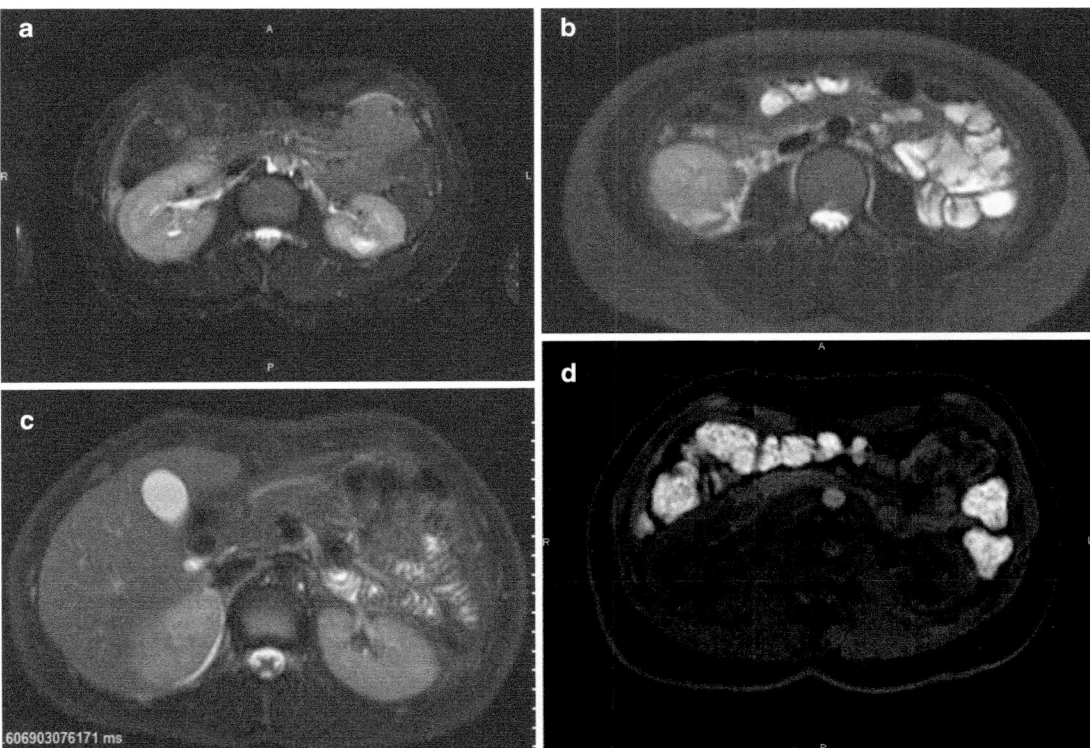

Fig. 11.1 (**a**) *Axial SPAIR SENSE* show right kidney enlargement due to edema. (**b**) *Axial SPAIR SENSE* show fat stranding around caudal right kidney pole. (**c**) *Axial SPAIR SENSE* show thin perirenal effusion. (**d**) *Axial 3D FFE T1w Dixon* show abnormal cortico medullary interface consistent in poor/absent delineation of cortical layer

• Alteration of corticomedullary delineation (reduced or absent) (Fig. 11.1d)

• Focal or diffuse parenchymal signal alteration, with isointensity at T1-weighted sequences and slight hyperintensity at T2-weighted images or heavy hyperintensity at T2-weighted images in abscess

• Hyperintensity *at the DWI sequences* with high b value and hypointensity in the same area on ADC maps, correlating with focal reduction of enhancement at T1-weighted sequences in the contrast-enhanced study (Fig. 11.2a, b)

After the administration of contrast medium (GE-MRI), on T1-weighted sequences:

- Reduction of parenchymal contrast enhancement in the affected area. Multiple areas can readily be affected, and in most cases lesions are well-defined, wedge-shaped areas with their bases at the periphery and apexes toward the

renal sinus, with the renal parenchyma sometimes demonstrating a striated appearance. These abnormalities indicate hypoperfusion secondary to arteriolar vasoconstriction and inflammatory response (Fig. 11.3a, b).
- Abscessed areas, as fluid lesions delineated by a peripheral halo dilation of the collecting system (mild, moderate, marked) (Fig. 11.3c, d, e, f).

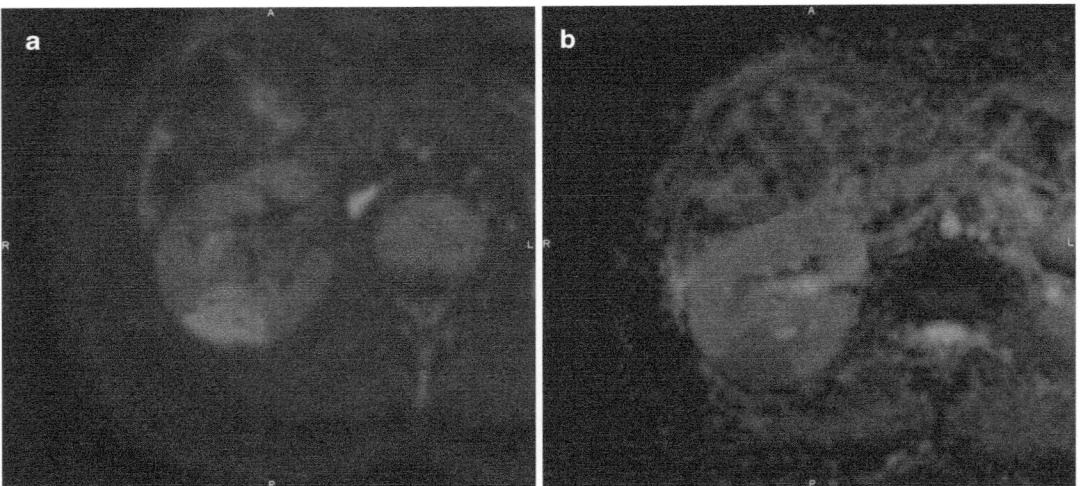

Fig. 11.2 (**a**) *Axial DWI SENSE* show wedge shaped corticomedullary focal hyperintensity. (**b**) *ADC map at high b value* show restricted ADC corresponding to DWI SENSE hyperintense lesion

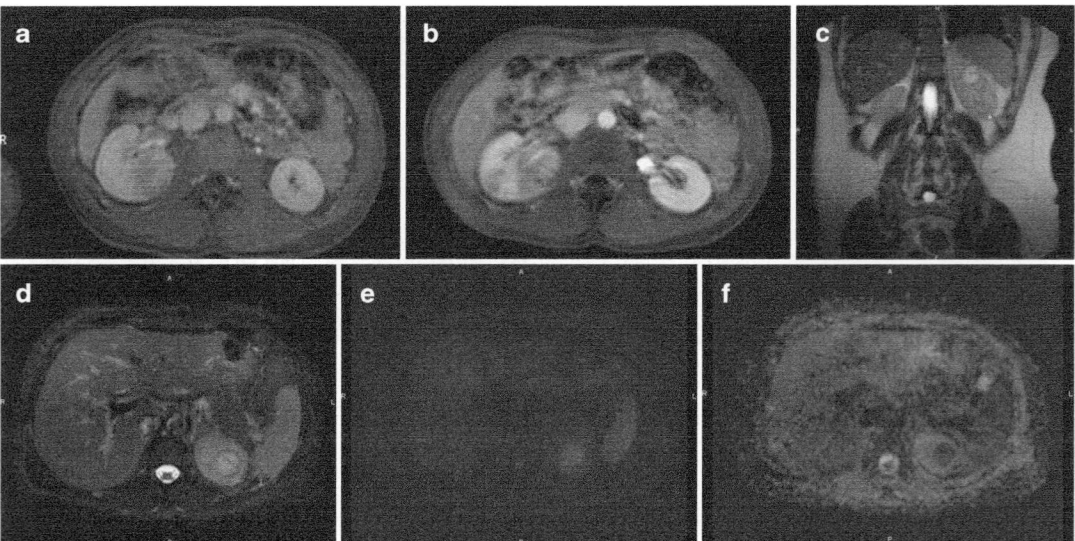

Fig. 11.3 (**a**) Axial 3D FFE T1w enhanced Dixon show reduction of parenchymal contrast enhancement in the affected wedge shaped area. (**b**) Axial 3D FFE T1w enhanced Dixon show multiple fluid filled lesion in the affected area consistent with microabscess. (**c, d**) Coronal TE_100 T2w SENSE and Axial SPAIR T2w show well defined superior left pole mass with intermediate T2w signal and thickened periferal wall, consistent in macroabscess. (**e, f**) Axial DWI (b800) show marked hyperintensity of the mass with clear restricted diffusion in ADC map

11.4 Role of MRI and DW-MRI in the Diagnostic Algorithm

APN is a topic that has remained relatively neglected in terms of imaging research, and its diagnosis is still a challenge. None of the clinical signs or laboratory biochemical markers at presentation allow discrimination between a few small lesions and multifocal or abscessed ones [15]. Thus, imaging techniques are needed to assess the severity of kidney involvement and to plan the antibiotic therapy. Diagnostic imaging plays a role in looking for previous occult structural or functional abnormalities that may require intervention, to assess those patients at significant risk of more life-threatening complications as in diabetic, elderly, or immunosuppressed patients, to balance the severity of the infection, and to evaluate the extent of organ damage subsequent to a resolved acute infection. Second-line imaging tests (CT or MRI) should be systematically used to define the presence, extent, and type of parenchymal lesions and to reveal complications (such as abscess or perirenal fluid collections), in order to tailor interventions to the specific clinical contexts [19, 20].

Our interest in APN originated from the observation of the increasing frequency of this disease and from the uncertain indications in the literature with regard to the opportunity to perform DW-MRI [21–25]. DWI provides information about the molecular translational motion of water, which can be affected by disease. This DW finding is probably secondary to compressive alterations due to edematous swelling and inflammatory parenchymal damage responsible for interstitial space reduction, with a resulting decrease in the diffusivity of water molecules. The degree of restricted diffusion is affected by various factors, including the type of pathogenic organism, the concentration of inflammatory cells and bacteria, the degree of viscosity, and the protein level [26–27]. ADC is a measure of the degree of molecular water motion. Lesions of high signal intensity on high-b-value images correspond to lesions of low signal intensity on the ADC map, and they represent restricted diffusion. Dealing with functional DW-MRI, in our series the mean ADC value was $2.38 \pm 0.14 \times 10^{-3}$ mm^2 s^{-1}, with a range of 1.99–2.76×10^{-3} mm^2 s^{-1}. In areas of affected parenchyma, ADC value in mm2/s was found to be consistently lower (mean 1.385; minimum 1.109, maximum 1.717) compared with healthy parenchyma (mean 2.383; minimum 1.989, maximum 2.763) (Fig. 4).

Comparing DW-MRI with gadolinium-enhanced (GE) MRI for diagnostic accuracy in APN in 163 patients with noncomplicated APN, we found DWI-MRI achieving 95.2% sensitivity, 94.9% specificity, a 96.9% positive predictive value, a 92.3% negative predictive value, and 94.6% accuracy.

Several other reports noted the utility of non-enhanced MRI, particularly DWI, in the diagnosis of APN. Kuniyoshi et al. used non-enhanced MRI with DWI to detect foci in children with APN, showing high-intensity lesions as well [28]. In another study, 39 children (mean age, 5.7 years) with suspected APN underwent MRI, including DWI and gadolinium-enhanced T1-weighted imaging (Gd-T1-WI). The sensitivity and specificity of the DWI were 100% (32/32) and 93.5% (43/46), respectively [29].

The high diagnostic agreement between DW-MRI and GE-MRI provided an interesting starting point for gaining a new perspective on the diagnostic management of APN. In fact, DW-MRI of the kidney seems to be a feasible, rapid, and reliable method as quantification of ADC values can be useful in diagnosing noncomplicated APN. The high diagnostic agreement between GE-MRI and DW-MRI offers new perspectives in diagnostic management, enabling monitoring of APN in a short time without use of ionizing radiation or administration of paramagnetic contrast medium. We can assume the use of DW-MRI, together with the performance of the usual basal sequences T1 and T2, in the acute phase, possibly in the ED, affecting minimally (negligible time is required) the workflow of the MRI service, thus allowing a timely therapeutic approach.

Thereafter, in case of hospitalization, an exam with paramagnetic contrast as first examination

Table 11.3 Diagnostic algorithm of acute pyelonephritis

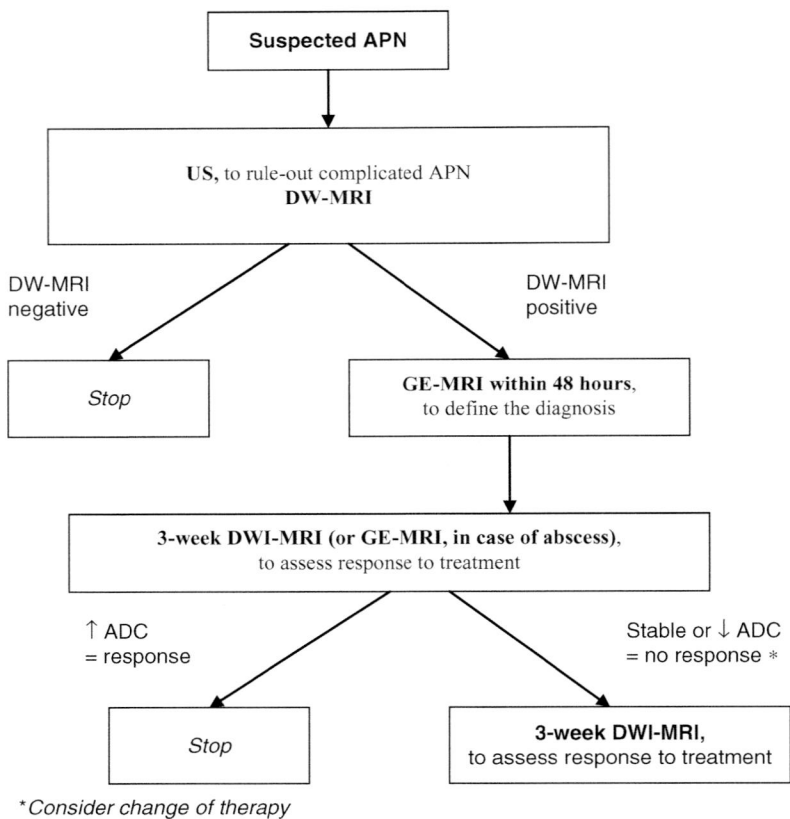

*Consider change of therapy

should be systematically used to better define the presence, extent, and type of parenchymal lesions and to reveal complications (such as abscess or perirenal fluid collections), in order to tailor interventions to the specific clinical contexts [19, 20].

The subsequent checks, performed about every 3 weeks until complete resolution of the inflammatory process, may instead be programmed with DWI alone (Table 11.3).

Additionally, DW-MRI is an alternative to dynamic investigation in all cases where there are contraindications to administration of iodinated and/or paramagnetic contrast medium, such as those patients with renal insufficiency and pregnant or lactating women. Actually, the short duration of the examination and the easy response and reproducibility of ADC values allow a proper diagnostic evaluation even in uncooperative sub-

jects or slightly sedated claustrophobic ones. Dealing with costs too, DW-MRI is an interesting tool for detecting noncomplicated APN, thanks to its inherent cost and its potential impact on the suitability and timeliness of treatment.

References

1. Craig WD, Brent JW, Travis MD (2008) From the archives of the AFIP, pyelonephritis: radiologic-pathologic review. Radiographics 28:255–276
2. Schappert SM, Rechtsteiner EA (2011) Ambulatory medical care utilization estimates for 2007. Vital Health Stat 13(169):1–38
3. Hooton TM, Stamm WE (1997) Diagnosis and treatment of uncomplicated urinary tract infection. Infect Dis Clin N Am 11:551–581
4. Ramakrishnan K, Schedi DC (2005) Diagnosis and management of acute pyelonephritis in adults. Am Fam Physician 71:933–942

5. Georgi A, Reddy YNV, Gautam G (2012) Diagnosis of acute pyelonephritis with recent trends in management. Nephrol Dial Transplant 27:3391–3394
6. Ramzan MM, Sandstrom CK (2016) Core curriculum illustration: acute pyelonephritis. Emerg Radiol:1–3. https://doi.org/10.1007/s10140-016-1474-2
7. Medical Research Council Bacteriuria Committee (1979) Recommended terminology of urinary tract infection: a report by the members of Medical Research Council Bacteriuria committee. Br Med J 2:717–719
8. Talner LB, Davidson AJ, Lebowitz RL, Dalla Palma L, Goldman SM (1994) Acute pyelonephritis: can we agree on terminology? Radiology 192:297–305
9. Dyer RB (1997) CT of renal inflammatory disease. Invited commentary. Radiographics 17:867–868
10. De Pascale A, Piccoli GB, Priola SM et al (2013) Diffusion-weighted magnetic resonance imaging: new perspectives in the diagnostic pathway of non-complicated acute pyelonephritis. Eur Radiol 23(11):3077–3086. https://doi.org/10.1007/s00330-013-2906-y
11. Soulen MC, Fishman EK, Goldman SM, Gatewood OM (1989) Sequelae of acute renal infection: CT evaluation. Radiology 173:423–426
12. Webb JAW (1987) The role of imaging in adult acute urinary tract infection. Eur Radiol 7:837–843
13. Parenti GC, Passari A (2001) Pielonefrite acuta: ruolo della diagnostica per immagini. Radiol Med 101:251–254
14. Majd M, Nussbaum Blask AR, Markle BM et al (2001) Acute pyelonephritis: comparison of diagnosis with 99mTc-DMSA, SPECT, spiral CT, MR imaging, and power Doppler US in an experimental pig model. Radiology 218:101–108. Diffusion-weighted magnetic resonance imaging: new perspectives in the diagnostic pathway of non-complicated acute pyelonephritis
15. Piccoli GB, Consiglio V, Deagostini MC et al (2011) The clinical and imaging presentation of acute "non complicated" pyelonephritis, a new profile for an ancient disease. BMC Nephrol 12:68–78
16. Martina MC, Campanino PP, Caraffo F et al (2010) Dynamic magnetic resonance imaging in acute pyelonephritis. Radiol Med 115:287–300
17. Nikken JJ, Krestin GP (2007) MRI of the kidney: state of the art. Eur Radiol 17:2780–2793
18. Hagmann P, Jonasson L, Maeder P, Thiran JP, Wedeen VJ, Meuli R (2006) Understanding diffusion MR imaging technique. Radiographics 26:S205–S223
19. Kawashima A, Sandler CM, Goldman SM (2000) Imaging in acute renal infection. BJU Int 86:70–79
20. Johansen TE (2004) The role of imaging in urinary tract infections. World J Urol 22:392–398
21. Muller MF, Prasad PV, Bimmler D, Kaiser A, Edelman RR (1994) Functional imaging of the kidney by means of measurement of the apparent diffusion coefficient. Radiology 193:711–715
22. Chow LC, Bammer R, Moseley ME, Sommer FG (2003) Single breath-hold diffusion-weighted imaging of the abdomen. J Magn Reson Imaging 18:377–382
23. Thoeny HC, De Keyzer F, Oyen RH, Peeters RR (2005) Diffusionweighted MR imaging of kidneys in healthy volunteers and patients with parenchymal diseases: initial experience. Radiology 235:911–917
24. Xu Y, Wang X, Jiang X (2007) Relationship between the renal apparent diffusion coefficient and glomerular filtration rate: preliminary experience. J Magn Reson Imaging 26:678–681
25. Carbone SF, Gaggioli E, Ricci V, Mazzei F, Mazzei MA, Volterrani L (2007) Diffusion-weighted magnetic resonance imaging in the evaluation of renal function: a preliminary study. Radiol Med 112:1201–1210
26. Fanning NF, Laffan EE, Shroff MM (2006) Serial diffusion-weighted MRI correlates with clinical course and treatment response in children with intracranial pus collections. Pediatr Radiol 36:26–37
27. Acyagi J, Odaka J, Kuroiwa Y, Nakashima N, Ito T, Sato T, Kanai T, Yamagata T, Momoi MY (2014) Utility of non-enhanced magnetic resonance imaging to detect acute pyelonephritis. Pediatr Int 56(3):e4–e6. https://doi.org/10.1111/ped.12312
28. Kuniyoshi Y, Kamura A, Yasuda A, Tashiro M (2011) Acute pyelonephritis diagnosed by diffusion-weighted whole body imaging with background signal suppression: three case reports. J Jpn Pediatr Soc 115:1919–1925
29. Vivier P-H et al (2014) MRI and suspected acute pyelonephritis in children: comparison of diffusion-weighted imaging with gadolinium-enhanced T1-weighted imaging. Eur Radiol 24:19–25

Cross-Sectional Imaging of Renal Cyst Infection

12

Massimo Tonolini

12.1 Background

Simple renal cysts (RCs) represent a common incidental finding on imaging studies performed for unrelated reasons in adult and elderly people. Nowadays, most radiologists increasingly do not report small- and moderate-sized sporadic RCs with characteristic sonographic, CT or MRI appearance as they do not require further investigation, follow-up or treatment.

On the other hand, multicystic renal disorders exist, either congenital or acquired. Autosomal dominant polycystic kidney disease (ADPKD) is the commonest inherited renal disorder, is found in 1:400–1:1000 individuals in white populations, results from progressive development of RCs originating from collecting ducts and nephrons and may have associated liver cysts and abnormalities in other organ systems. ADPKD causes progressive enlargement of the kidneys and development of hypertension and ultimately leads to decreased function in more than 70% of cases, thus accounting for 10–15% of all patients on renal replacement therapy. Acquired cystic kidney disease (ACKD) refers to the progressive, secondary development of multiple RCs in patients with chronic renal failure from different, primarily non-cystic kidney disorders, which is

reported to occur in 50 and 90% of patients after 3–5 years and 5–10 years of dialysis, respectively [1, 2].

Renal enlargement from multiple RCs commonly causes chronic flank discomfort or pain. Furthermore, serious complications such as cyst haemorrhage, rupture and infection sometimes occur in patients with hereditary or acquired polycystic renal disorders and occasionally in those with large and/or multiple sporadic RCs [3].

12.2 Clinical Features and Diagnosis of Renal Cyst Infection

Renal cyst infection (RCI) may result from ascending urinary tract infection or, more rarely, from haematogenous dissemination. In the general population, RCI is considered exceptional, although in our experience it may be encountered in patients with pre-existing sporadic RCs during bacteraemia. Conversely, in patients with inherited multicystic disorders, RCI reaches an annual incidence of approximately 0.01 episodes/patient, with age, female gender and recent urinary tract instrumentation as risk factors. It has been estimated that at least 30% of patients with ADPKD experience at least one infectious episode during their lifetime and that RCI is responsible for 15% of all hospitalisations in people with ADPKD [3–5].

M. Tonolini, M.D.
Radiology Department, "Luigi Sacco" University
Hospital, Via G.B. Grassi 74, Milan 20157, Italy
e-mail: mtonolini@sirm.org

© Springer International Publishing AG 2018
M. Tonolini (ed.), *Imaging and Intervention in Urinary Tract Infections and Urosepsis*,
https://doi.org/10.1007/978-3-319-68276-1_12

Most usually, RCI manifests acutely with fever, lumbar pain and flank tenderness and elevated serum inflammatory markers such as leukocytes and C-reactive protein (CRP). Alternatively, imaging findings suggestive of RCI may be unexpectedly encountered in patients with urinary or unexplained sepsis. In either case, RCI usually represents a potentially life-threatening situation which requires aggressive treatment including percutaneous or surgical drainage to eradicate infection [3–5].

The only specific and gold standard criterion for diagnosing RCI is represented by cyst aspiration yielding bacteria and neutrophils, but is commonly not performed unless when percutaneous drainage is felt indispensable. Urine and blood cultures are frequently negative, even in confirmed cases. In the majority of situations, the diagnosis is challenging and relies on consistent clinical and laboratory features plus imaging exclusion of cystic bleeding [3–5].

12.3   Cross-Sectional Imaging of Renal Cyst Infection

When assessing patients with urosepsis or suspected renal infection, radiologists should thoroughly search for abnormalities of the characteristic, well-known appearance of uncomplicated RCs. The latter appear anechoic with posterior through transmission at ultrasound, homogeneous with water-like CT attenuation and markedly T1-hypointense and T2-hyperintense MRI signal intensity. Suspicious features such as mural thickening or irregularities, calcifications or peripheral or septal contrast enhancement should be absent [6–8].

The diagnosis of RCI should be suggested when faced with size increase or changed mural or intraluminal features of a benign cyst known from previous imaging or reports. Sonographically, infected cysts show highly variable echogenicity, often resulting in complex collections with through transmission, and are thus unreliably differentiated from haematomas and tumours. In our experience, in most cases the diagnosis of RCI is made during CT, which represents the mainstay technique to comprehensively investigate patients with suspected renal

or systemic infection. In this setting, enhancement by intravenous contrast medium (CM) is generally warranted unless contraindicated. However, particularly in patients with ADPKD and ACKD, the degree of renal function should be carefully assessed, and the potential benefits of a comprehensive CM-enhanced CT examination should be weighed against the concern for CM-induced nephrotoxicity. As most European radiologists do, we strongly suggest to follow the indications found in the most recent European Society of Urogenital Radiology (ESUR) guidelines [3, 4, 9].

At CT, infected renal cysts are depicted as uni- or multilocular hypoattenuating renal collections with an enhancing peripheral rim of variable thickness (Figs. 12.1 and 12.2). Indeed, RCI are indistinguishable from renal abscesses resulting from other mechanisms including haematogenous spread, extension from extra-urinary inflammation and ascending urinary infection. A possible diagnostic pitfall is represented by misinterpretation of compressed functioning renal parenchyma as an abnormal 'rim' enhancement surrounding a fluid collection. Although exceptional, the presence of gas is highly specific for bacterial infection. Furthermore, renal abscesses may variably extend into the perirenal and sometimes even pararenal spaces [3, 10–13].

In this setting, the aims of cross-sectional imaging include:

(a) To exclude cystic haemorrhage
(b) To differentiate RCI from parenchymal infection (acute pyelonephritis)
(c) To identify pyocysts within polycystic kidneys
(d) To detect hydronephrosis and infected pyonephrosis, which require emergency urinary drainage

However, according to some authors, CT allows a confident diagnosis of RCI in only a minority (less than 20%) of cases, and unremarkable findings are observed in approximately one-half of patients with consistent clinical and laboratory features [4].

Although its accuracy has not been precisely quantified, MRI probably offers supe-

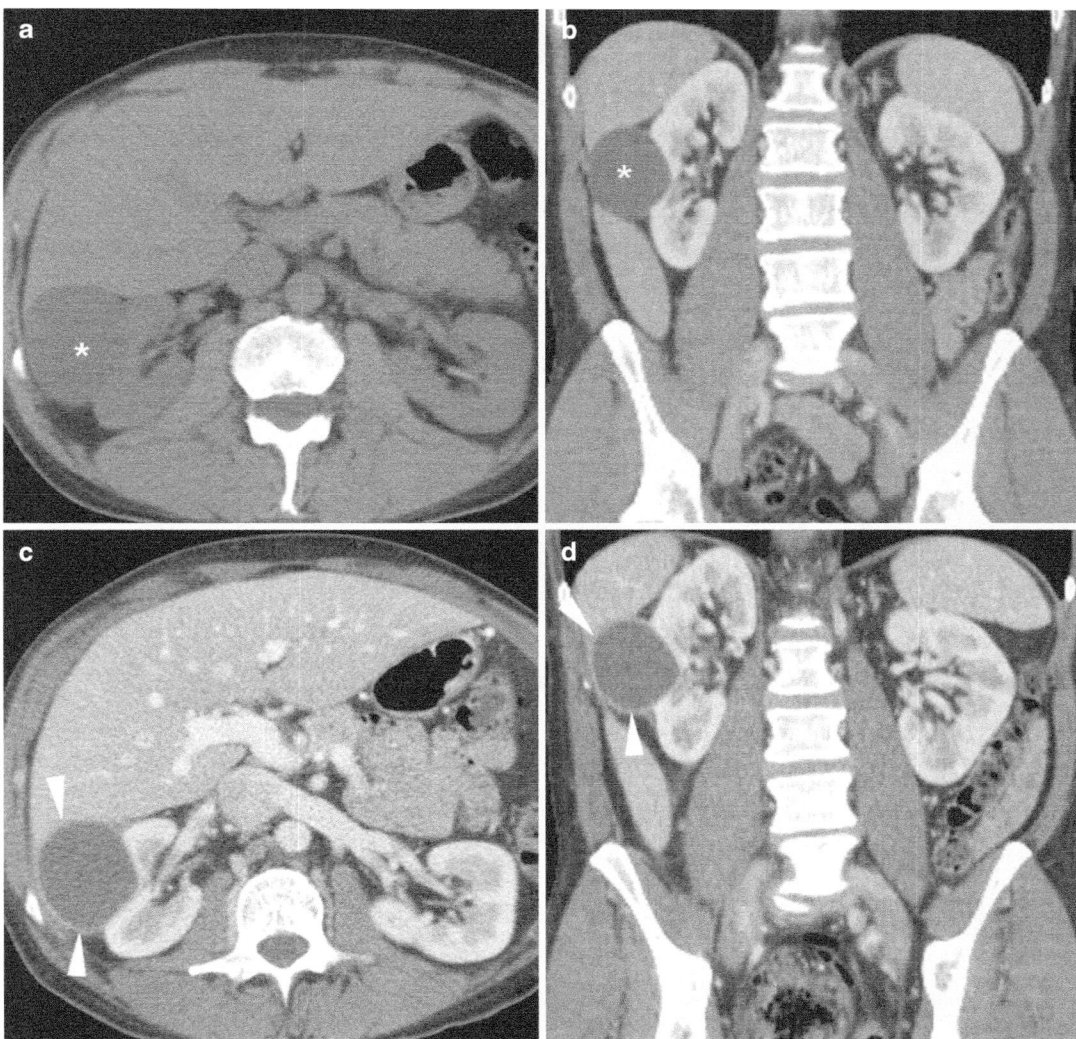

Fig. 12.1 Unenhanced (**a**) and portal-venous phase contrast-enhanced (**b**) CT study previously performed for reasons unrelated to the urinary tract in a 39-year-old female depicted a 4-cm, predominantly exophytic simple cyst (*) at the middle third of the right kidney, with characteristic features including round shape, well-demarcated contour, homogeneous fluid attenuation and absence of enhancing walls or septa. More than 2 years later, the patient suffered from right abdominal and flank pain: in the emergency department, clinical and laboratory features were consistent with a diagnosis of acute pyelonephritis. She had no significant predisposing factors for a complicated urinary tract infection. Compared to the previous study, repeated contrast-enhanced CT (**c, d**) showed the known renal cyst with unchanged size and shape, and with appearance of a thin, enhancing peripheral rim (*arrowheads*). In absence of CT signs of renal parenchymal infection, superinfected cyst from probable ascending infection was diagnosed and successfully treated with intravenous antibiotics

rior diagnostic capability compared to CT in the diagnosis of RCI. Renal abscesses are consistently depicted at MRI as T1-hypointense, heterogeneously T2-hyperintense collections, with characteristic thickened and enhancing walls and septa (Fig. 12.3) [3, 10, 11]. Furthermore, the implementation of diffusion-weighted imaging (DWI) may improve differentiation of infected from uncomplicated cysts on the basis of abnormal DWI signal intensity

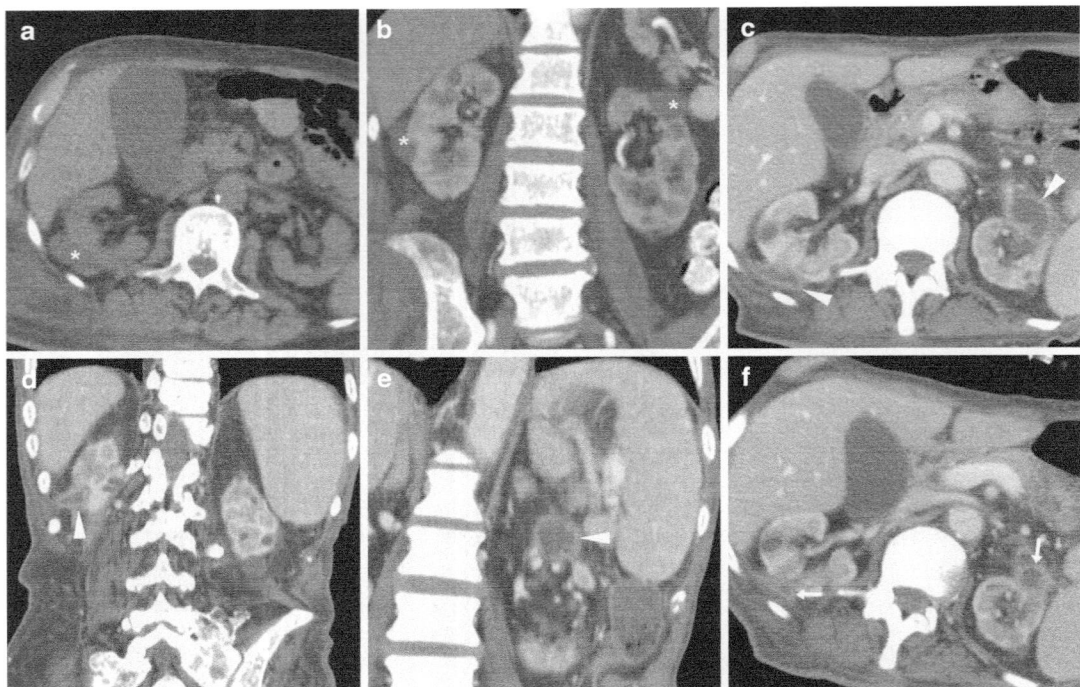

Fig. 12.2 A 79-year-old male with comorbidities including ischemic cardiomyopathy and chronic kidney disease had a few non-enhancing renal cysts (*), as previously depicted during aortic CT angiography (an unenhanced scan, **b** arterial phase acquisition). Months later, during hospitalisation for unexplained septic fever, contrast-enhanced CT (**c–e**) showed development of abscess-like collections with enhancing periphery (*arrowheads*) in the same site of the dominant cysts of each kidney. Follow-up CT after intravenous antibiotics (**e**) showed decreased size of the infected cysts (*arrows*)

and decreased apparent diffusion coefficient (ADC) values: in fact the non-enhancing purulent content made up of inflammatory exudate, bacteria and necrosis shows marked diffusion restriction (Fig. 12.3) [14, 15].

More recently, as further discussed in the following chapter of this book, (18)-fluorodeoxyglucose positron-emission computed tomography (18F-FDG PET/CT) has been increasingly reported as the most reliable modality to diagnose RCI [4, 16].

12.4 Differential Diagnosis of Renal Cyst Infection

Clinically, in patients with known cystic renal disorders, particularly if hereditary or extensive, the sudden onset of flank pain mostly suggests cystic

haemorrhage or renal colic from coexistent urolithiasis. The majority (approximately 80%) of patients with ADPKD experience acute flank pain at least once during their lifetime. Although its true incidence is unknown, cyst bleeding is more common than RCI and may be further complicated by rupture with pericystic and/or retroperitoneal haemorrhage. Spontaneous renal bleeding typically presents with acute lumbar or abdominal pain, signs of haemodynamic impairment and laboratory evidence of blood loss palpable mass and hypovolemic shock, which warrant immediate investigation. Alternatively, manifestations may be nonspecific with variable degrees of haemodynamic compromise [3, 17, 18].

To the radiologist's eye, the hallmark of recent haemorrhage is represented by the identification of high-attenuation effusion (in the range 40–90 Hounsfield units, HU) blood compared to

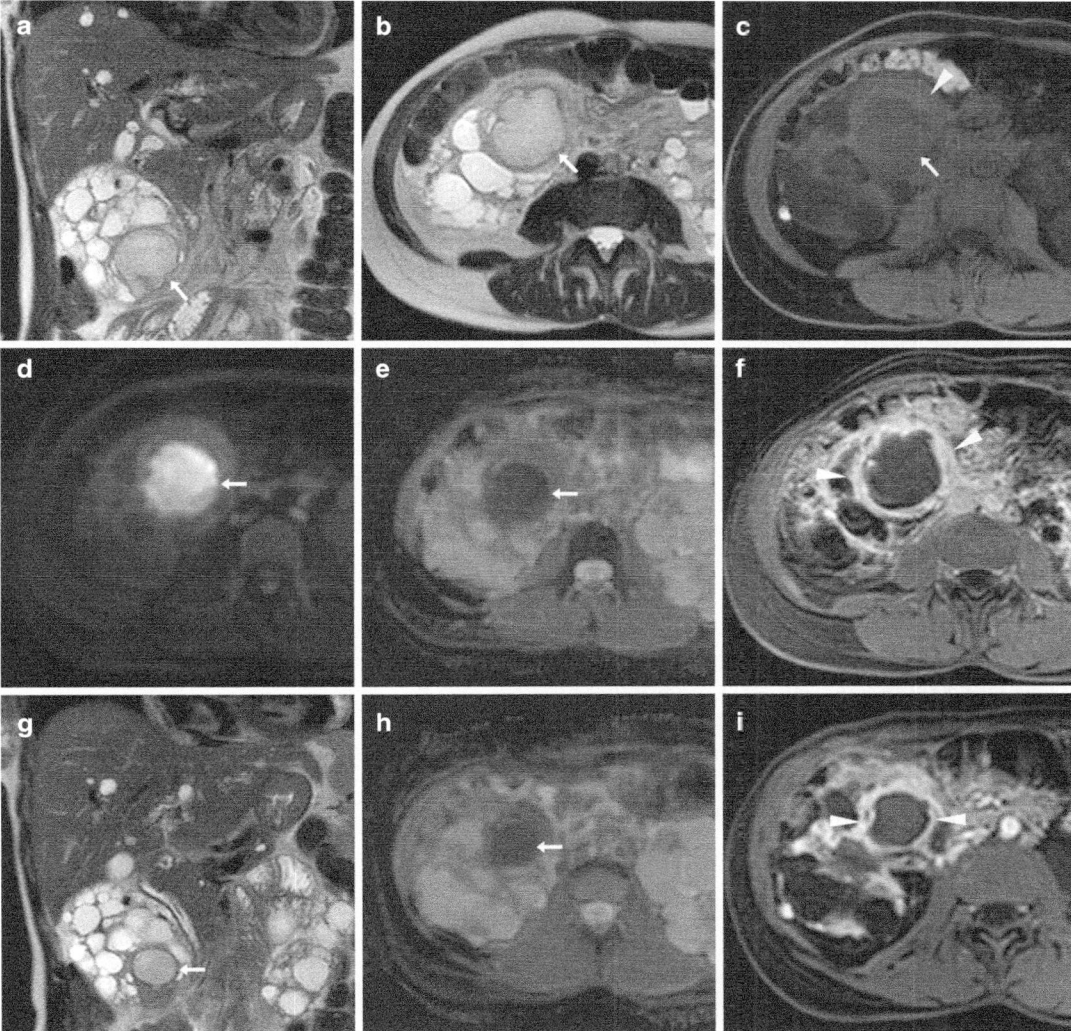

Fig. 12.3 A 47-year-old female with polycystic kidney suffered from lumbar pain, pyuria and persistent fever despite empiric antibiotic therapies. Initial MRI (**a–f**) showed a 6-cm lower right pole cyst (arrows) with heterogeneously abnormal signal intensity compared to the other fluid cysts on both T2- (**a, b**) and precontrast T1-weighted (**c**) acquisitions, marked hyperintensity on high b-value (800 s/mm^2) diffusion-weighted imaging (DWI, **d**) and visually low apparent diffusion coefficient (ADC, **e**) indicating restricted diffusion, and thickened wall (arrowheads) with strong enhancement after gadolinium contrast (**f**). Cyst superinfection was confirmed and treated with percutaneous aspiration. Follow-up MRI (**g–i**) showed decreased size (3 cm) of the infected cyst (arrows) with unchanged signal intensity (**g**) and restricted diffusion (**h**), reduced thickness of enhancing wall (arrowheads in **i**).

the renal parenchyma on precontrast CT acquisition, sometimes with an internal fluid-fluid level. CT has absolute sensitivity for detection of subcapsular and perinephric haematomas. However, the identification of collections with more or less heterogeneous, hyperattenuating internal 'debris' is confusing and does not allow confident differentiation between blood and pus. The role of ultrasound is limited by the unreliable differentiation of clotted blood from dense pus and from solid tissue. Conversely, MRI reliably detects recent blood with high T1 signal intensity accompanied by variable signal changes on T2-weighted sequences corresponding to haemoglobin degradation products [3, 17–19].

Infectious inflammatory masses with or without perirenal extension often appear as complex indeterminate (Bosniak category III) cystic lesions. Furthermore, misinterpretation of abscesses ad necrotic or cystic tumours is not uncommon, particularly because of the concern for increased incidence of renal cell carcinoma (RCC) in patients with ADPKD and ACKD. When confronted with a heterogeneously enhancing lesion, helpful clinical discriminating features include:

(a) The acute clinical context
(b) Laboratory changes consistent with infection
(c) History of benign cyst in the same location
(d) Coexistent imaging signs of acute infectious pyelitis or pyelonephritis

At CT or MRI imaging, abscess is favoured over tumour by the identification of perirenal fat inflammatory stranding and thickened Gerota's fascia and by markedly restricted diffusion (similar to brain abscesses) compared to areas of cystic degeneration within RCC [2, 3, 7, 8].

References

1. Thomsen HS, Levine E, Meilstrup JW et al (1997) Renal cystic diseases. Eur Radiol 7:1267–1275
2. Degrassi F, Quaia E, Martingano P et al (2015) Imaging of haemodialysis: renal and extrarenal findings. Insights Imaging 6(3):309–321
3. Tonolini M, Rigiroli F, Villa F et al (2014) Complications of sporadic, hereditary, and acquired renal cysts: cross-sectional imaging findings. Curr Probl Diagn Radiol 43:80–90
4. Jouret F, Lhommel R, Devuyst O et al (2012) Diagnosis of cyst infection in patients with autosomal dominant polycystic kidney disease: attributes and limitations of the current modalities. Nephrol Dial Transplant 27:3746–3751
5. Migali G, Annet L, Lonneux M et al (2008) Renal cyst infection in autosomal dominant polycystic kidney disease. Nephrol Dial Transplant 23:404–405
6. Israel GM, Bosniak MA (2004) MR imaging of cystic renal masses. Magn Reson Imaging Clin N Am 12:403–412
7. Israel GM, Bosniak MA (2008) Pitfalls in renal mass evaluation and how to avoid them. Radiographics 28:1325–1338
8. Hindman N (2016) Cystic renal masses. Abdom Radiol 41:1020–1034
9. European Society of Urogenital Radiology (2016) ESUR guidelines on contrast media 9.0. Available at: "www.esur.org/guidelines"
10. Craig WD, Wagner BJ, Travis MD (2008) Pyelonephritis: radiologic-pathologic review. Radiographics 28:255–277. quiz 327-258
11. Demertzis J, Menias CO (2007) State of the art: imaging of renal infections. Emerg Radiol 14:13–22
12. Stunell H, Buckley O, Feeney J et al (2007) Imaging of acute pyelonephritis in the adult. Eur Radiol 17:1820–1828
13. Erkoc R, Sayarlioglu H, Ceylan K et al (2006) Gas-forming infection in a renal cyst of a patient with autosomal dominant polycystic kidney disease. Nephrol Dial Transplant 21:555–556
14. Kita Y, Soda T, Terai A (2009) Diagnosis and localization of infected renal cyst by diffusion-weighted magnetic resonance imaging in polycystic kidney disease. Int J Urol 16:918–919
15. Goyal A, Sharma R, Bhalla AS et al (2013) Diffusion-weighted MRI in inflammatory renal lesions: all that glitters is not RCC! Eur Radiol 23:272–279
16. Lantinga MA, Drenth JP, Gevers TJ (2015) Diagnostic criteria in renal and hepatic cyst infection. Nephrol Dial Transplant 30:744–751
17. Diaz JR, Agriantonis DJ, Aguila J et al (2011) Spontaneous perirenal hemorrhage: what radiologists need to know. Emerg Radiol 18:329–334
18. Tonolini M, Ierardi AM, Carrafiello G (2015) Letter to the editor: spontaneous renal haemorrhage in end-stage renal disease. Insights Imaging 6:693–695
19. Chicoskie C, Chaoui A, Kuligowska E et al (2001) MRI isolation of infected renal cyst in autosomal dominant polycystic kidney disease. Clin Imaging 25:114–117

Nuclear Medicine in the Management of Patient with Kidneys Intracystic Infection

13

Daniele Penna, Vincenzo Militano,
Vincenzo Arena, Angelina Cistaro,
and Ettore Pelosi

13.1 Introduction

Infections, abscesses, and other inflammatory process are a major concern to the clinician and to the patient. Inflammatory imaging requires a multidisciplinary approach to accurately diagnose, stage, and follow up infectious processes. Inflammation acts as the initial host defense against invasive pathogens and other inciting stimulus. It plays an important role in tissue repair and elimination of harmful pathogens. Although the inflammatory response is essential for host defense, it is very much a double-edged sword. Inappropriate inflammatory reaction or delay in the resolution of inflammation will damage adjacent normal cells in the tissue.

Timely diagnosis and localization of infection is a critical step in the appropriate clinical management of this group of diseases. Radiological imaging modalities such as computed tomography (CT), magnetic resonance imaging (MRI), and ultrasonography (US) are all being currently used for the evaluation of infection. These imaging techniques are, however, based on morphological changes and are therefore of limited value in the early stage of the infectious process, which may show only insignificant structural infection-related tissue mocifications or none at all.

Nuclear medicine plays an important role in the evaluation of infection. Scintigraphic tests are excellent noninvasive modalities of whole-body scanning that allow diagnosis of infectious foci and assessment cf the extent of disease in any part of the body. Nuclear medicine procedures have been the tool of choice for assessment of musculoskeletal infections such as osteomyelitis, infected prosthetic joint implants, and diabetic foot. These functional imaging modalities are also used for the evaluation of patients presenting with fever of unknown origin. Infection-seeking radiotracers are used for diagnosis and localization of suspected abdominal abscesses, vascular graft infection, and pulmonary infection [1].

Nuclear medicine provides unique information on pathophysiological and patho-biochemical processes—as opposed to other imaging procedures such as CT, MRI, and US, which supply high-resolution data cn morphological changes that take place as a result of a specific disease. Because they provide a different type of information, scintigraphic and anatomical imaging modalities play a complementary role in many clinical settings,

D. Penna • V. Arena (✉) • A. Cistaro • E. Pelosi
PET/CT Center, Affidea IRMET, Torino, Italy
e-mail: daniele.penna@affidea.it;
vincenzo.arena@affidea.it;
angelina.cistaro@affidea.it;
ettore.pelosi@affidea.it

V. Militano
Nuclear Medicine Department, Central Manchester University Hospitals Foundation Trust,
Manchester, UK
e-mail: vinmilitano@gmail.com

© Springer International Publishing AG 2018
M. Tonolini (ed.), *Imaging and Intervention in Urinary Tract Infections and Urosepsis*,
https://doi.org/10.1007/978-3-319-68276-1_13

including the assessment and management of patients with infectious processes.

13.1.1 Devices

13.1.1.1 Gamma Camera

The vast majority of all clinical nuclear medicine studies are based on the imaging of the internal distribution of one or more radiopharmaceuticals with a gamma camera. The term gamma camera refers to a device that can image the distribution of a gamma-emitting radionuclide.

For many years, nuclear medicine procedures have been performed using a gamma camera. Originally, multiple planar projections were acquired to provide diagnostic information, but, more recently, the techniques of SPECT (Single Photon Emission Computed Tomography) have been utilized. Conventional planar images generally suffered from poor contrast due to the presence of overlying and underlying activity that interferes with imaging of the region of interest. The resulting planar image is low in contrast due to the effect of the superposition of depth information.

This effect can be reduced by collecting images from multiple positions around the distribution and producing an image of a transverse slice through the distribution.

The resulting tomographic image is of higher contrast than the planar image due to the elimination of contributions of activity above and below the region of interest. This is the goal of SPECT to provide images of slices of radionuclide distributions with image contrast that is higher than that provided by conventional techniques. Currently with the new hybrid tomograph, SPECT/CT images could be performed with a more accurate localization.

13.1.1.2 PET/CT

Positron emission tomography (PET) is a nuclear medicine functional imaging technique that is used to observe metabolic processes in the body. The system detects pairs of gamma rays emitted indirectly by a positron-emitting radionuclide (tracer), which is introduced into the body on a biologically active molecule. Three-dimensional

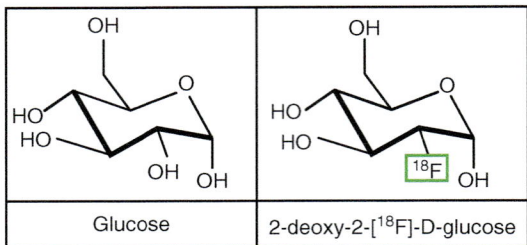

Fig. 13.1 Difference between glucose and FDG

images of tracer concentration within the body are then constructed by computer analysis. In modern PET/CT scanners (Fig. 13.1), three-dimensional imaging is often accomplished with the aid of a CT performed on the patient during the same session, in the same machine [2]. Currently, it is principally used for oncology purpose (almost 90% of the scan), but there is a continuous rise of the use in the field of neurology, cardiology, and infectious disease. It is clear that the different types of tests that we can do with the PET depend on the type of tracer rather than from the tomograph; it follows that the variation of the tracer will change the function studied. However there are tracers which have a major versatility, compared to others, and can be used for different purpose.

13.1.2 Tracers

The detection and localization of inflammation and infection with nuclear medicine techniques has been studied using different methods of conventional nuclear medicine since the 1970s. The ideal characteristics of an infection-imaging radiopharmaceutical are well synthesized in Table 13.1.

Currently there are several SPECT and PET tracers in general use. The common tracers are being gallium-67 (67Ga)-, indium-111 (111In)-, and 99mTechnetium (99mTc)-labeled white blood cells (WBCs), labeled antigranulocyte antibody (LeukoScan), and fluorine-18-fluorodeoxyglucose (18F-FDG). The sensitivity and specificity of these tracers depend on the clinical scenario and the organ involved.

Table 13.1 Inflammation tracer caracteristics

Ideal characteristics of an infection-imaging radiopharmaceutical
– High sensitivity and specificity
– Differentiates infection and inflammation
– Differentiates acute and chronic infection
– Rapid clearance from circulation/background
– No significant normal uptake in liver, spleen, intestine, bone, bone marrow, kidneys, and muscle
– Easy to prepare, low cost, and easily available
– No toxicity and free of immune reaction

13.1.2.1 ^{67}Ga-Citrate

^{67}Ga-citrate (Ga) has been used for imaging infection for almost four decades, since its discovery in the early 1970s [3]. Ga was used for the investigation of fever of unknown origin, acute or chronic osteomyelitis, and the diagnosis of infections in immunocompromised patients. Although Ga scintigraphy shows high sensitivity in detection of both acute and chronic infections, it has several drawbacks that limit its clinical application. Its specificity is relatively low because of early physiologic excretion through the urinary system and delayed excretion through the bowel and because of the normal biodistribution to the liver. Ga is a bone-seeking tracer, accumulating in areas of bone remodeling. It is also a tumor-seeking agent, accumulating in such tumors as lymphoma or hepatoma. Physiological hepatic, bowel, and renal uptake can either mimic or mask foci of infection localized inside or in the vicinity of these organs. Optimal Ga imaging may therefore require delayed imaging of up to a few days after injection, a disadvantage when diagnosing acute infectious processes that may require rapid therapeutic interventions [3, 4].

13.1.2.2 Radiolabeled Leukocytes

Labeled WBC imaging using either 99mTc or 111In has been shown to perform excellently in detecting acute and chronic infections. This test has become the nuclear medicine modality of choice in a variety of clinical settings when the suspicion of an infectious process exists. Clinical indications for labeled leukocytes scintigraphy include osteomyelitis, especially in cases where infected joint prosthesis or posttraumatic osteomyelitis is suspected.

Scintigraphic assessment, however, lacks anatomical landmarks, rendering the topographic localization of sites of abnormal tracer uptake difficult. In this clinical setting, the precise localization achieved with SPECT/CT in a single imaging step and with greater diagnostic accuracy may provide a tool for guiding invasive tissue sampling procedures and further treatment planning.

A study aimed at investigating the potential advantage of 111In-labeled WBC-SPECT/CT compared with SPECT alone evaluated 14 patients with various sites of suspected infection. The authors concluded that SPECT/CT improved the accuracy of anatomic localization of foci of abnormal WBC uptake and led to modification in clinical management [5].

13.1.2.3 Labeled Antigranulocyte Antibodies

The preparation of radiolabeled leukocytes is laborious, requires specialized staff and dedicated expensive equipment, and can be hazardous because of blood-product handling.

The advantages of radioimmunoscintigraphy over techniques involving labeled autologous leukocytes for imaging infection have to do mainly with the simplicity of its use due to the fact that there is no need for blood-product handling. Indications for labeled antigranulocyte antibody scintigraphy include the suspicion of osteomyelitis, fever of unknown origin, abdominal infections, and vascular graft infections [6–8].

Correlation of results from this scintigraphic technique to anatomical imaging modalities is considered mandatory for accurate diagnosis. False-positive studies may be the result of increased vascular permeability. Increased uptake of labeled antibodies has been observed in perivascular hematomas and contusions, especially in the delayed phase images obtained 24 h after injection. With the additional anatomical information it provides, SPECT/CT can be of value in excluding or confirming the presence of a hematoma as the cause of abnormal tracer uptake. Similar to the performance capabilities of other nuclear medicine procedures, the precise localization of the infected site may be difficult on scintigraphy alone. A study investigating the value of SPECT/CT in chronic osteomyelitis assessed 27 patients with 29 sites of suspected bone infection and compared planar and SPECT/CT imaging after injection of 99mTc-labeled antigranulocyte antibodies [9]. SPECT/CT was able to correctly localize all positive foci detected on planar and SPECT images. SPECT/CT also allowed the differential diagnosis of soft tissue infection, septic arthritis, and osteomyelitis. Furthermore, following the diagnosis of bone involvement, hybrid imaging was also able to differentiate between cortical, corticomedullar, and subperiosteal foci of disease involvement. The authors concluded that combined SPECT/CT imaging improves the accuracy of radioimmunoscintigraphy for diagnosis of soft tissue infection and osteomyelitis [9].

13.1.2.4 FDG

Fluorodeoxyglucose (FDG) is currently mainly used in oncology, neurology, and cardiology and in the study of infectious and inflammatory disease.

FDG has been approved by US Food and Drug Administration (FDA) and European Medicines Agency (EMEA) and authorized as a diagnostic radiopharmaceutical in the diagnosis of infection. Fluorine-18 (18F) is a cyclotron-produced radioisotope with a half-life of 109.7 min that undergoes positron decay. [^{18}F]FDG is an analogue of glucose, whereby the 2-carbon hydroxyl group of glucose is substituted with a fluorine atom (Fig. 13.1).

Like glucose, [^{18}F]FDG is taken up by cells via the glucose transporter (GLUT1) and phosphorylated by hexokinase II (HKII) to form [^{18}F]FDG-6-PO$_4$; however, unlike glucose, further metabolism is prevented due to the absence of the required 2-carbon hydroxyl, and hence [^{18}F]FDG remains trapped within the cell (Fig. 13.2). [^{18}F]FDG-6-PO$_4$ accumulates in cells over time, leading to signal amplification and making this imaging agent a suitable indicator of hexokinase II activity as well as a cell's need for glucose [10].

FDG rapidly accumulates at the sites of infection and inflammation with high target-to-background ratio. The mechanism of FDG localization in infection is that cells involved in infection and inflammation, especially neutrophils and the monocyte/macrophage, are able to express high levels of glucose transporters, especially GLUT1. The common indications of FDG-PET/CT in infection and inflammation included the following in descending order of accuracy: sarcoidosis, osteomyelitis, spondylodiscitis, fever of unknown origin, vasculitis, diabetic foot, prosthesis (especially hip), and vascular grafts. Also it is used for assessing the extent of fungal infection and evaluation of therapy in infectious or inflammatory diseases [11].

Mechanism of uptake of SPECT and PET	
SPECT and PET tracer	Mechanism of uptake
67Ga-citrate and 99mTc-HMPAO migration of leukocytes	Transferrin and lactoferrin receptor binding
99mTc-HMPAO-WBC	Migration of leukocytes
111In-oxine-WBC	Cellular migration of leukocytes
LeukoScan (Tc-anti-NCA-90 FAB antigranulocyte antibody)	Increased vascular permeability and binding and migration of antibody-labeled granulocytes
18F-FDG	Glucose uptake by activated inflammatory cells

13.2 Diagnosis of Cyst Infection

Cyst infection is a diagnostic challenge in patients with autosomal dominant polycystic kidney disease (ADPKD) because of the lack of specific manifestations and limitations of conventional imaging procedures [12]. ADPKD represents the most common inherited kidney disease [13]. It is characterized by the development of fluid-filled cysts in kidney and liver parenchyma, derived from various renal tubular segments and biliary ducts. Cyst growth causes organ enlargement leading to abdominal and/or loin discomfort. Liver cysts are not associated with hepatic dysfunction, whereas kidney cysts cause end-stage renal disease (ESRD) in more than 70% of ADPKD patients. Also, cysts carry significant

Fig. 13.2 18F-FDG metabolism

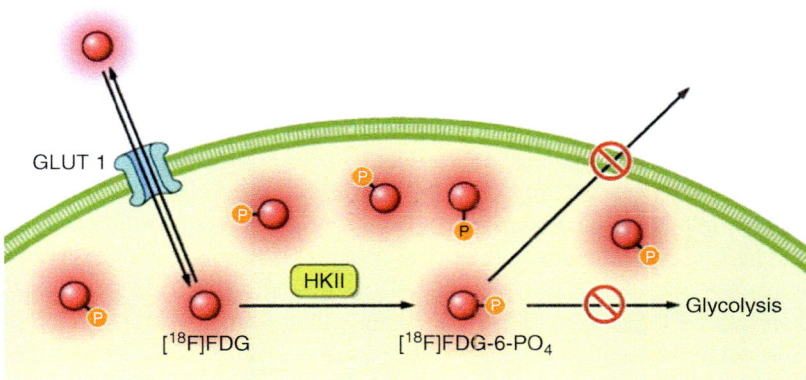

morbidity, including bleeding and infection. Cyst infection is a serious complication of ADPKD. Its incidence is 0.01 episode/patient/year, according to a retrospective monocentric series of Sallée et al. [14]. Predisposing conditions include age, female gender, and recent instrumentation of the urinary tract. In the chronic hemodialysis population, the prevalence of renal infection is significantly higher in ADPKD patients than in controls [15]. In the renal transplant recipient (RTR) population, the prevalence of urinary tract infections in patients with ADPKD does not appear to be increased [16]. Cyst infection is the cause of hospitalizations for 15% of ADPKD patients [14, 17]. Most common pathogens are enteric flora, *Escherichia coli*. The retrograde route via the ureters is the presumed mechanism of cyst infection in the kidney. The identification of the germ is lacking in more than half of cases, similar to the rate observed in the general population with severe sepsis. Although the identification of the infectious agent is essential for tailoring the antibiotic therapy, the diagnosis of cyst infection is not easy because of the various, most often nonspecific, clinical manifestations and the limitations of conventional imaging techniques. Proving the presence of cyst infection requires cyst fluid analysis. However, this is not always possible or indicated, so that diagnosis relies practically on a constellation of concurrent clinical, biological, and radiological parameters.

Conventional imaging procedures, such as CT and magnetic resonance imaging (MRI), were largely discussed on the previous chapter.

13.2.1 WBC

Radiolabeled-leukocyte scintigraphy in the diagnosis of kidney cyst infection is a complement of the radiological procedures in the assessment of infectious site localization. Particularly, ^{111}In leukocyte scanning allowed the identification of renal cyst infection in ADPKD patients in whom other noninvasive imaging procedures had failed. [111]In leukocyte scanning requires the handling of blood derivatives and in vitro labeling process, as well as a 24-h delay imaging. [111]In scintigraphy is characterized by poor spatial resolution, low sensitivity, high radiation activity, and significant interobserver variability. Hexamethylpropyleneamine oxime (HMPAO) represents an alternative lipophilic chelator for efficient labeling of leukocytes with 99mtechnetium (99mTc). Radiation characteristics of 99mTc-HMPAO are more favorable for imaging than those of ^{111}In, particularly for single-photon emission computed tomography (SPECT). Furthermore, the dual modality technique combining CT with SPECT using radiolabeled WBC has been associated with a diagnostic yield of 85% of cases with abdominal infections. The relevance of SPECT/CT to cyst infection diagnosis in ADPKD patients is currently unknown [12].

13.2.2 FDG-PET/CT

In the general population, 18FDG-PET/CT imaging represents a reliable tool for the detection of tissue infection on the basis of the high metabolic activity and increased uptake of the radiolabeled glucose analogue, 18FDG, by inflammatory cells [22]. Importantly, 18FDG is not nephro- or hepatotoxic and has been successfully used in patients with renal function ranging from mildly reduced GFR to ESRD [14, 23]. First, 18FDG-PET alone proved helpful in identifying or excluding renal and hepatic cyst infection in case reports and two retrospective series [14, 20, 24]. To further improve the localization of infectious sites, PET was combined with CT to integrate metabolic data from PET with anatomical information from CT [22]. In our series, 18FDG-PET/CT yielded positive results in 87% of cyst infection cases [17]. PET/CT was considered as positive for cyst infection when the uptake of 18FDG was focally increased around at least one cyst in comparison with the physiological accumulation in the parenchyma and was located at distance from the pelvicalyceal excretion. PET/CT yielded two false-negative results in a diabetic RTR during the immediate posttransplantation period and in a 62-year-old nondiabetic woman with stage IV CKD. By contrast, three liver pyocysts could be percutaneously drained only after localization by PET/CT. The median delay between the onset of symptoms and PET/CT imaging was 9 days, and the mean maximal standardized uptake value (SUV_{max}) reached 5.1 ± 1.7 g/mL. The measurement of SUV_{max} allows standardized quantification of the inflammatory process in addition to the visual evaluation [23]. Repeated measurements of SUV_{max} may help follow up the inflammatory process over time. Piccoli et al. [18] reported on the clinical management of ten patients with suspected cystic infection, which was tailored upon 18FDG-PET/CT results. PET/CT identified five kidney and one liver cyst infections. The mean SUV_{max} reached 8.4 ± 5.4 g/mL on initial PET/CT images. The follow-up of four patients included a comparative PET/CT performed 3–6 weeks later, which showed a visual reduction of pathological 18FDG uptake but no significant change of SUV_{max}. Three patients underwent a third PET/CT 7–9 weeks after the initial imaging, which disclosed no residual 18FDG uptake. Of note, the normalization of serum CRP levels preceded

PET/CT normalization. The clinical relevance of persistent altered PET/CT images to treated infectious diseases remains unclear. The literature in oncology supports that the follow-up by 18FDG-PET/CT of therapeutic responses to chemo- or radiotherapy varies from 3 to 12 weeks depending upon the type of cancer and the administered therapy. However, the pathophysiology of infection is intrinsically different from neoplasia, and cyst infection is associated with the additional challenge of antibiotic diffusion into a chronically damaged organ and a cystic cavity. Consequently, 18FDG-PET/CT probably represents an optimal tool for the detection and localization of pyocysts in ADPKD patients, but its role in the follow-up after antibiotic therapy remains uncertain. PET/CT in ADPKD patients with suspected cyst infection offers the additional advantage of entirely scanning the abdominal cavity, thereby occasionally identifying non-cystic inflammatory disorders and adjusting the therapy. PET/CT results significantly changed the management of 26% of cases [17]. Moreover, PET/CT confirmed two kidney cyst infections, although both patients did not meet all four of the standardized criteria [19]. The advantages of 18FDG-PET/CT are rapid imaging, minimal labor intensity, high target-to-background ratio, high interobserver agreement, and a simultaneous coregistration with low-dose CT without administration of contrast medium [23]. Limitations of PET/CT include its cost, restricted availability, and relative inability to reliably distinguish infectious from noninfectious inflammation or malignancy. The differentiation of 18FDG accumulation in residual functional renal parenchyma from that in inflammatory cells lining pyocysts remains debatable. The distinction between cyst infection and pyelonephritis may not be easy. The PET/CT pattern of pyelonephritis usually includes a diffuse 18FDG uptake in an edematous cortex and locoregional hypermetabolic adenopathies, which contrasts with the focally increased uptake of 18FDG lining the pyocyst. Besides infectious processes, 18FDG uptake can be increased in other conditions, such as cancer. The actual risk of malignancy in ADPKD patients does not seem to be increased [25]. Liver cystadenocarcinoma is very uncommon, and most kidney tumors show low-grade malignancy leading to low 18FDG uptake. However, "false-positive" rate of 18FDG-PET/CT in cyst infection diagnosis remains to be prospectively investigated. Finally, PET/CT has not been evaluated in intracystic bleeding, the main differential diagnosis of cyst infection in ADPKD patients. Accumulation of 18FDG has been reported in the setting of extrarenal hematoma [26]. In conclusion the 18FDG-PET is a very useful method for increasing the accuracy of the diagnosis of the infected cyst with a sensitivity of 77%, a specificity of 100%, and a negative predictive value of 77% [27].

13.2.3 Cases Presentation

13.2.3.1 Case 1

An 81-year-old woman, suffering from polycystic hepatorenal disease, was hospitalized for onset of fever of unknown origin. Following investigations, because of the suspect of left acute multifocal pyelonephritis, the patient was treated with ceftriaxone and amikacin. The abdominal CT examination showed the presence of a renal cyst with diameter of 80 × 90 mm and characterized by homogeneous fluid content and slightly and uniformly thickened walls in the absence of nodular lesions. Then therapy was later stopped due to the persistence of symptoms and high levels of inflammatory markers. The patient was thus treated with ertapenem getting better results but not a complete response. She was therefore aimed at our center to perform an 18F-FDG-PET/CT scan. This functional examination showed the presence of an abnormal FDG uptake at the level of the left kidney cyst walls (Fig. 13.3).

The pathological presence of radiotracer at this level, indicative of an active inflammatory process, suggested the continuation of antibiotic treatments. After 37 days a second PET scan showed a good response to the treatment documented by a significant reduction in the extent and intensity of the abnormal uptake of radiotracer (Fig. 13.4).

During the follow-up a second CT scan showed the persistence of the right renal cysts although dimensionally significantly reduced compared to the previous control. In the absence of a definitive imaging judgment of complete response, a third PET scan was performed. PET showed the complete disappearance of the abnormal uptake of the radiopharmaceutical at the walls of the kidney cysts, still present from a morphological point of view (Fig. 13.5).

In this clinical case, the PET examination, together with clinical parameters, seems to have helped, both in the correct diagnosis and in response assessment to the treatment.

13.2.3.2 Case 2

A 55-year-old patient with hepatorenal polycystic disease went to the hospital for pain in the left lumbar region associated with fever. Biochemical examinations showed a high CRP value (188.3 mg/L), and a possible left renal cyst with hemorrhagic aspects was detected by contrast-enhanced CT in the suspect of an active inflammatory process in this site; the patient was subjected to antibiotic therapy with amoxicillin. One month later the symptoms disappeared almost completely, and the PCR values were significantly reduced although not yet in standard levels, while a second CT scan showed no more signs of active left kidney inflammation. In consideration of the difficult judgment of treatment response, the patient was sent to our clinic for a PET/CT examination. The examination showed an abnormal uptake of radiotracer at the lower portion of the known left renal cyst, with a SUV_{max} 2.9 (Fig. 13.6).

In the following months, the patient underwent further antibiotic therapy and was monitored with multiple diagnostic tests. It was interesting to note that PET scan was the only imaging examination able to identify the persistent focus of the disease. This finding was further reduced by size and fixation in the subsequent PET control, showing a SUV_{max} of 2.4 (Fig. 13.7).

A further reduction in this finding was found in the third PET examination, showing a SUV_{max} of 2.0 (Fig. 13.8).

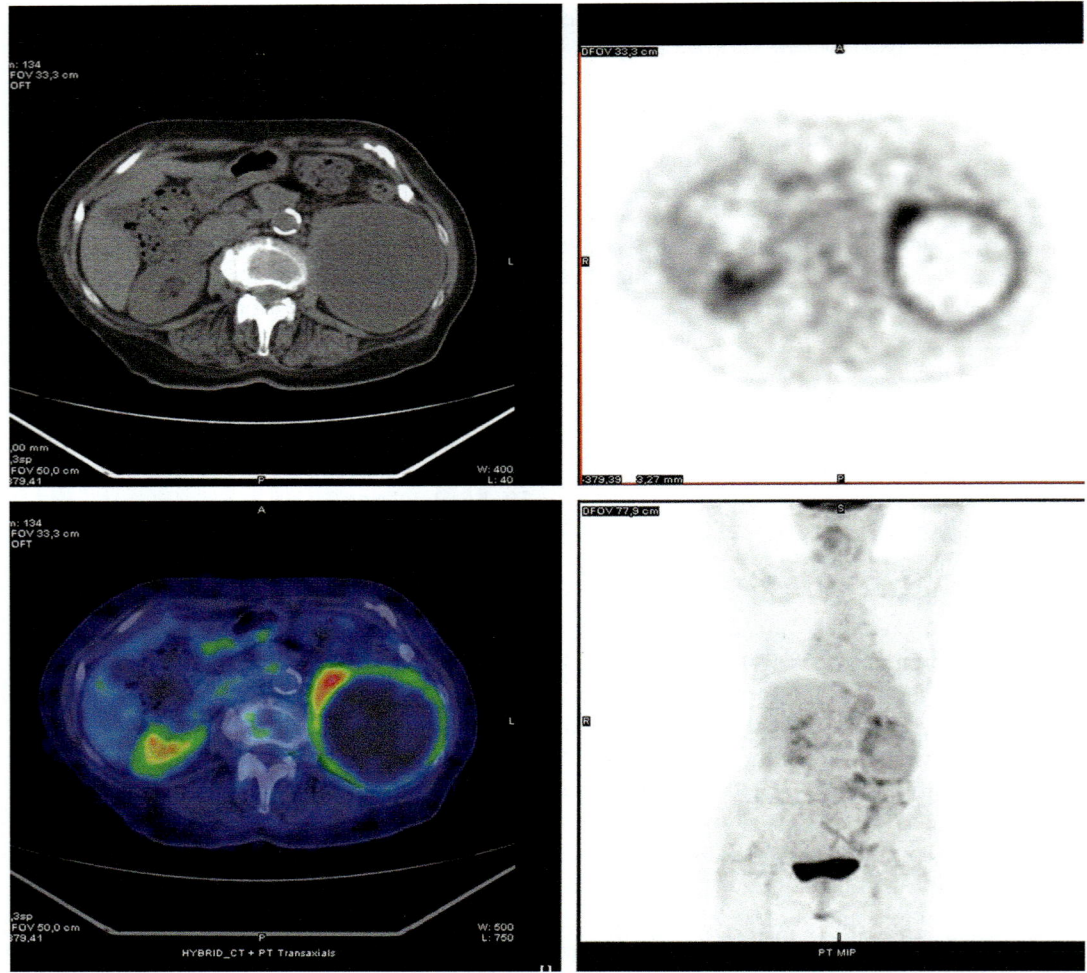

Fig. 13.3 PET/CT scan (CT, PET, Fusion, Transaxial and MIP images): diffuse abnormal uptake of 18F-FDG at the walls of a large kidney cyst indicative of a high presence of inflammatory active cells at this level

One last PET scan was performed when the patient showed total normalization of inflammatory indices and a complete resolution of the symptoms. This last examination showed the complete disappearance of the radiotracer uptake (Fig. 13.9).

In this clinical case, PET has proven to be a good diagnostic tool in evaluating minimal persistence of inflammatory disease. PET scan, used during the treatment, has helped clinicians decide on the type and duration of therapy.

13.3 Future Development

In addition to glucose metabolism, a variety of targets for inflammation imaging are being discovered and utilized, some of which are considered superior to FDG for imaging inflammation. We summarize the potential inflammation imaging targets and corresponding PET tracers and the applications of PET in major inflammatory disease.

18F-FDG-PET imaging of inflammation tends to give false-positive results, especially in

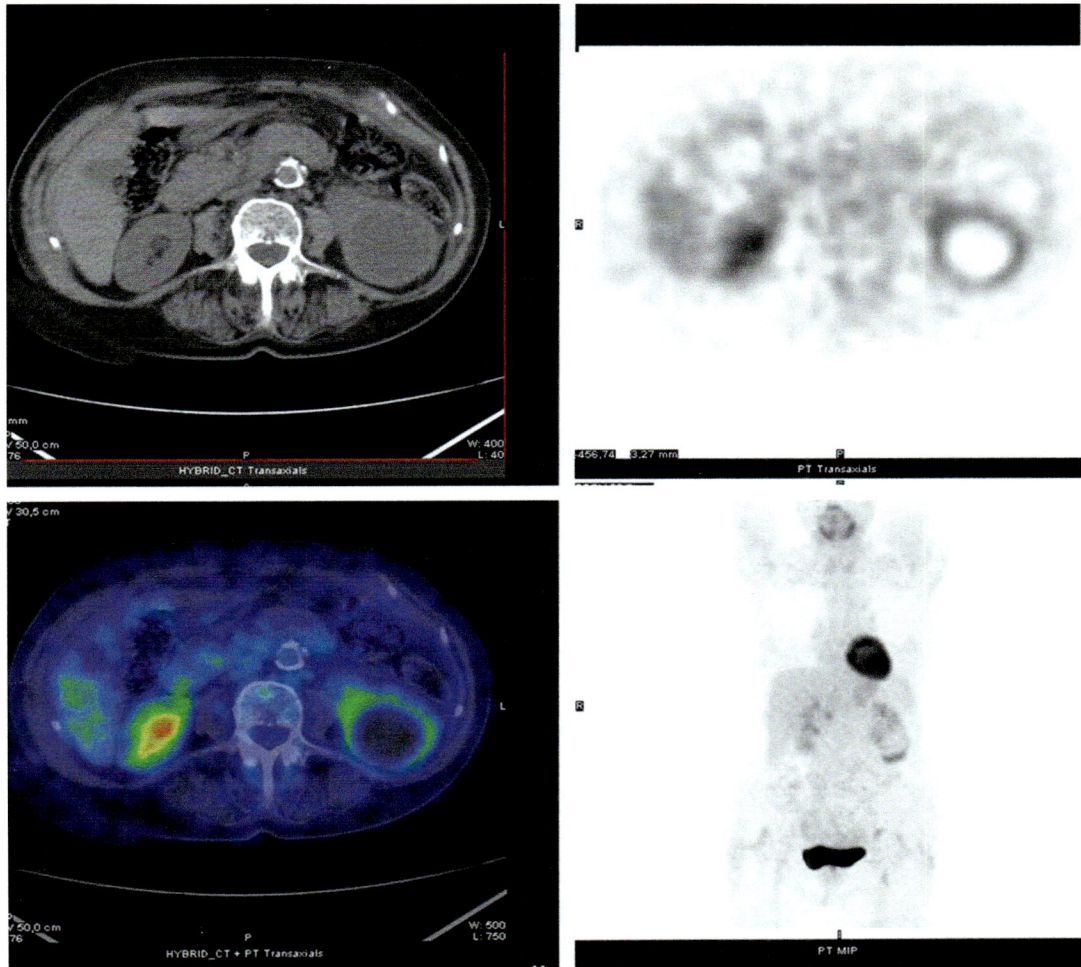

Fig. 13.4 PET/CT scan (CT, PET, Fusion, Transaxial and MIP images): significant reduction of the abnormal uptake of radiotracer at the renal cyst wall, indicative of good response to antibiotic treatment

patients with cancer. Moreover, the high tracer accumulation in the heart and brain makes it difficult to detect inflammatory foci near those organs or tissues. Consequently, new imaging tracers and targets for more specific inflammation detection and therapy evaluation are under intensive investigation. PET imaging with these new tracers greatly improved our understanding of the mechanism of inflammation and increased the diagnostic specificity and accuracy of inflammatory foci. As summarized in Fig. 13.10, various radiopharmaceuticals have been devel-

oped for PET imaging of inflammation, targeting different biomarkers from macrophages to angiogenesis.

A small survey of the new tracer potentially available in the next future.

13.3.1 Translocator Protein (TSPO)

Formerly known as peripheral benzodiazepine receptor (PBR), TSPO is ubiquitously expressed in peripheral tissues but is only min-

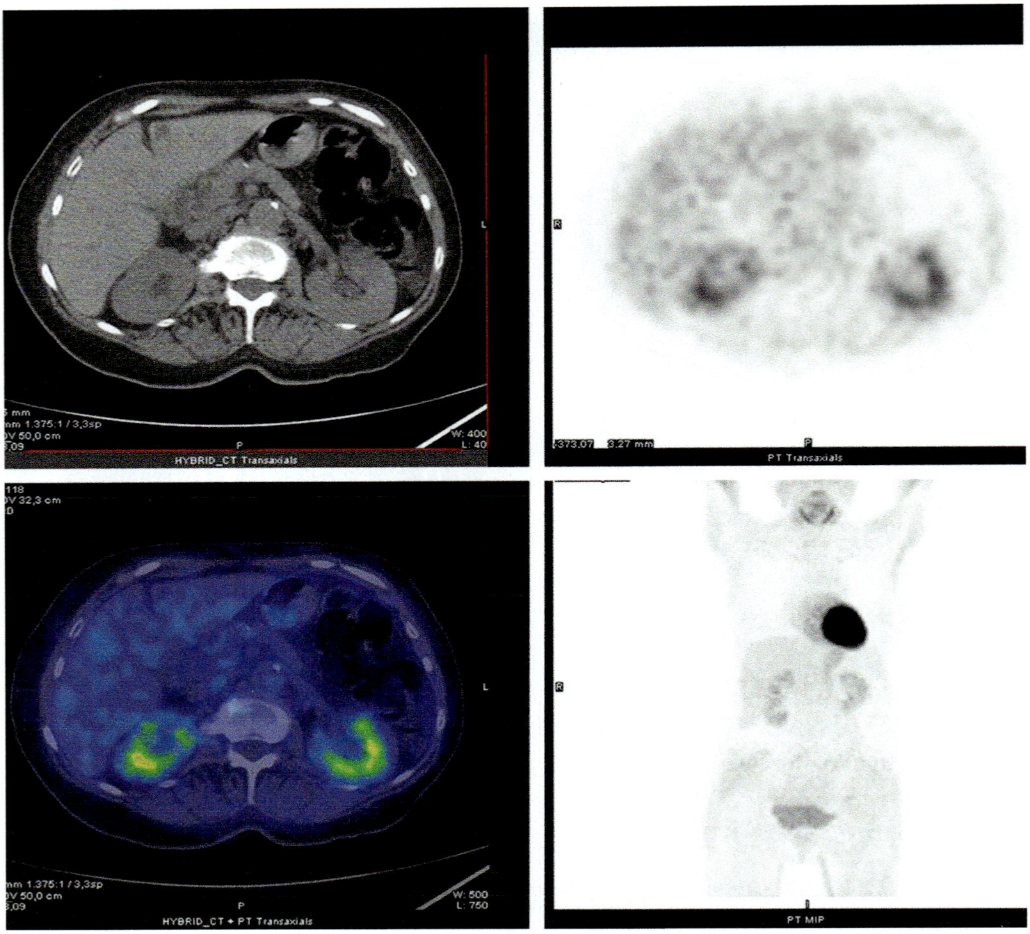

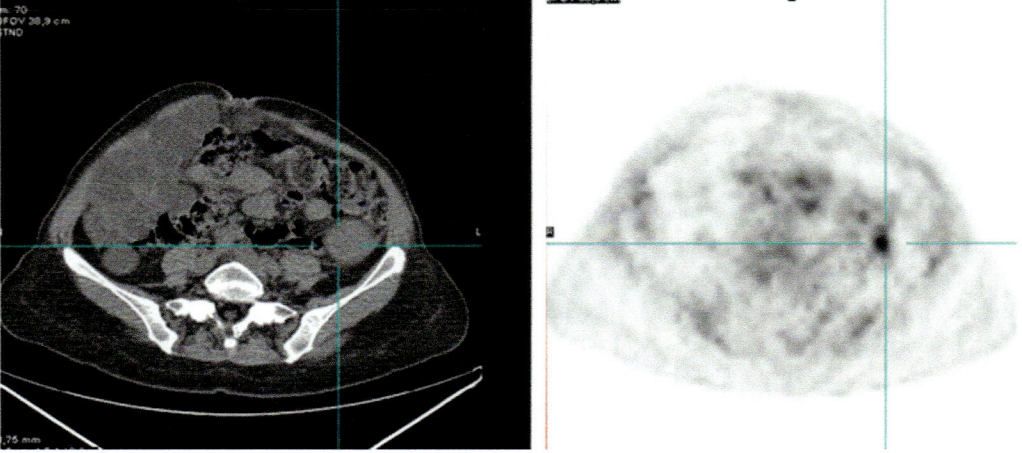

Fig. 13.5 PET/CT scan (CT, PET, Fusion, Transaxial and MIP images): complete disappearance of the abnormal radiotracer uptake at the renal cyst level, after further antibiotic treatment

Fig. 13.6 PET/CT scan (CT and PET Transaxial images): focal abnormal uptake of 18F-FDG at the level of the lower portion of a left kidney cyst, due to the presence of active inflammatory cells

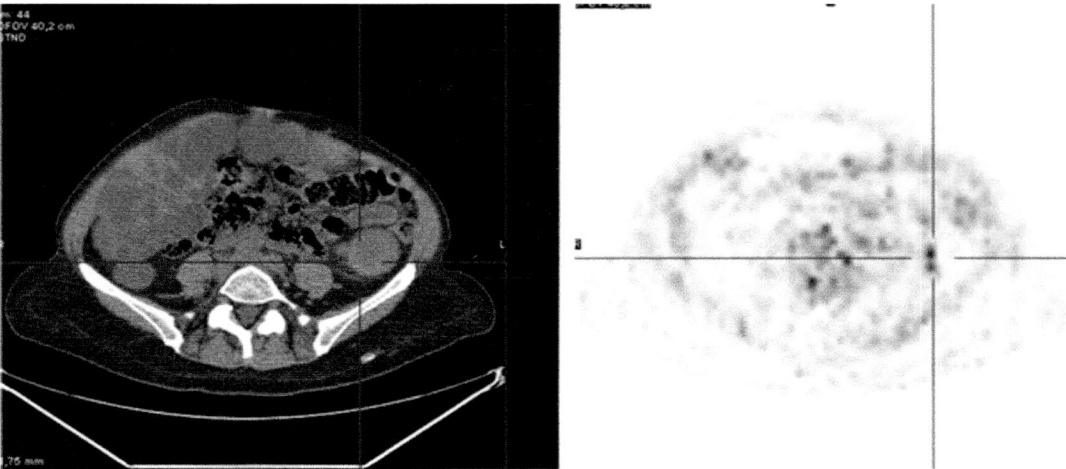

Fig. 13.7 PET/CT scan (CT and PET Transaxial images): reduction of the abnormal uptake of radiotracer at the left kidney cyst after antibiotic treatment

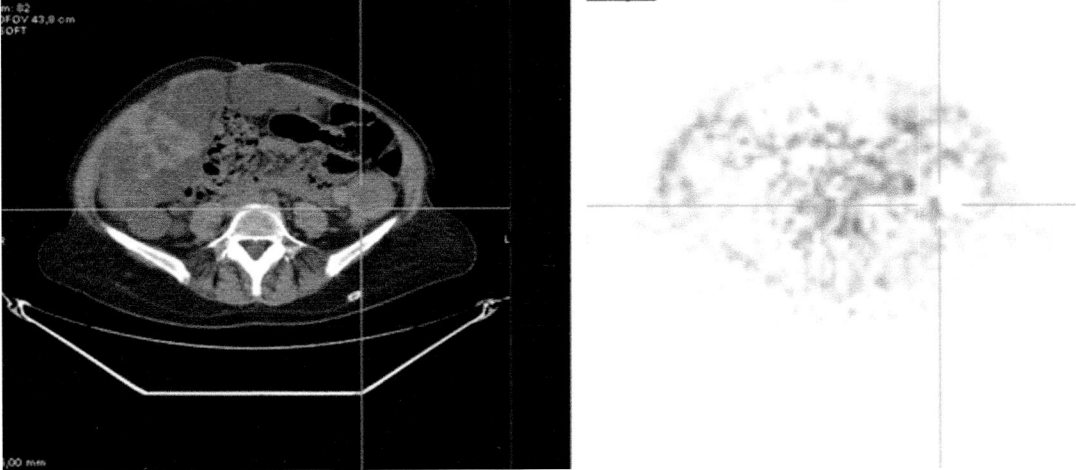

Fig. 13.8 PET/CT scan (CT and PET Transaxial images): further reduction of radiotracer uptake during antibiotic therapy

imally expressed in the healthy human brain. Previous studies found high TSPO expression in macrophages, neutrophils, lymphocytes [28–30], activated microglia, and astrocytes [31–35]. PET imaging using TSPO as an inflammation biomarker has also been reported for atherosclerosis detection with promising results [31, 32, 36, 37]. TSPO PET has also been used to image inflamed lung and liver diseases [30, 38, 39].

13.3.2 Type 2 Cannabinoid Receptor (CB2R)

There are at least two subtypes of CBRs in the endocannabinoid system. The first in vivo PET of brain CB2R was performed in 2010 by Horti and his group [40]. Promising results on CB2R targeted PET imaging warrant further applications in a wide range of neuroinflammatory diseases and evaluation of the therapeutic value of novel

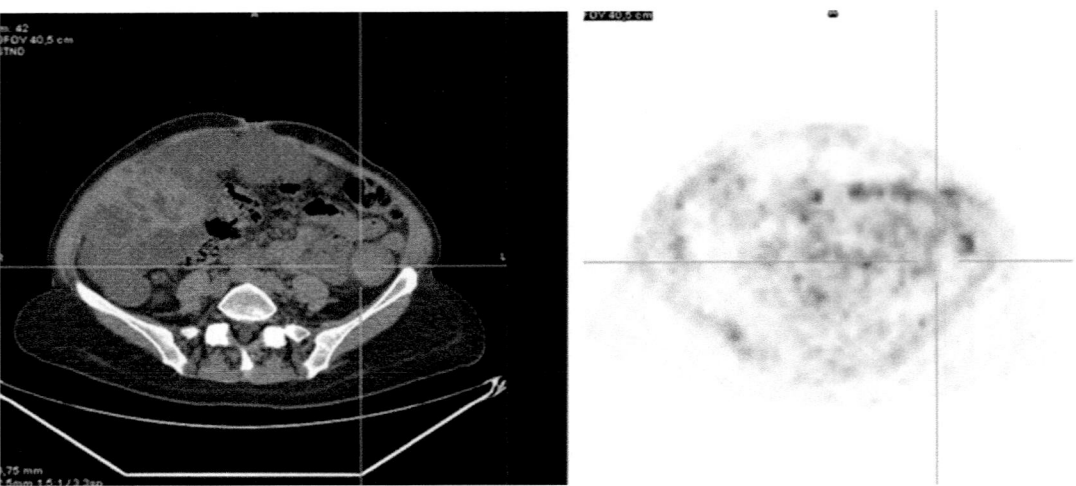

Fig. 13.9 PET/CT scan (CT and PET Transaxial images): total disappearance of the 18F-FDG cystic uptake, indicative of complete metabolic response to the treatment

CB2R-related drugs. However, the exact role of CB2R in CNS still remains to be fully elucidated, and more in vivo studies using relevant disease models should be conducted to get a better understanding.

13.3.3 Formyl Peptide Receptor (FPR)

FPR is a type of G-protein-coupled receptor expressed on neutrophils, responsible for the leukocyte migration cascade in the inflammation process. PET using cFLFLFK-PEG-64Cu as FPR-specific ligand could visualize inflammatory foci within the lung in an animal model of lung inflammation induced by *Klebsiella pneumoniae* [41].

13.3.4 Cyclooxygenase (COX)

COX is the target of nonsteroidal anti-inflammatory drugs (NSAIDs) [42]. In addition, COX is an integral membrane glycoprotein which can be induced by acute and chronic inflammatory stimulations. Thus far, three COX subtypes (COX-1, 2, and 3) have been identified. Among them, the inducible isoform COX-2 plays a piv-

otal role in cancer, cardiac/cerebral ischemia, Alzheimer's/Parkinson's disease, and response to inflammatory stimuli, especially neuroinflammation [43, 44]. Celecoxib is broadly used as a selective COX-2 inhibitor to treat inflammatory diseases. Imaging tracers have also been developed using celecoxib and some other COX inhibitors by radiolabeling them with either 18F or 11C. They have been used to image neuroinflammations [45], tumors, or experimental skin inflammation [46, 47]. However, most of the tracers showed unsatisfactory ex vivo or in vivo properties due to either nonspecific bindings or low sensitivity in inflammatory foci or both.

13.3.5 Interleukin-2 (IL-2)

IL-2 is a small single-chain glycoprotein synthesized and secreted by activated T lymphocytes seen in many types of inflammatory diseases, such as inflammatory degenerative diseases, graft rejection, tumor inflammation, organ-specific autoimmune diseases, and adipose inflammatory insulin resistance [48]. Previously, 123I and 99mTc-labeled IL-2 have been used in many chronic inflammatory diseases, such as autoim-

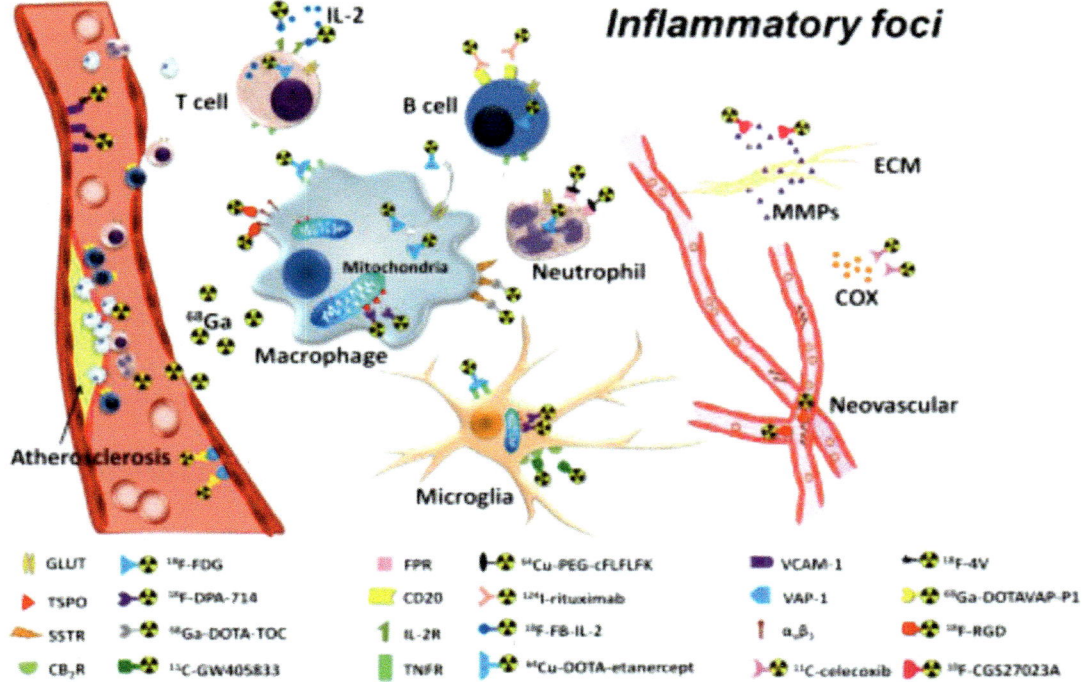

Fig. 13.10 PET imaging of Inflammation Biomarkers

mune diseases [49], celiac disease [50], and vulnerable atherosclerotic plaques [51] via SPECT imaging. However, routine application of this technique was limited because the labeling procedures are complex and the spatial resolution of SPECT is not high enough. Recently, Gialleonardo et al. reported the labeling of IL-2 with *N*-succinimidyl 4-18F-fluorobenzoate (18F-SFB) for the synthesis of 18F-FB-IL-2 to detect activated T lymphocytes in inflammation [52].

13.3.6 Tumor Necrosis Factor-α (TNF-α)

TNF-α is a cytokine that can contribute to cell apoptosis and organ dysfunction [53]. Many studies show that TNF-α is important in acute immune response to infection, injury, autoimmune, and chronic inflammatory disorders such as rheumatoid arthritis [54] and psoriasis [55]. Previously,

some group used a PET tracer 64Cu-DOTA-etanercept, to image acute inflammatory process induced by 12-O-tetradecanoylphorbol-13-acetate (tetradecanoylphorbol acetate, TPA) [56].

So far, many inflammation-related biomarkers have been identified and investigated as imaging or therapy targets, including inflammatory cell metabolism, membrane markers, cytokines, and vascular changes during inflammation. After intensive preclinical studies, some of these targets have been tested in humans. However, very few of them are considered to be inflammation specific. With better understanding of the inflammatory reaction in each disease type, more sensitive and specific biomarkers will be identified, and potential new imaging probes may be developed to target these biomarkers. Moreover, multiplexed imaging with tracers targeting different biomarkers and multimodal imaging by incorporating PET with other imaging modalities will also contribute to improved visualization and quantification of the inflammatory diseases.

References

1. Jamar F, Buscombe J, Chiti A, Christian PE, Delbeke D, Donohoe KJ, Israel O, Martin-Comin J, Alberto S (2013) EANM/SNMMI guideline for 18F-FDG use in inflammation and infection. J Nucl Med 54(4):647–658

2. Bailey DL et al (2005) Positron emission tomography: basic sciences. Springer-Verlag, Secaucus

3. Boerman OC, Rennen H, Oyen WJ et al (2001) Radiopharmaceuticals to image infection and inflammation. Semin Nucl Med 31:286–295

4. Love C, Palestro CJ (2004) Radionuclide imaging of infection. J Nucl Med Technol 32:47–57

5. Mirtcheva RM, Kostakoglu SJ, Goldsmith SJ (2003) SPECT/CT fusion imaging in 111In WBC scintigraphy. J Nucl Med 44:341

6. Becker W, Meller J (2001) The role of nuclear medicine in infection and inflammation. Lancet Infect Dis 1:326–333

7. Hakki S, Harwood SJ, Morrissey MA et al (1997) Comparative study of monoclonal antibody scan in diagnosing orthopaedic infection. Clin Orthop 335:275–285

8. Palestro CJ, Kipper SL, Weiland FL et al (2002) Osteomyelitis: diagnosis with (99m)Tc-labeled antigranulocyte antibodies compared with diagnosis with (111)In-labeled leukocytes—initial experience. Radiology 223(3):758–764

9. Horger M, Eschmann SM, Pfannenberg C et al (2003) The value of SPET/CT in chronic osteomyelitis. Eur J Nucl Med Mol Imaging 30(12):1665–1673

10. James ML, Gambhir SS (2012) A molecular imaging primer: modalities, imaging agents, and applications. Physiol Rev 92(2):897–965

11. Farghaly H, Nasr H, Al Qarni A (2015) Role of FDG PET/CT in infection and inflammation. J Nucl Med 56(supplement 3):1954

12. Jouret F, Lhommel R, Devuyst O, Annet L, Hassoun Z, Kanaan N (2012) Diagnosis of cyst infection in patients with autosomal dominant polycystic kidney disease: attributes and limitations of the current modalities. Nephrol Dial Transplant 27(10):3746–3751

13. Torres VE, Harris PC, Pirson Y (2007) Autosomal dominant polycystic kidney disease. Lancet 369(9569):1287–1301

14. Sallée M, Rafat C, Zahar JR et al (2009) Cyst infections in patients with autosomal dominant polycystic kidney disease. Clin J Am Soc Nephrol 4(7):1183–1189

15. Christophe JL, van Ypersele de Strihou C, Pirson Y (1996) Complications of autosomal dominant polycystic kidney disease in 50 haemodialysed patients. A case-control study. The U.C.L. collaborative group. Nephrol Dial Transplant 11(7):1271–1276

16. Jacquet A, Pallet N, Kessler M et al (2011) Outcomes of renal transplantation in patients with autosomal dominant polycystic kidney disease: a nationwide longitudinal study. Transpl Int 24(6):582–587

17. Jouret F, Lhommel R, Beguin C et al (2011) Positron-emission computed tomography in cyst infection diagnosis in patients with autosomal dominant polycystic kidney disease. Clin J Am Soc Nephrol 6(7):1644–1650

18. Piccoli GB, Arena V, Consiglio V et al (2011) Positron emission tomography in the diagnostic pathway for intracystic infection in ADPKD and 'cystic' kidneys. A case series. BMC Nephrol 12:48

19. Telenti A, Torres VE, Gross JB Jr et al (1990) Hepatic cyst infection in autosomal dominant polycystic kidney disease. Mayo Clin Proc 65(7):933–942

20. Migali G, Annet L, Lonneux M et al (2008) Renal cyst infection in autosomal dominant polycystic kidney disease. Nephrol Dial Transplant 23(1):404–405

21. Ichioka K, Saito R, Matsui Y et al (2007) Diffusion-weighted magnetic resonance imaging of infected renal cysts in a patient with polycystic kidney disease. Urology 25(1):1219

22. Keidar Z, Gurman-Balbir A, Gaitini D et al (2008) Fever of unknown origin: the role of 18F-FDG PET/CT. J Nucl Med 49(12):1980–1985

23. Boellaard R, O'Doherty MJ, Weber WA et al (2010) FDG PET and PET/CT: EANM procedure guidelines for tumour PET imaging. Eur J Nucl Med Mol Imaging 42:328–354

24. Bleeker-Rovers CP, de Sevaux RG, van Hamersvelt HW et al (2003) Diagnosis of renal and hepatic cyst infections by 18-F-fluorodeoxyglucose positron emission tomography in autosomal dominant polycystic kidney disease. Am J Kidney Dis 41(6):E18–E21

25. Bonsib SM (2009) Renal cystic diseases and renal neoplasms: a mini review. Clin J Am Soc Nephrol 4(12):1998–2007

26. Repko BM, Tulchinsky M (2008) Increased F-18 FDG uptake in resolving atraumatic bilateral adrenal hemorrhage (hematoma) on PET/CT. Clin Nucl Med 33(9):651–653

27. Bobot M, Ghez C, Gondouin B, Sallée M, Fournier PE, Burtey S, Legris T, Dussol B, Berland Y, Souteyrand P, Tessonnier L, Cammilleri S, Jourde-Chiche N (2016) Diagnostic performance of [(18)F] fluorodeoxyglucose positron emission tomography-computed tomography in cyst infection in patients with autosomal dominant polycystic kidney disease. Clin Microbiol Infect 22(1):71–77

28. Bird JL, Izquierdo-Garcia D, Davies JR, Rudd JH, Probst KC, Figg N et al (2010) Evaluation of translocator protein quantification as a tool for characterising macrophage burden in human carotid atherosclerosis. Atherosclerosis 210(2):388–391

29. Gaemperli O, Shalhoub J, Owen DR, Lamare F, Johansson S, Fouladi N et al (2012) Imaging intraplaque inflammation in carotid atherosclerosis with 11C-PK11195 positron emission tomography/computed tomography. Eur Heart J 33(15):1902–1910

30. Hatori A, Yui J, Yamasaki T, Xie L, Kumata K, Fujinaga M et al (2012) PET imaging of lung inflam-

mation with [18F]FEDAC, a radioligand for translocator protein (18 kDa). PLoS One 7(9):e4506

31. Hannestad J, Gallezot JD, Schafbauer T, Lim K, Kloczynski T, Morris ED et al (2012) Endotoxin-induced systemic inflammation activates microglia:[11C]PBR28 positron emission tomography in nonhuman primates. NeuroImage 63(1):232–239

32. Roeda D, Kuhnast B, Damont A, Dollé F (2012) Synthesis of fluorine-18-labelled TSPO ligands for imaging neuroinflammation with positron emission tomography. J Fluor Chem 134:107–114

33. Ching AS, Kuhnast B, Damont A, Roeda D, Tavitian B, Dolle F (2012) Current paradigm of the 18-kDa translocator protein (TSPO) as a molecular target for PET imaging in neuroinflammation and neurodegenerative diseases. Insights Imaging 3(1):111–1119

34. Oh U, Fujita M, Ikonomidou VN, Evangelou IE, Matsuura E, Harberts E et al (2011) Translocator protein PET imaging for glial activation in multiple sclerosis. J Neuroimmune Pharmacol 6(3):354–361

35. Papadopoulos V, Lecanu L (2009) Translocator protein (18 kDa) TSPO: an emerging therapeutic target in neurotrauma. 2009. Exp Neurol 219:53–57

36. Pugliese F, Gaemperli O, Kinderlerer AR, Lamare F, Shalhoub J, Davies H et al (2010) Imaging of vascular inflammation with [11C]-PK11195 and positron emission tomography/computed tomography angiography. J Am Coll Cardiol 56(8):653–661

37. Lamare F, Hinz R, Gaemperli O, Pugliese F, Mason JC, Spinks T et al (2011) Detection and quantification of large-vessel inflammation with 11C-(R)-PK11195 PET/CT. J Nucl Med 52(1):33–39

38. Hardwick MJ, Chen MK, Baidoo K, Pomper MG, Guilarte TR (2005) In vivo imaging of peripheral benzodiazepine receptors in mouse lungs: a biomarker of inflammation. Mol Imaging 4(4):432–438

39. Xie L, Yui J, Hatori A, Yamasaki T, Kumata K, Wakizaka H et al (2012) Translocator protein (18kDa), a potential molecular imaging biomarker for non-invasively distinguishing non-alcoholic fatty liver disease. J Hepatol 57(5):1076–1082

40. Horti AG, Gao Y, Ravert HT, Finley P, Valentine H, Wong DF et al (2010) Synthesis and biodistribution of [11C]A-836339, a new potential radioligand for PET imaging of cannabinoid type 2 receptors (CB2). Bioorg Med Chem 18(14):5202–5207

41. Locke LW, Chordia MD, Zhang Y, Kundu B, Kennedy D, Landseadel J et al (2009) A novel neutrophil-specific PET imaging agent: cFLFLFK-PEG-64Cu. J Nucl Med 50(5):790–797

42. Hawkey CJ (1999) COX-2 inhibitors. Lancet 353(9149):307–314

43. Katori M, Majima M (2000) Cyclooxygenase-2: its rich diversity of roles and possible application of its selective inhibitors. Inflamm Res 49(8):367–392

44. Minghetti L (2004) Cyclooxygenase-2 (COX-2) in inflammatory and degenerative brain diseases. J Neuropathol Exp Neurol 63(9):901–910

45. de Vries EFJ, Doorduin J, Dierckx RA, van Waarde A (2008) Evaluation of [11C]rofecoxib as PET tracer for cyclooxygenase 2 overexpression in rat. Nucl Med Biol 35(1):35–42

46. Uddin MJ, Crews BC, Ghebreselasie K, Huda I, Kingsley PJ, Ansari MS et al (2011) Fluorinated COX-2 inhibitors as agents in PET imaging of inflammation and cancer. Cancer Prev Res (Phila) 4(10):1536–1545

47. Wuest F, Kniess T, Bergmann R, Pietzsch J (2008) Synthesis and evaluation in vitro and in vivo of a 11C-labeled cyclooxygenase-2 (COX-2) inhibitor. Bioorg Med Chem 16(16):7662–7670

48. Kintscher U, Hartge M, Hess K, Foryst-Ludwig A, Clemenz M, Wabitsch M et al (2008) T-lymphocyte infiltration in visceral adipose tissue: a primary event in adipose tissue inflammation and the development of obesity-mediated insulin resistance. Arterioscler Thromb Vasc Biol 28(7):1304–1310

49. Signore A, Picarelli A, Annovazzi A, Britton KE, Grossman AB, Bonanno E et al (2003) 123I-Interleukin-2: biochemical characterization and in vivo use for imaging autoimmune diseases. Nucl Med Commun 24(3):305–316

50. Signore A, Chianelli M, Annovazzi A, Rossi M, Maiuri L, Greco M et al (2000) Imaging active lymphocytic infiltration in coeliac disease with iodine-123-interleukin-2 and the response to diet. Eur J Nucl Med 27(1):18–24

51. Annovazzi A, Bonanno E, Arca M, D'Alessandria C, Marcoccia A, Spagnoli LG et al (2006) 99mTc-interleukin-2 scintigraphy for the in vivo imaging of vulnerable atherosclerotic plaques. Eur J Nucl Med Mol Imaging 33(2):117–126

52. Di Gialleonardo V, Signore A, Glaudemans AW, Dierckx RA, De Vries EF (2012) N-(4-18F-fluorobenzoyl)interleukin-2 for PET of human-activated T lymphocytes. J Nucl Med 53(5):679–686

53. Cairns CB, Paracek EA, Harken AH, Banerjee A (2000) Bench to bedside:tumor necrosis factor-alpha: from inflammation to resuscitation. Acad Emerg Med 7(8):930–941

54. Maki-Petaja KM, Elkhawad M, Cheriyan J, Joshi FR, Ostor AJ, Hall FC et al (2012) Anti-tumor necrosis factor-alpha therapy reduces aortic inflammation and stiffness in patients with rheumatoid arthritis. Circulation 126(21):2473–2480

55. Bissonnette R, Tardif JC, Harel F, Pressacco J, Bolduc C, Guertin MC (2013) Effects of the TNF alpha antagonist adalimumab on arterial inflammation assessed by positron emission tomography in patients with psoriasis: results of a randomized controlled trial. Circ Cardiovasc Imaging 6(1):83–90

56. Cao Q, Cai W, Li ZB, Chen K, He L, Li HC et al (2007) PET imaging of acute and chronic inflammation in living mice. Eur J Nucl Med Mol Imaging 34(11):1832–1842

Part III

Imaging of Lower Urinary and Male Genital Tract Infections

Ultrasound of Lower Urinary Tract Infections

14

Emilio Quaia, Antonio G. Gennari, and Maria A. Cova

14.1 Bladder

Acute bladder infection and inflammation (cystitis) is the most common infection of all UTI counting 0.70 episodes per person-year in young women starting a new contraceptive method and 0.07 episodes per person-year in postmenopausal women [1]. Moreover cystitis has a high recurrence rate with 25% of women experiencing further episodes within 6 months, and rate increases with more than one prior UTI [1]. A cystitis occurring in healthy premenopausal, non-pregnant women with no suspects of abnormalities of the urinary tract is generally classified as uncomplicated, rarely progresses to severe disease, so do not necessitate further investigations other than a short-course antibiotic treatment [1]. A gram-negative organism is isolated in the vast majority of patients, with *Escherichia coli* being the most common organism encountered. Other pathogens such as *Klebsiella pneumoniae* and *Proteus mirabilis* and gram-positive organisms of *Enterococcus* species are isolated less frequently

and sometimes may raise suspicions about culture contamination [1, 2]. Up to two-thirds of the episodes of recurrent cystitis involves the same strain of bacteria that caused the initial infection [1]. There are several associated risk factors for uncomplicated sporadic and recurrent cystitis such as irritating hygiene products, sexual intercourse, reaction to certain drugs, use of diaphragms or spermicides, previous UTI, a new sex partner (within the past year) and a history of UTI in a first-degree female relative [1]. Older populations often have predisposing factors, such as diabetes mellitus, urinary retention due to an enlarged prostate. increased exposure to interventions such as catheterisation and menopause which are associated to an increased susceptibility to infection [2]. Symptoms of cystitis are dysuria; nocturia, with or without urinary frequency and urgency; suprapubic discomfort; and, occasionally, gross haematuria.

Cystitis is a clinical diagnosis, so imaging usually is not required.

14.1.1 Recurrent Bladder Infection/ Chronic Cystitis

Chronic cystitis (CC) is a recurrent bladder infection. As previously said the most common cause of recurrent bladder infection is reinfection. CC is more common in women than in men, particularly in women over 30 years old and even more

E. Quaia (✉)
Edinburgh Imaging facility, Queen's Medical Research Institute, University of Edinburgh, 47 Little France Crescent, Edinburgh EH16 4TJ, UK
e-mail: equaia@exseed.ed.ac.uk

A.G. Gennari • M.A. Cova
Department of Radiology, Cattinara Hospital, University of Trieste, Strada di Fiume 447, Trieste 34149, Italy

© Springer International Publishing AG 2018
M. Tonolini (ed.), *Imaging and Intervention in Urinary Tract Infections and Urosepsis*,
https://doi.org/10.1007/978-3-319-68276-1_14

frequent in women over their 50s. Reinfection does not require a specific urologic evaluation and is managed conservatively with the same therapy as acute cystitis. Symptoms and bacteria are the same as the ones detailed for acute bladder infection.

CC is a clinical diagnosis, and management is not dependent on imaging, particularly in sporadic cases. However in cases of several repeated episodes, imaging helps in defining the underlying cause of symptoms, such as tumours, bladder outlet obstruction and bladder calculi. Typical findings are non-specific and shared with several other forms of cystitis. Plain film allows imaging bladder calculi. At US evaluation are a focal or diffuse mucosal thickening, irregularities and mucosal ulceration of varying intensity. In patients with a mass protruding in the bladder lumen, attached to the mucosal surface, it is important to modify patient decubitus and use colour Doppler evaluation to correctly differentiate thrombus from bladder cancer. A thrombus generated by a small ulceration modifies its position, contrary to tumour that does not. Contrast-enhanced ultrasound (CEUS) may better demonstrate the absence of internal contrast typical of thrombus.

14.1.2 Emphysematous Cystitis

Emphysematous cystitis (EC) is a potentially life-threatening condition, defined as air within the bladder lumen or in the bladder wall, and requires prompt diagnosis and treatment. Prevalence and incidence are unknown; however it is more frequent in middle-aged women, with a man-to-women ratio of 1.8:1 [3]. Moreover EC is highly related to diabetes mellitus; in fact two-thirds of patients had it. Predisposing factors are chronic UTI, indwelling urethral catheters, urinary tract outlet obstruction and neurogenic bladder [3, 4]. Symptoms may vary ranging from sepsis to incidental diagnosis. The most frequent ones are dysuria, haematuria, abdominal pain and urinary urgency and frequency, which are similar to the symptoms of uncomplicated cystitis [4]. The presence of pneumaturia is highly suspicious of EC, but it could be also related to colovesical fistula, bladder instrumentation, Crohn's disease or carcinoma

of the colon or bladder [3, 4]. The most prevalent pathogen isolated in urine culture of EC patients is *E. coli* (58% of cases); anyhow various other bacterial and fungal organisms proved to be related with EC such as *K. pneumoniae*, *Pseudomonas aeruginosa*, *P. mirabilis*, *Candida albicans* and many more [3, 4]. Several theories have been postulated to explain gas formation. In one the combination of high tissue glucose level, gas-forming pathogens and poor tissue vascularisation is all related to emphysematous infection. The high-glucose tissue concentration allows bacteria to produce carbon dioxide through natural fermentation process [3]. In another, used to explain EC in non-diabetic patients, albumin is the substrate for gas production. An impaired host response to pathogens, due to vascular compromise and impaired catabolism in the tissue, is another theory proposed [3]. When left untreated, mortality rate is as high as 7%.

Diagnosis relies on radiographic procedures rather than in clinical ones. If EC is suspected, a simple plain radiography of the abdomen should be ordered [4]. Typical findings are a curvilinear radiolucency outlining the bladder wall with or without luminal gas associated. US of the bladder may reveal an abnormal ticked bladder wall with dirty shadowing associated. However US findings are not specific for EC.

14.1.3 Schistosomiasis

The pathogenesis, symptoms and pathologic modification related with schistosomiasis have been elucidated in the previous chapter. As previously said the bladder, together with the intestine, is involved in the final part of the life cycle of the *Schistosoma haematobium* during oviposition. There, a granulomatous response to infection develops.

When bladder lesions heal, they often calcify, determining the typical linear opacity in plain X-ray exams. However at least 100,000 calcified eggs per cubic millimetre are needed to be detected at radiography [5]. Initially lesions have patchy nature and may spare relatively healthy mucosa, but with chronic infection they tend to coalesce, and the bladder mucosa calcification is more homogeneous. So at plain films, the appearance is various: may encircle the bladder or may affect only parts of it or one side more than another [5]. Moreover submucosa and muscle layer involvement and fibrosis determine a reduction in bladder capacity due to contraction of the bladder [6]. The 'bladder neck obstruction' is a condition related to eggs entering the muscle creating a sort of hyperplasia that later evolves in fibrosis [5]. This condition is typically described in Egypt [5]. At IVU the formation of submucosal oedema and pseudotubercles determines haziness of the bladder outline with a nodular bladder wall thickening. Chronic bladder wall irritation determines also urothelium penetration and proliferation in the lamina propria, creating buds (von Brunn nests) [5]. These buds evolve into cystic deposits. The latter stage is the formation of cystitis cystica, or cystitis glandularis, when intestinal columnar mucin-secreting glands (goblet cells) are present [5].

14.1.4 Tuberculosis

The pathogenesis, symptoms and pathologic modification related with tuberculosis have been elucidated in the previous chapter. Since the genitourinary tract is frequently involved and tuberculosis of the bladder is present in 10–45.6% of patients with urogenital tuberculosis, this possibility must be kept in mind. In fact, tuberculosis bacilli reach the urinary bladder from the infected kidney through the ureters. Granulomatous lesion produces tumour-like mass or ulcer. The extensive fibrosis produced by chronic infection determines a shrunken, small, urinary bladder (thimble bladder) (see Fig. 3 in Chap. 17). That is why recurrent UTI associated with pus, in absence of positive urine culture for usual pathogens, should always raise the suspicion of urinary tract tuberculosis.

Multiple irregular mucosal masses may be seen at US determined by coalescing tubercles with ulceration and oedema, diffuse wall thickening and trabeculation [7]. IVU demonstrates an irregular bladder mucosa, with associated ureteral strictures. The vesicoureteric junction orifice could be thickened and obstructed, resulting in vesicoureteric reflux [7]. A contracted, thick-walled bladder is detected in chronic stages when there is bladder fibrosis. Bladder wall calcifica-

tion is not a frequent finding and is seen only after healing allowing an easy differential diagnosis with schistosomiasis [7].

14.2 Prostate

Acute prostatitis is a severe, potentially life-threatening systemic infection [2]. Clinical manifestations are simple and include fever and perineal pain or tenderness, symptoms of lower UTI such as urgency, frequency or nocturia and, occasionally, obstructive uropathy. It is encountered in both young sexually active men and in older ones with predisposing risk factors such as bladder voiding outlet obstruction usually due to benign prostatic hyperplasia (BPH). Moreover the rate of progression to chronic prostatitis is approximately 5%. Several theories proved to define the exact aetiology; however, intraprostatic urinary reflux is the most widely accepted. The infection is generated by infected urine reflux into the ejaculatory and prostatic ducts. Since ducts draining the peripheral zone are positioned more horizontally than others, most infections occur in the peripheral zone. However acute prostatitis may be also related with sexual intercourse, instrumentation and prolonged catheterisation. Acute bacterial prostatitis is usually generated by a single pathogen that in the majority of cases is *E. coli*, but *P. mirabilis*, *Klebsiella* species, *Enterobacter* species, *P. aeruginosa* and *Serratia* species may also produce prostatitis. Symptoms may vary and depend on the severity of the case but usually include fever, chills, pelvic pain, dysuria, haematuria, urinary frequency, a painful ejaculation, haematospermia and pain localised at genitals, testicles or rectum. An uncommon but threatening complication of acute prostatitis is prostatic abscess. It usually occurs in immunocompromised or diabetic patients or in ones with prolonged indwelling urethral catheters.

Imaging techniques are not mandatory to diagnose acute prostatitis; however transrectal US (TRUS) shows an enlarged prostate gland with homogeneous hypoechoic parenchyma due to oedema. Colour Doppler and power Doppler US demonstrate a diffuse increased blood signal [8]. TRUS may be helpful in the evaluation of complication of acute prostatitis such as prostatic abscess. It manifests as a defined round hypoechoic or anechoic mass with increased flow signal around it at colour Doppler evaluation enlargement [8]. Moreover TRUS may guide abscess drainage.

14.2.1 Chronic Prostatitis

Chronic bacterial prostatitis is quite common and may manifest as recurring UTI that lasts for at least 3 months. It will affect about two men in ten at some point during their life; however it is more common in men between the ages of 30 and 50 but may affect men of any age. Chronic prostatitis is sustained by the same bacterial strains isolated in acute bacterial prostatitis [2] and is not a sexually transmitted infection. Bacteria eradication is very difficult and challenging due to limited diffusion of antibiotic agents into the gland or to the presence of colonised prostate stones [2]. Moreover migration of pathogens persisting in the prostate, in the bladder and in the urethra may determine recurrent cystitis. Symptoms are similar to the ones of acute bacterial prostatitis, but they wax and wane and usually are less severe compared to that of acute bacterial prostatitis. The most frequent symptom is a persistent discomfort or pain in the pelvic region, mainly at the base of the penis and around the anus.

At TRUS the main features of chronic prostatitis are the presence of prostatic calcifications and calculi. Prostatic calcifications are easily encountered in older men and are not a specific finding of chronic prostatitis; contrary, prostate calculi are more frequent in patients with chronic prostatitis than in general population and could be easily identified with TRUS but could be detected also on plain film [9]. Moreover an increased colour Doppler blood flow was defined as a marker to identify chronic prostatitis [9].

14.3 Seminal Vesicles

Acute seminal vesiculitis is usually secondary to prostatitis. Chronic vesiculitis is rare and challenging to diagnose since symptomatology is usually non-specific. Anyhow, the reproductive health is strictly related to a correct diagnosis. Abscess formation is related to low drug concentration within the seminal vesicles (SV) due to low vascularity and is more frequent in patients undergoing instrumentation or surgery or in diabetic patients [10]. Moreover it is often paired with a prostatic abscess. In endemic areas, tuberculosis and schistosomiasis should be considered as possible aetiologies.

Typical imaging findings of vesiculitis on US include diffuse wall thickening [10]. Cystic dilation of the seminal vesicles is frequent in acute and subacute phase and may be seen at US.

In the initial phase, seminal vesicles are enlarged with destruction of convolutions and hypoechoic areas on US (see Fig. 14.14 of Chap. 14) [11]. Abscess formation follows with caseation, cavitation (Fig. 14.1) and fibrosis and may eventually result in a calcified mass [11].

In endemic areas of schistosomiasis, postmortem studies have demonstrated parasite eggs in the SV of approximately 58% of the male cadavers [11]. Seminal vesiculitis is due to *Schistosoma* eggs deposited into the wall of the SV and may lead to SV dilatation and wall calcifications, best seen on CT or US [11].

14.4 Scrotal Infections

Scrotum is a complex anatomical male reproductive structure composed of a dual chamber sac each of which could be divided into an inner portion composed by the testis, epididymis and ductus deferens and an outer portion, the scrotal wall. Both the inner and the outer portion may be infected by pathogens. Even though clinical examination may guide the diagnosis, symptoms are shared with other pathological entities such as testicular torsion that represents a urological emergency.

14.4.1 Epididymitis, Orchitis and Epididymo-Orchitis

Epididymo-orchitis (EO) and epididymitis are the most common causes of scrotal pain. Even though

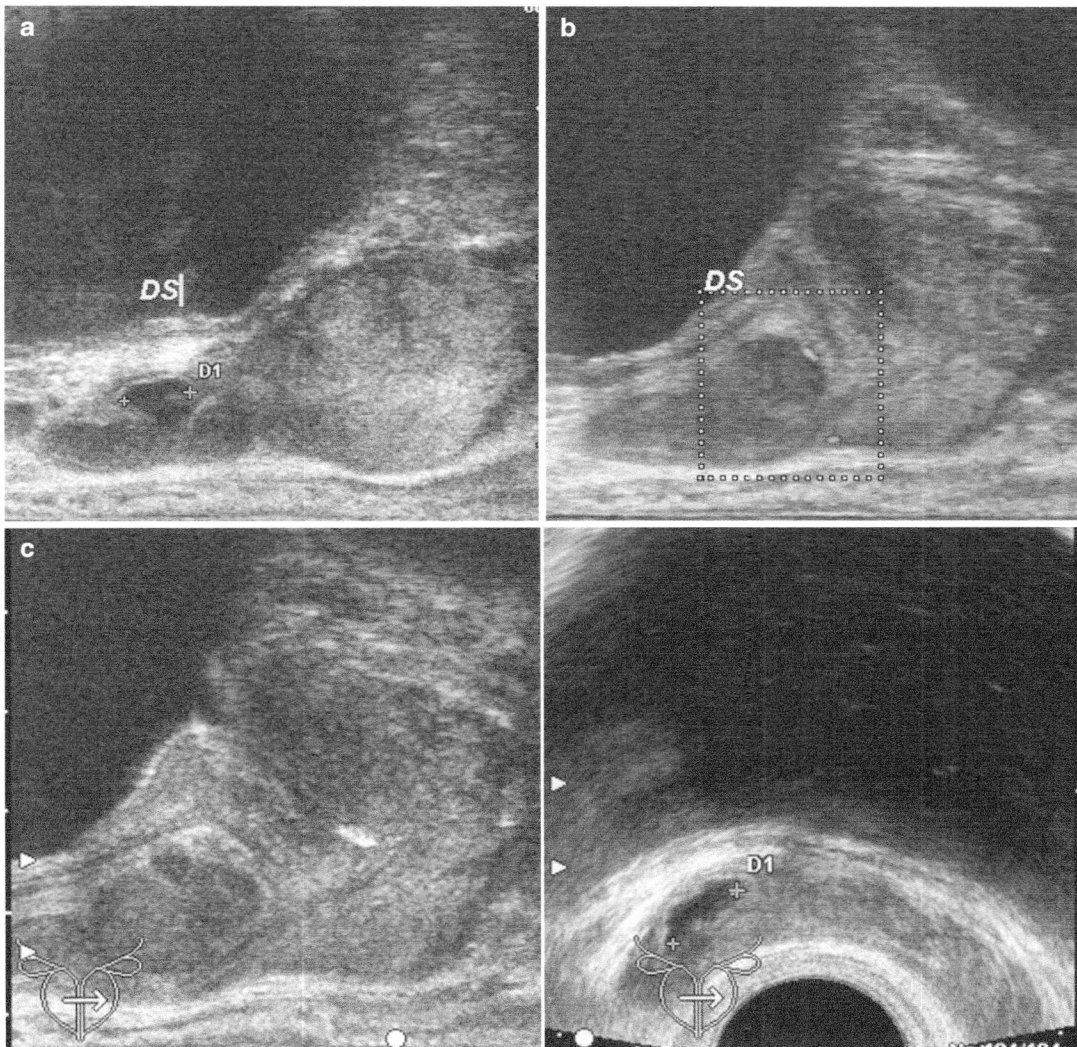

Fig. 14.1 In a 50-year-old HIV-positive male with hae-mospermia, longitudinal (**a**, **b**) and transverse (**c**) transrectal ultrasound images showed chronic infection of the right seminal vesicle, which appeared as hypoechoic, poorly vascularised (colour Doppler image in **b**) enlargement containing an anechoic liquefied focus (calipers)

UTI is not so frequent in males, epididymitis results from retrograde bacteria seed and infection of the epididymis via the urethra through the urinary and reproductive system. Epididymis is directly connected with the prostate and SV through the ductus deferens, so it is the first site of infection. Bacteria could spread further reaching testis and generating an EO. Isolated orchitis is less frequent and usually related with mumps virus. Bloodstream route of infection is unusual. Acute epididymitis and EO are more common in young and middle-aged (35–50 years old), sexu-ally active men. The most frequent pathogens encountered are *Chlamydia trachomatis* that accounts for two-thirds of acute cases, *Neisseria gonorrhoeae* and *E. coli*. The latter one, which represents enteric flora, is commonly encountered in older patients and homosexuals. Tuberculosis and brucellosis infection are encountered in immu-nosuppressed patients. Schistosomiasis may gen-erate EO, in tropical countries. Clinically patient presents with pain, tenderness and swelling of a single scrotum and its content. The most important differential diagnosis that has to be made is with testicular torsion that represents a urologic emergency. The clinical hallmark of testicular torsion is a higher position of the testis within the scrotal sac, contrary to EO testicle will hang low in the scrotum. Moreover in EO the cremasteric reflex is present, and Prehn's sign (the relief of scrotal pain during elevation of the testicle) may aid in the differential diagnosis, although non-specific. Complications of epididymitis and EO include abscesses, testicular ischaemia and pyocele formation. Testicular ischaemia is generated by the obstruction of venous outflow, related to the testicular enlargement and engorgement, and produces impairment of the arterial blood supply. Testicular ischaemia may evolve in segmental or global testicular infarction [12]. In chronic epididymitis, a disease that lasts for over 3 months, patients have had symptoms for over 5 years. Palpation may reveal an indurated epididymis with or without irregular shape. The differential diagnosis includes causes of chronic scrotal pain such as testicular cancer and varicocele.

US is definitely the imaging modality of choice in the evaluation of the acute scrotum. An entirely or partially enlarged hypoechoic or hyperechoic (thought to be related to haemorrhage) epididymis is a frequent finding [13, 14]. Diffuse or focal epididymis and testicular enlargement associated with a focal or a global uneven echotexture are findings suggesting concurrent epididymitis or orchitis [13–15]. These areas are usually hypoechoic compared to the adjacent normal parenchyma. At colour Doppler evaluation, EO and epididymitis demonstrate hyperaemia and hypervascularisation of the involved areas. It is well established that colour Doppler demonstrates a high sensitivity in detecting scrotal inflammation (see Figs. 4, 5 and 6 of Chap. 15) [13, 14]. In acute epididymitis, the spectral analysis of arterial flow demonstrates a reduced resistive index (below 0.7) compared to normal ones. Also the spectral analysis of testicular arterial flow is usually lower (below 0.5). A thickening of scrotal tunica and the presence of hydrocele, an anechoic fluid collection that surrounds the anterolateral aspects of the testis [13], are frequent associated findings. Pyocele may be present in more serious cases. At US it can be visualised as cystic lesions with internal septations and loculations. Scrotal skin thickening, an enlarged epididymis characterised by increased echogenicity and calcifications, on the other hand, are findings that indicate chronic epididymitis [14]. Furthermore US may be used to correctly differentiate EO from testicular torsion and diagnose EO complications such as abscess formation and testicular ischaemia. In high-grade testicular torsion, the testis is completely avascular, and a twisting of the spermatic cord may be depicted. Contrary to low-degree testicular torsion, in which intratesticular arteries demonstrate high-resistance flow signal at spectral analysis [12]. Abscesses present as hypo- or anechoic areas of fluid collection, with irregular borders with hypoechoic edges [13]. Sometimes intra-abscess gas is visualised as focal hyperechoic spot with posterior shadowing. At colour Doppler evaluation, the inner part of abscesses is not vascularised; contrary, the outer part demonstrates perilesional hyperaemia [13]. An enlarged testis with reduced vascularisation compared to the contralateral one is the hallmark for testicular ischaemia [13]. Moreover spectral analysis demonstrates increased resistive index compared to normal. CEUS is useful in the evaluation of tissue vascularity, so it helps in differentiating necrotic from viable, hypoperfused testis [12]. Moreover CEUS allows to follow up patients and monitor the restoration of parenchymal vascularisation during therapy or progression to global infarction. Anyhow an enlarged, irregularly hypoechoic testis is not specific for orchitis. In fact lymphoma, which represents the most frequent testicular malignancy in middle-aged patients, may present with similar features. Lymphoma has an infiltrative growth pattern, so at US evaluation, it may present as single or multiple areas of reduced echogenicity or as a diffuse enlarged hypoechoic testis without loss of testicular shape [12]. Moreover vascularity may be increased, and testicular vascular anatomy is normal. Those cases are challenging, and accurate evaluation of patient symptoms and laboratory and clinical examination is mandatory. MR is useful in complicated or inadequately treated patients and in ones with unusual US appearance.

14.4.2 Fournier's Gangrene

Fournier's gangrene (FG) is a polymicrobial necrotising fasciitis that involves the perineal, perianal or genital regions and constitutes a urologic emergency with a potentially high mortality rate (7–50%) [16, 17]. Accurate incidence rates are not known, but the disease is relatively rare. Usually FG affects middle-aged patients (50–60 years old) with a male-to-female ratio of roughly 10:1; however, the diagnosis in females is underreported. The Parisian venereologist Jean Alfred Fournier originally described FG in 1883, without any underlying clear aetiology. Nowadays, the relationship between FG and the impaired local blood supply, the subsequent vascular thrombosis of cutaneous and subcutaneous tissues due to oedema and inflammation induced by an infection is well established. Primary bacterial sources include anorectal, genitourinary and cutaneous sources. Urethral strictures, chronic UTI, neurogenic bladder, recent instrumentation and epididymitis are all suspected causes of urologic sources of FG [17]. On the other hand, anal fissures and colonic perforations are the ones claimed for anorectal sources. The most commonly encountered pathogens are *E. coli*, *Bacteroides*, *Streptococcus*, *Staphylococcus*, *Clostridium* and *Klebsiella*. Predisposing factors are immunosuppression, steroid therapy, diabetes, alcohol abuse, malignancies and hepatic and renal impairment. Early diagnosis is mandatory due to the high rate of perifascial dissection with subsequent spread of bacteria and progression to gangrene (up to 2–3 cm per hour) [16]. Necrotising fasciitis may spread along Colles fascia, Buck fascia or dartos fascia and reach neighbours' tissues. Scrotal swelling, pain, crepitus, fever and hyperaemia are the most common symptoms. Crepitus is encountered in up to 64% of patients and is produced by insoluble gas produced by anaerobic bacteria in the soft tissues [16, 17]. The differential diagnoses include cellulitis, testicular torsion and epididymitis. Broad-spectrum antibiotic therapy and rapid surgical debridement of all necrotic tissues are the treatment of choice.

At plain films, scrotal swelling and hyperlucencies (representing soft tissues gas) may be depicted before the crepitus is present at physical examination. However these are rare findings [17]. Beside US may be helpful and consistent in demonstrating a thickened, oedematous, scrotal wall (Fig. 14.2a–c) with hyperechoic foci with reverberation artefact inside representing the gas [16–18]. Moreover US may precede clinical findings and exclude differential diagnosis such as inguinal hernia or the ones previously detailed due to the normal greyscale appearance of the testes and epididymis. Vascularisation of scrotal wall is related to the pudendal arteries, branches of femoral arteries; contrary, testicular arteries arise directly from aorta, so testes and epididymis vascularisation is preserved.

14.4.3 Scrotal Wall Cellulitis and Scrotal Wall Abscess

Scrotal wall cellulitis is more frequent in obese, diabetic or immunocompromised patients; however scrotal wall abscess may occur also in young men due to infected hair follicles and infections of scrotal lacerations. Scrotal wall abscess may be the evolution of untreated scrotal cellulitis. Patient presents with signs of inflammation and pain in scrotal region. Even though the diagnosis seems easy thanks to the history and physical examination (absence of Prehn's sign and the testis hanging low in the scrotal sac), however, the pain could be so important to mimic testicular torsion or EO. The scrotum is often erythematous and oedematous, and a scrotal fluctuance may be palpable.

US may be used to confirm diagnosis in non-obvious cases. The most important findings are the absence of any pathologic imaging alteration of epididymis and testis. Scrotal wall thickness is increased, and hypoechoic areas with increased blood flow seen at colour Doppler may be depicted. As previously described in epididymitis and EO orchitis subchapter, abscesses (Fig. 14.2D) are hypo-anechoic well-loculated areas, with irregular borders, and may contain debris [14].

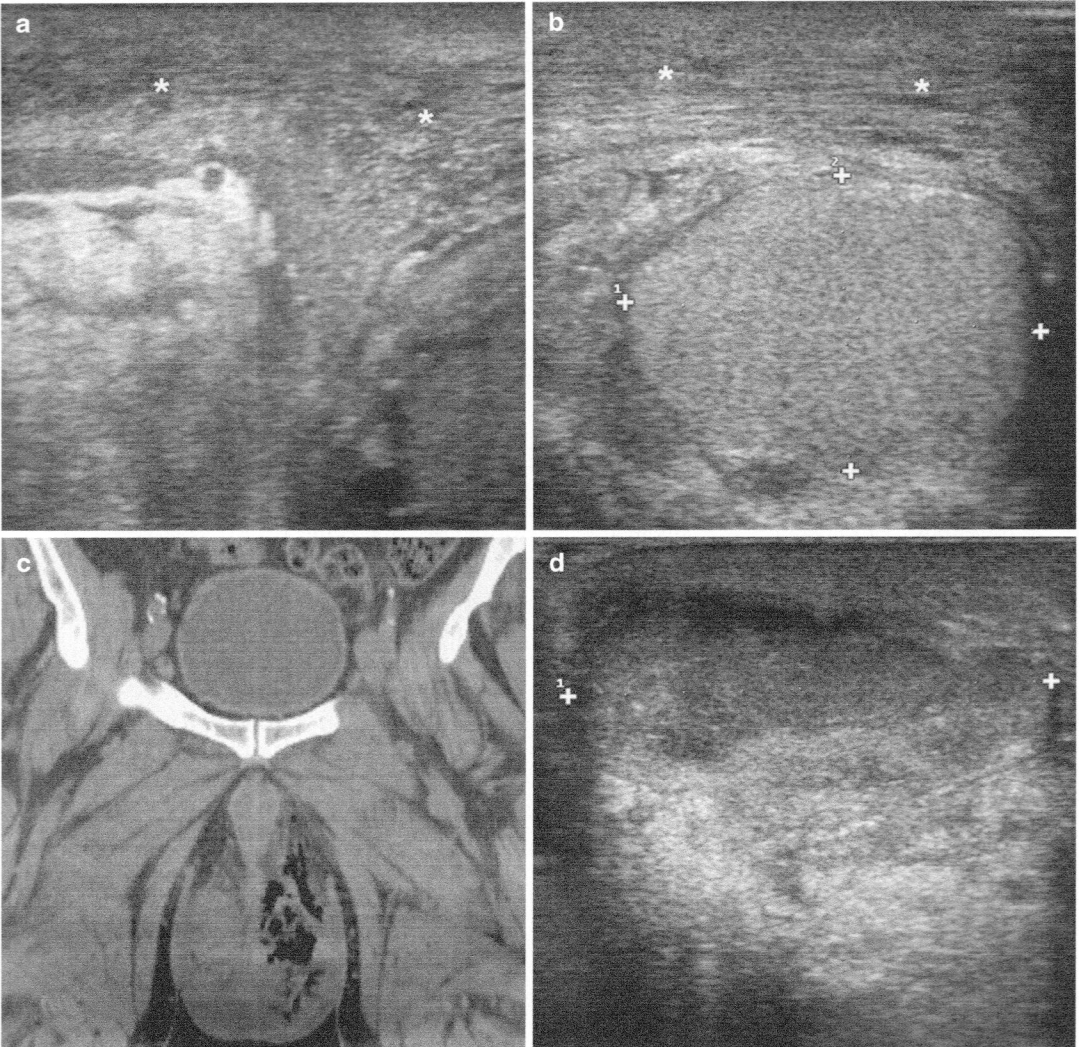

Fig. 14.2 In a 60-year-old male with diabetes, recurrent urinary tract infections and left-sided scrotal swelling, ultrasound (**a**, **b**) showed marked oedematous thickening of the superficial tissues (*), without hydrocele and signs of acute orchitis (testis is indicated by calipers), which ultimately corresponded to clinically unsuspected Fournier's gangrene as better demonstrated by CT (**c**) detection of intrascrotal gas. In a different male patient, ultrasound (**d**) depicted an elongated, hypo-anechoic abscess (between calipers) of the scrotal wall

References

1. Hooton T (2012) Uncomplicated urinary tract infection. N Engl J Med 2012 366:1028–1037
2. Solomon CG, Schaeffer AJ, Nicolle LE (2016) Urinary tract infections in older men. N Engl J Med 374(6):562–571
3. Thomas AA, Lane BR, Thomas AZ, Remer EM, Campbell SC, Shoskes DA (2007) Emphysematous cystitis: a review of 135 cases. BJU Int 100(1):17–20
4. Eken A, Alma E (2013) Emphysematous cystitis: the role of CT imaging and appropriate treatment. J Can Urol Assoc 7(11–12):11–13
5. Shebel HM, Elsayes KM, Abou El Atta HM, Elguindy YM, El-Diasty TA (2012) Genitourinary schistosomiasis: life cycle and radiologic-pathologic findings. Radiographics 32:1031–1046
6. Barsoum RS (2013) Urinary schistosomiasis: review. J Adv Res 4(5):453–459
7. Wong-you-Cheong JJ, Woodward PJ, Maria A, Davis CJ (2006) From the archives of the AFIP inflammatory and

nonneoplastic bladder masses: radiologic-pathologic correlation. Radiographics 1595(4):2006

8. Seung-Hyup K, Min-Hoan M, Byung-Kwan P (2002) Clinical applications of transrectal ultrasound in the prostate and seminal tract. J Med Ultrasound 10(4):181–190

9. Wee A, Shoskes DA (2008) Ultrasound findings in patients with chronic prostatitis/chronic pelvic pain syndrome. Curr Prostate Rep 6:182–184

10. Kim B, Kawashima A, Ryu J-A, Takahashi N, Hartman RP, King BF (2009) Imaging of the seminal vesicle and vas deferens. Radiographics 29(4):1105–1121

11. Reddy MN, Verma S (2014) Lesions of the seminal vesicles and their MRI characteristics. J Clin Imaging Sci 4(4):61

12. Bertolotto M, Cantisani V, Valentino M, Pavlica P, Derchi LE (2016) Pitfalls in imaging for acute scrotal pathology. Semin Roentgenol 51(1):60–69

13. Pavlica P, Barozzi L (2001) Imaging of the acute scrotum. Eur Radiol 11(2):220–228

14. Gottlieb RH, Oka M (2003) Sonography of the scrotum. Radiology i(1):18–36

15. Schull A, Monzani Q, Bour L, Barry-Delongchamps N, Beuvon F, Legmann P et al (2012) Imaging in lower urinary tract infections. Diagn Interv Imaging 93(5):500–508

16. Kim DJ, Kendall JL (2013) Fournier's Gangrene and its characteristic ultrasound findings. J Emerg Med 44(1):1–3

17. Levenson RB, Singh AK, Novelline RA (2008) Fournier gangrene: role of imaging. Radiographics 28:519–528

18. Feldman MK (2009) US Artifacts 1. Radiographics 29:1179–1189

Cross-Sectional Imaging of Urinary Bladder, Prostate and Seminal Vesicle Infections

15

Massimo Tonolini

As discussed in the previous chapter of this book, ultrasound with colour Doppler represents the mainstay first-line technique to investigate the lower urogenital tract, particularly in patients with acute conditions involving the urinary bladder, prostate, penis and scrotum [1–3].

However, during the last decade, the dramatic technical advances in multidetector computed tomography (CT) and magnetic resonance imaging (MRI) have increasingly provided a comprehensive multiplanar assessment of genitourinary structures and disorders with high spatial and contrast resolution. This chapter reviews the CT and MRI techniques and imaging appearances of urinary tract infections (UTIs) affecting the urinary bladder, prostate and seminal vesicles, with an emphasis on their differential diagnosis [3–5].

15.1 CT Technique and Indications in the Lower Urogenital Tract

State-of-the-art multidetector CT provides a panoramic visualisation of the entire abdomen and pelvis and is recommended by the World Society of Emergency Surgery (WSES) as the mainstay modality to comprehensively search for intra-abdominal infections in the majority of situations [6]. Compared to ultrasound, CT consistently detects:

(a) Inflammatory changes in the perivisceral fat
(b) Abnormal gaseous, fluid, abscessual or haemorrhagic collections
(c) Calcific lithiasis in the kidneys and along the urinary tract
(d) Implanted medical devices
(e) More or less subtle thickening and abnormal contrast enhancement of the pyeloureteral and bladder wall
(f) Renal and excretory functional information from contrast enhancement [3–5, 7]

As discussed in the appropriate chapter of this book, in patients with urosepsis or sepsis from unknown source, CT offers a proven benefit in detecting the infectious focus and the possible underlying structural abnormalities of the urinary tract. The main indications for obtaining CT include:

(a) Suspected or confirmed urinary sepsis
(b) Unexplained sepsis
(c) High or persistent clinical suspicion of lower urogenital tract infection despite inconclusive ultrasound findings
(d) Suspected or culture-proven complicated UTI, particularly those associated with the usual risk factors such as diabetes, immunosuppression, nephropathy, obstructive uropathy and urologic instrumentation [4, 6, 8, 9]

M. Tonolini, M.D.
Radiology Department, "Luigi Sacco" University Hospital, Via G.B. Grassi 74, Milan 20157, Italy
e-mail: mtonolini@sirm.org

© Springer International Publishing AG 2018
M. Tonolini (ed.), *Imaging and Intervention in Urinary Tract Infections and Urosepsis*,
https://doi.org/10.1007/978-3-319-68276-1_15

Indwelling (Foley-type or suprapubic) catheters should be closed before CT, in order to achieve adequate urinary bladder distension which allows assessing the true mural thickness. However, this is usually difficult to obtain, since most patients with chronic lower urinary tract dysfunction poorly tolerate bladder filling [4].

In our experience, the CT protocol should include a preliminary unenhanced acquisition, which is generally withheld in young patients to limit the erogated radiation dose and when urolithiasis has been ruled out on clinical or imaging grounds. Enhancement by intravenous iodinated contrast medium (CM) is warranted, unless contraindicated by history of allergy or impaired renal function. Particularly in septic or dehydrated patients with limited urine output, according to the European Society of Urogenital Radiology (ESUR) guidelines, special care in ensuring adequate hydration before and after CT is recommended, both to improve urinary tract opacification and prevent CM nephrotoxicity [10, 11].

In the setting of suspected or confirmed UTI, a single breath-hold nephrographic CT acquisition is acquired using a 75–85 s delay, which should encompass the abdomen, pelvis and perineum. An optional excretory phase acquired 5–20 min after CM injection visualises the opacified urinary collecting systems, ureter and bladder. Strategies for dose reduction such as automated tube current modulation or, if available, iterative reconstruction from raw CT data are recommended. Modern double- or triple-bolus CT-urography protocols are appealing to radiologists since they provide a comprehensive corticomedullary, nephrographic and excretory imaging with reduced effective radiation dose in a single volumetric acquisition; however CT-urography may be misleading in the investigation of suspected UTI since densely opacified urine in the collecting systems, ureters and bladder easily masks the subtle urothelial enhancement which is one of the key signs of active infection [12–14].

To elucidate the lower urogenital anatomy, multidetector CT studies tailored to the urinary tract are routinely visualised along axial, coronal and sagittal planes [4].

In selected patients, performing multidetector CT-cystography is beneficial to visualise or otherwise exclude urinary bladder leaks (such as those resulting from surgery, obstetric injuries or instrumentation) and fistulas. At our Department of Radiology, CT-cystography is performed, after preliminary bladder emptying, using slow retrograde administration by gravity of CM diluted 1:10 in saline through the Foley catheter, until the patient complains of intolerable bladder distension, flow stops or at least 300 mL is injected. Then, volumetric CT of the pelvis is acquired with an adequately distended, uniformly opacified urinary bladder and visualised along multiple planes at CT angiography window settings (width 600–900 HU, level 150–300 HU) and optionally with additional maximum intensity projection (MIP) or volume rendering techniques [15–17].

15.2 MRI Role and Technique

Up to a few years ago, the use of MRI to investigate acute abdominal conditions was largely limited by scanner time availability, lengthy examination, and need for patient cooperation: since then, state-of-the-art scanners have now significantly decreased most of these limitations. Compared to CT, MRI provides multiplanar visualisation of the pelvic, genital and perineal structures with superior contrast resolution and thus allows better tissue characterisation: for instance, fat-suppressed T2-weighted sequences easily show detected oedematous changes without the use of intravenous contrast. However, MRI is insensitive for calcifications and gas. Albeit increasingly appealing to avoid irradiation of the reproductive organs, MRI may still be contraindicated by claustrophobia, early pregnancy, metallic foreign body in vital sites, cardiac pacemaker or other non-MRI compatible implanted devices [18–20].

In our experience, MRI is increasingly established as a problem-solving modality to investigate disorders of the urinary bladder, prostate and seminal vesicles after inconclusive sonographic and CT findings or as a first-line examination in younger patients. On current high-magnetic field strength MRI scanners, pelvic studies are routinely acquired using phased-array coils. The patient is positioned supine on the scanner table;

in males a folded towel is positioned between the legs to elevate the scrotum, with the penis secured at the midline hypogastrium. Most MRI acquisition protocols heavily rely on multiplanar high-resolution T2-weighted sequences, centred in the region of interest, with spectral fat suppression or short-tau inversion recovery (STIR) in at least one plane to detect parenchymal or perivisceral oedematous changes (Fig. 15.1). Optional MR urography sequences using heavily T2-weighted sequences sensitive to static fluid may provide a panoramic view of the entire urinary collecting systems without the use of intravenous contrast. Albeit contraindicated in patients with severely decreased renal function (glomerular filtration rate below 30 mL/min), the injection of gadolinium-based CM provides a comprehensive examination including information on enhancement, generally with acquisition of three-dimensional fat-suppressed gradient-echo T1-weighted sequences such as THRIVE, LAVA or VIBE (Fig. 15.1): however, in our expe-

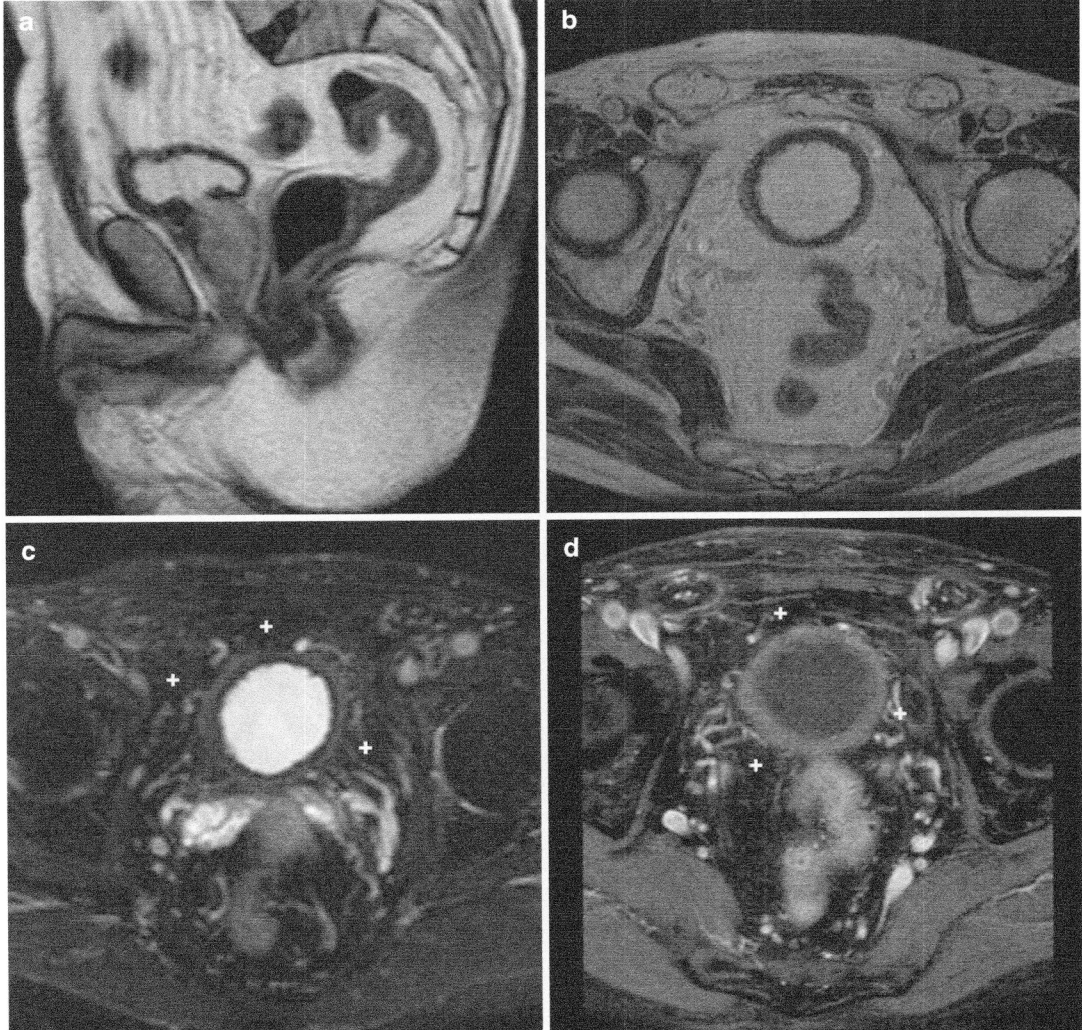

Fig. 15.1 Usual MR appearance of senile urinary bladder with detrusor hypertrophy, in a patient without ongoing infectious or neoplastic processes. Sagittal (**a**) and axial (**b**) T2-weighted images show moderately distensible bladder filled with urine, with mild circumferential mural thickening and minimal uniform irregularities along the mucosal surface. The fat-saturated STIR image (**c**) and post-gadolinium T1-weighted (**d**) images exclude oedematous changes and abnormal contrast enhancement in the bladder wall and perivesical fat planes (+)

rience unenhanced MRI is frequently sufficient to provide the key information on the lower urogenital structures [3, 4].

15.3 Cross-Sectional Imaging of Urinary Bladder Infections

15.3.1 Infectious Cystitis

The cross-sectional imaging diagnosis of acute infectious cystitis (AIC) is suggested by a combination of three features:

(a) Oedematous mural bladder thickening
(b) Inflammation of the surrounding fat planes
(c) Urothelial hyperenhancement

Concerning the first feature, a circumferential wall thickening is commonly encountered on CT studies performed for investigation of suspected UTI or sepsis, since most patients experiencing complicated UTIs have a poorly distensible, thickened urinary bladder from underlying chronic conditions such as detrusor hypertrophy and recurrent infections (Fig. 15.1). However, in our experience a diffuse wall thickening may correspond to acute UTI, particularly when:

(a) Marked (over 1 cm)
(b) Increased compared to previous studies
(c) With hypoenhancing dominant muscular layer corresponding to intramural oedema (Figs. 15.2 and 15.3)

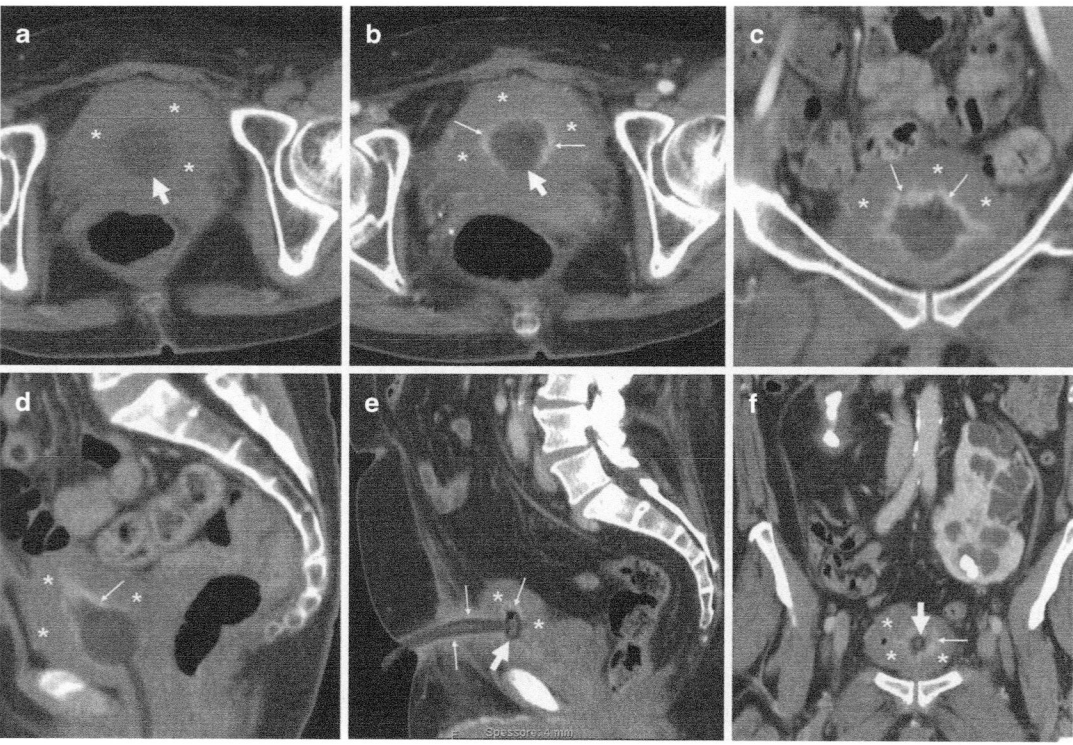

Fig. 15.2 Active infectious cystitis in a 52-year-old diabetic female with dehydration, pelvic and flank pain, pyuria and elevated C-reactive protein (CRP). Unenhanced (**a**) and contrast-enhanced (**b–d**) multidetector CT images showed contracted urinary bladder with Foley catheter (thick arrows), marked circumferential mural thickening (*) with hypoenhancing oedematous wall and urothelial hyperenhancement (thin arrows). Urine cultures revealed polymicrobial infection including *Staphylococcus aureus* and multiresistant extended-spectrum beta-lactamase (ESBL)-positive *Escherichia coli* (Reproduced from Open Access Ref.no. [4]). Similarly, in a different male patient, post-contrast CT (**e, f**) showed contracted bladder with marked diffuse bladder wall thickening (*) and urothelial hyperenhancement (thin arrows) which extended along the suprapubic catheter (thick arrows) track

Additionally, suspicion of AIC is suggested or reinforced by the identification of "hazy" increased attenuation corresponding to inflammation of the extraperitoneal perivesical fat planes (Fig. 15.3) [4].

The third, more characteristic sign of AIC is represented by mild, circumferential and generally uniform thickening and hyperenhancement of the urothelium which lines the inner aspect of the urinary bladder (Figs. 15.2 and 15.3). Analogous to the inflammatory urothelial enhancement often encountered in acute pyelo-ureteritis, this appearance is sometimes encountered in CT studies performed for different or unrelated indications,

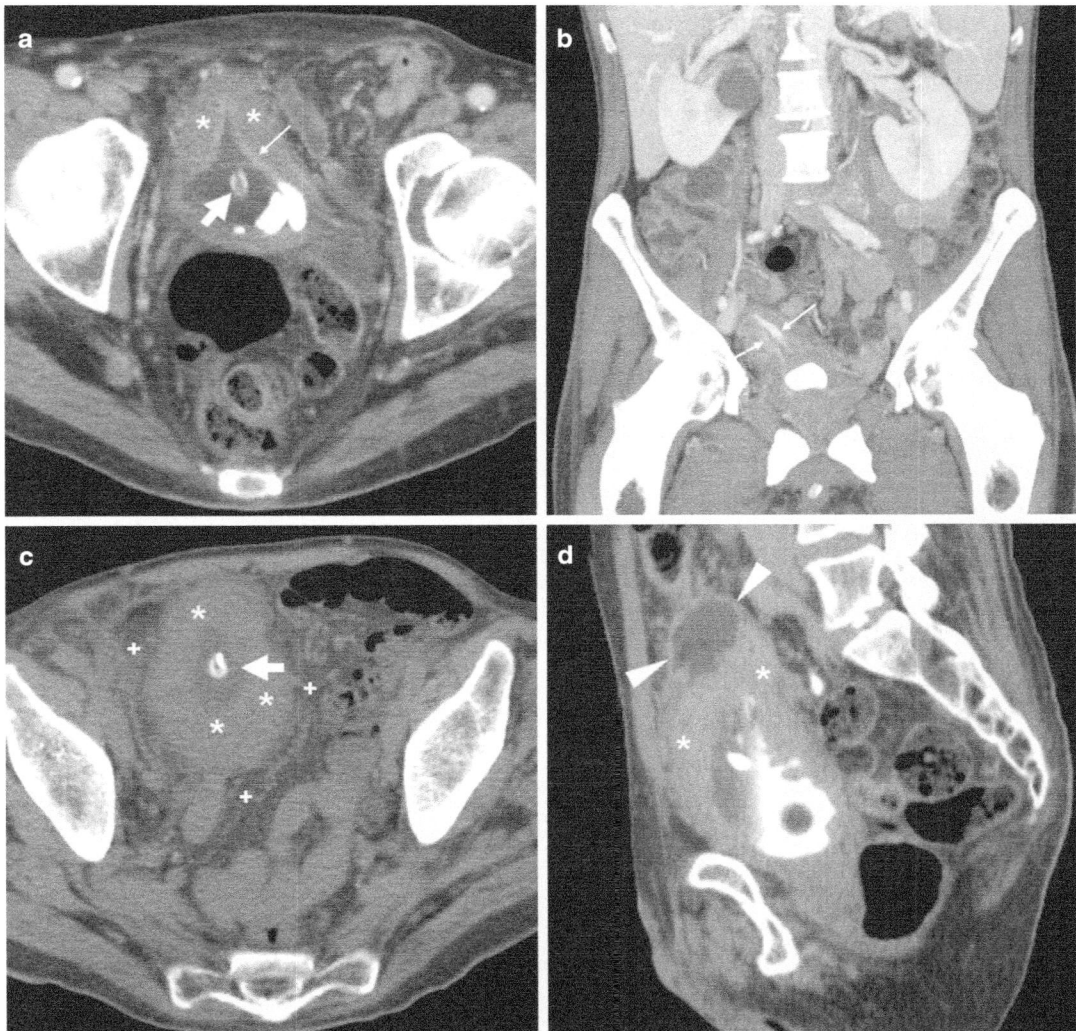

Fig. 15.3 Polymicrobial urinary tract infection (UTI) complicated by mural bladder abscess in a 67-year-old male with benign prostatic hyperplasia and indwelling catheter (thick arrows). Four months earlier, contrast-enhanced CT (**a, b**) revealed contracted urinary bladder with calcific lithiasis, circumferential mural thickening (*) from detrusor hypertrophy and urothelial hyperenhancement (thin arrow in **b**) consistent with active UTI. Currently, urgent CT (**c, d**) requested to investigate urosepsis showed increased mural thickening of the urinary bladder (*), appearance of inflammatory stranding of the perivesical fat planes (+) and development of a sizeable (over 6 cm) collection attached to the bladder dome (arrowheads) with nonenhancing hypoattenuating (10–15 Hounsfield units, HU) content and enhancing peripheral rim, consistent with abscess which required surgical drainage (Partially reproduced from Open Access Ref. no. [4])

should not be overlooked albeit rather subtle, may be confirmed by performing slab MIP reconstructions (Fig. 15.3b) and should be reported as consistent with AIC [3, 4, 21].

Emphysematous cystitis (EC) is a rare peculiar form of complicated UTI, most usually occurring in diabetics, in which gas-forming micro-organisms cause the formation of characteristic air-attenuation linear changes within the bladder wall (Fig. 15.4). The key differential diagnosis of EC is intraluminal air from catheterisation or urologic instrumentation, alternatively from enterovesical fistulisation [4, 7].

Compared to CT, MRI provides a superior assessment of the urinary bladder wall even without intravenous gadolinium CM. In patients with AIC, MRI shows:

(a) Focal or diffuse intramural oedematous regions with increased T2-weighted signal (Fig. 15.5) compared to the usual, uniformly low signal intensity corresponding to the detrusor muscle

(b) Inflammatory-type T2 hypersignal of the perivesical fat (Fig. 15.6), which is best appreciable with fat-suppression techniques

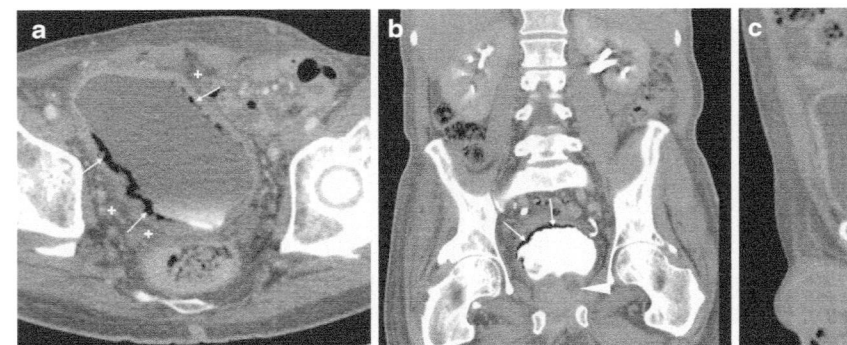

Fig. 15.4 Emphysematous cystitis in a 69-year-old male with diabetes, congestive heart failure and chronic obstructive lung disease, suffering from urinary frequency and pain. Multidetector CT-urography (a–c) revealed distended urinary bladder with linear gas attenuation changes (thin arrows) along the right lateral and upper posterior walls, with associated inflammatory stranding (+) of the perivesical fat planes. Additionally a small-sized fluidlike intraprostatic abscess collection (arrowhead in c) was noted. Emphysematous cystitis resolved after prolonged antibiotic therapy (Partially reproduced from Open Access Ref. no. [4])

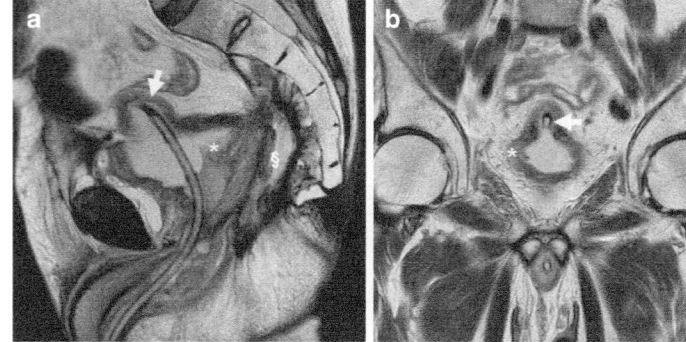
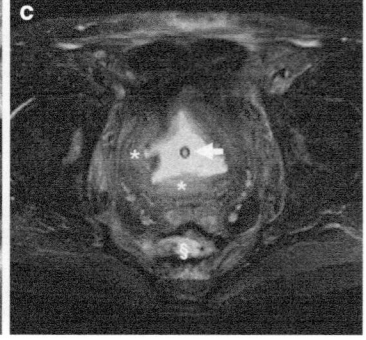

Fig. 15.5 Acute infectious cystitis in a 66-year-old bed-ridden male with urosepsis. After inconclusive abdomino-pelvic CT (not shown), unenhanced MRI including sagittal (a), axial (b, c) T2-weighted sequences showed contracted bladder with Foley catheter (thick arrows) and diffused mural thickening with multifocal high-signal oedematous regions best appreciated with fat saturation (c) (Reproduced from Open Access Ref.no. [4])

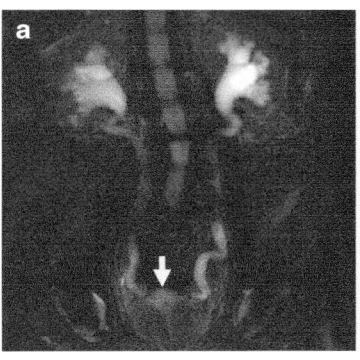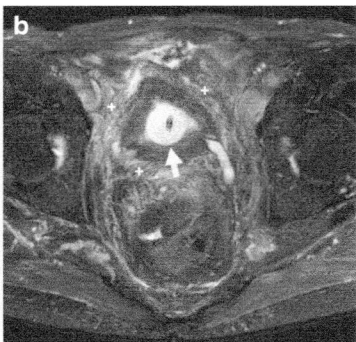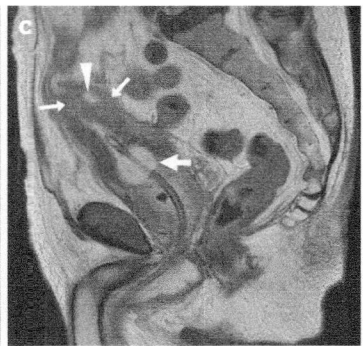

Fig. 15.6 Acute infectious cystitis with mural bladder abscess in an 89-year-old male with acute urinary retention, fever, leucocytosis and impaired renal function. Unenhanced MRI including MR-pyelographic (**a**) and axial fat-suppressed (**b**) images revealed bilateral hydronephrosis, contracted bladder and prominent inflammatory changes (+) of the surrounding extraperitoneal fat planes. Additionally, sagittal T2-weighted image (**c**) showed a focal thickening (arrows) at the bladder dome with intramural fluid collection (arrowhead). Repeated CT (not shown) after medical treatment revealed disappearance of abnormal mural changes (Reproduced from Open Access Ref.no. [4])

(c) Thin urothelial hyperenhancement lining the inner bladder aspect on optional post-gadolinium sequences [3–5, 7]

15.3.2 Urinary Bladder Abscess

Sometimes AIC may be further complicated by the formation of a mural bladder abscess, which characteristically develops at the upper bladder aspect and therefore is best visualised on sagittal and coronal CT or MRI images. The hallmark of a bladder abscess is an intramural or exophytic collection with internal hypoattenuating (10–15 Hounsfield units, HU) nonenhancing content and irregular, often thick peripheral enhancement (Figs. 15.2 and 15.6) [4, 7].

Avoiding misinterpretation of a bladder abscess is crucial since long-term catheterisation plus drainage (either percutaneous or surgical) is required to relieve the septic focus. The two differential diagnoses are:

(a) Infected diverticulum, which may have an appreciable communication with the bladder lumen
(b) Bladder carcinoma with perivesical invasion [4, 22–24]

15.3.3 Differential Diagnosis of Infectious Bladder Changes

The main concern for both radiologist and urologists is differentiating AIC from urinary bladder cancer. Other differential diagnoses include:
(a) Post-chemotherapy and postirradiation changes
(b) Infections such as tuberculosis and schistosomiasis
(c) Some rare non-neoplastic disorders such as nephrogenic adenoma, malacoplakia, cystitis cystica, cystitis glandularis and eosinophilic cystitis

Notably, all the above-mentioned entities have similar clinical manifestations including signs of lower urinary dysfunction, proteinuria and haematuria and may have unspecific imaging appearance as an abnormal bladder with multifocal or diffuse wall thickening, decreased distensibility or intraluminal vegetations [25–27].

Iatrogenic bladder changes are generally diagnosed on the basis of consistent history of symptoms developing after treatment of pelvic tumours. Post-chemotherapy cystitis is mostly encountered after cyclophosphamide or ifosfamide therapy and with intravesical use of mitomycin C. The bladder mucosa suffers from

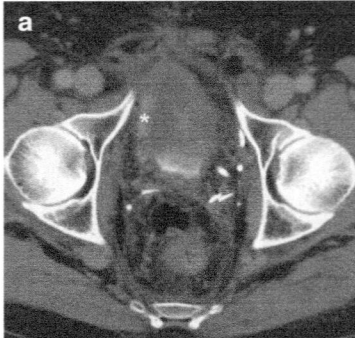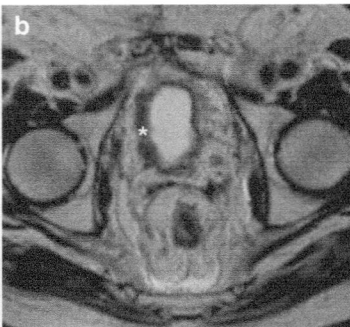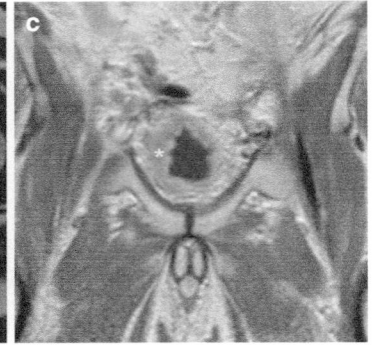

Fig. 15.7 A 73-year-old male with previous radical prostatectomy plus adjuvant radiotherapy for prostate cancer and dorsolumbar spine metastases. Contrast-enhanced CT (**a**) showed contracted bladder with asymmetric mural thickening, more pronounced and enhancing (*) on the right side. MRI confirmed moderately distended bladder; the asymmetric mural thickening (*) showed diffuse T2-hypointense signal (**b**) consistent with fibrosis and homogeneously enhancing after intravenous gadolinium contrast (**c**). Cystoscopy and biopsies excluded neoplastic changes, thus confirming the diagnosis of radiation cystitis

hyperaemia, ulcerations, haemorrhage and necrosis. At MRI, the diffuse or focal bladder wall thickening may show high T2 signal intensity consistent with inflammation, but abnormal contrast uptake is usually not apparent [25].

Albeit rare compared to the past decade, radiation cystitis may occur following external, interstitial or intracavitary irradiation of pelvic neoplasms [28]. The acute form manifests from 4–6 weeks up to 4 months after therapy, involves mucosal ulceration and mixed acute and chronic inflammatory cell infiltrate in the submucosa, but is usually self-limiting and conservatively treated. Conversely, chronic radiation cystitis usually manifests 1–4 years (occasionally even later) after radiation and is generally seen at imaging as a contracted bladder with circumferential thickening. MRI may support this diagnosis by showing T2-hypointense mural signal corresponding to the predominant interstitial fibrosis; mural enhancement may be persistently observed even years after treatment (Fig. 15.7) [26, 27, 29, 30].

Infections such as genitourinary tuberculosis and schistosomiasis should be suspected in patients from endemic countries. As discussed in the appropriate chapter of this book, tuberculous cystitis develops at a later stage after renal involvement, and the diagnosis is suggested by clinical history and supported by a characteristic constellation of imaging findings. Albeit declining, schistosomiasis

(bilharziasis) from *S. haematobium* worms' infection is still highly prevalent in sub-Saharan Africa and is acquired through human contact with contaminated water in rural areas. Frequently asymptomatic, schistosomiasis mostly affects the urinary bladder and distal ureters (60–70%), followed by male (prostate, seminal vesicles, testicles and epididymis) and female (vulva) genital organs. The schistosoma eggs incite a chronic granulomatous intramural inflammation, which ultimately leads to a contracted, thick-walled bladder with more or less nodular appearance and frequent mural calcifications (Fig. 15.8a, b) [31, 32]. Furthermore, bilharziasis has a well-established association with squamous cell bladder carcinoma, which occurs in younger (mean age 40–49 years) patients with a striking (5–6:1) male predominance. Therefore, in patients from endemic countries, an enhancing mural mass should raise suspicion of cancer (Fig. 15.8c, d) [33–36].

At CT, transitional cell carcinoma of the urinary bladder appears as uni- or multifocal, generally asymmetric wall thickening which enhances most prominently at a 60-s delay (Fig. 15.9). Tumour is suggested over infection when a soft-tissue density irregularity is detected at the interface between mural thickening and perivesical fat. Perivesical invasion is obvious when the neoplasia shows overt growth beyond the outer bladder wall contour [37, 38].

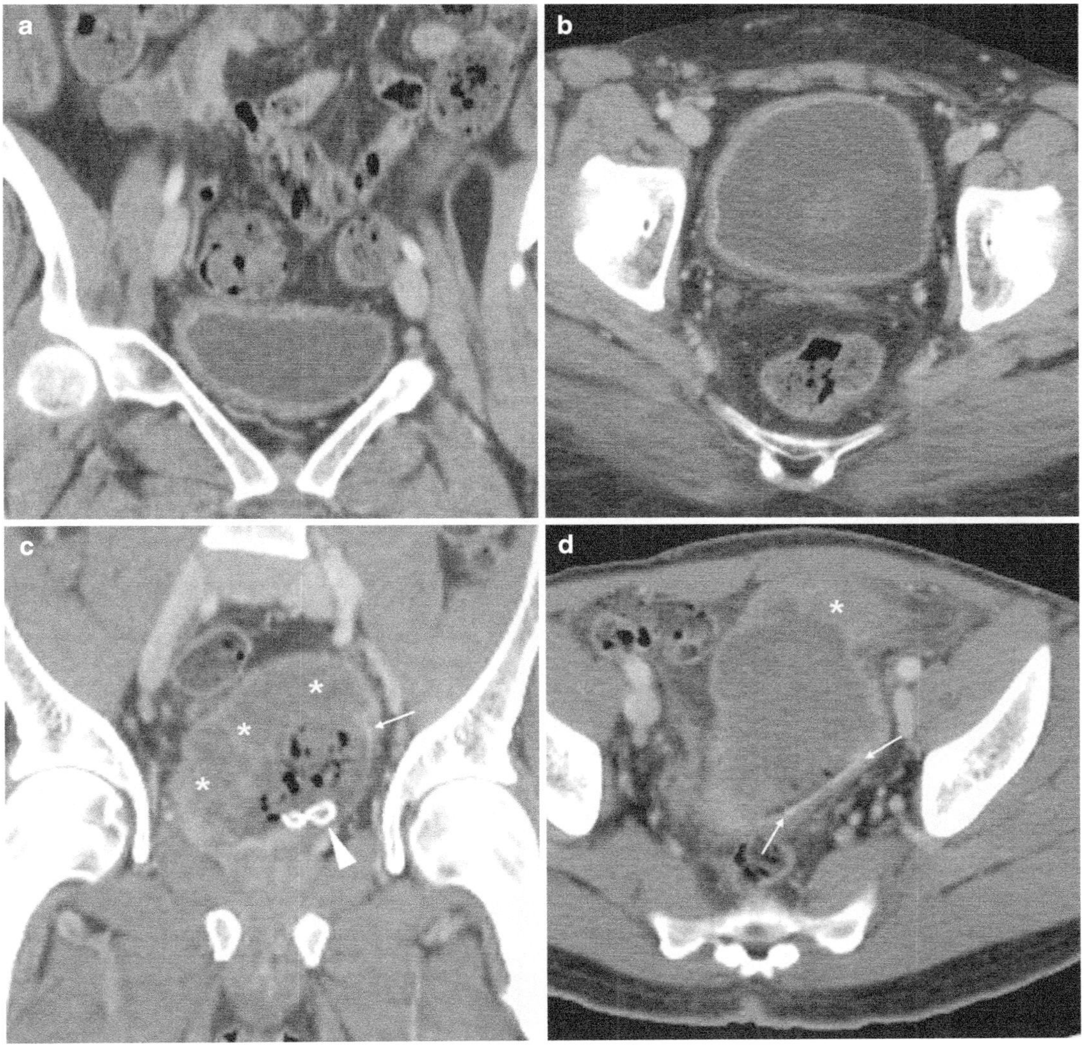

Fig. 15.8 Uncomplicated schistosomiasis in a 46-year-old male from Egypt, being hospitalised for unrelated reasons. Contrast-enhanced CT (**a, b**) showed mild, uniform thickening of the entire bladder wall, without macroscopic calcifications and intraluminal vegetations. In a 48-year-old Gambian male with pelvic pain and tenderness, dysuria and difficult urination, post-contrast (**c, d**) CT images showed marked, asymmetric solid mural thickening (*) with heterogeneous enhancement along the anterior, right lateral and superior bladder aspects, plus thin calcifications (thin arrows) along the left posterolateral bladder wall, and intraluminal stones (arrowhead). Final diagnosis was extensive squamous carcinoma superimposed on schistosomiasis (Partially reproduced from Open Access Ref.no. [4])

Finally, nephrogenic adenoma and malacoplakia of the urinary bladder mostly occur in diabetics or immunocompromised individual such as those with long-standing HIV infection. Whereas the latter is a rare chronic granulomatous condition, the former results from long-term irritation from calculi, infection, injury or previous surgery causing urothelial metaplasia. Both entities cannot be reliably differentiated from chronic UTI or bladder carcinoma on the basis their unspecific cross-sectional imaging features and therefore generally represent incidental diagnoses on endoscopic biopsies [4, 26]

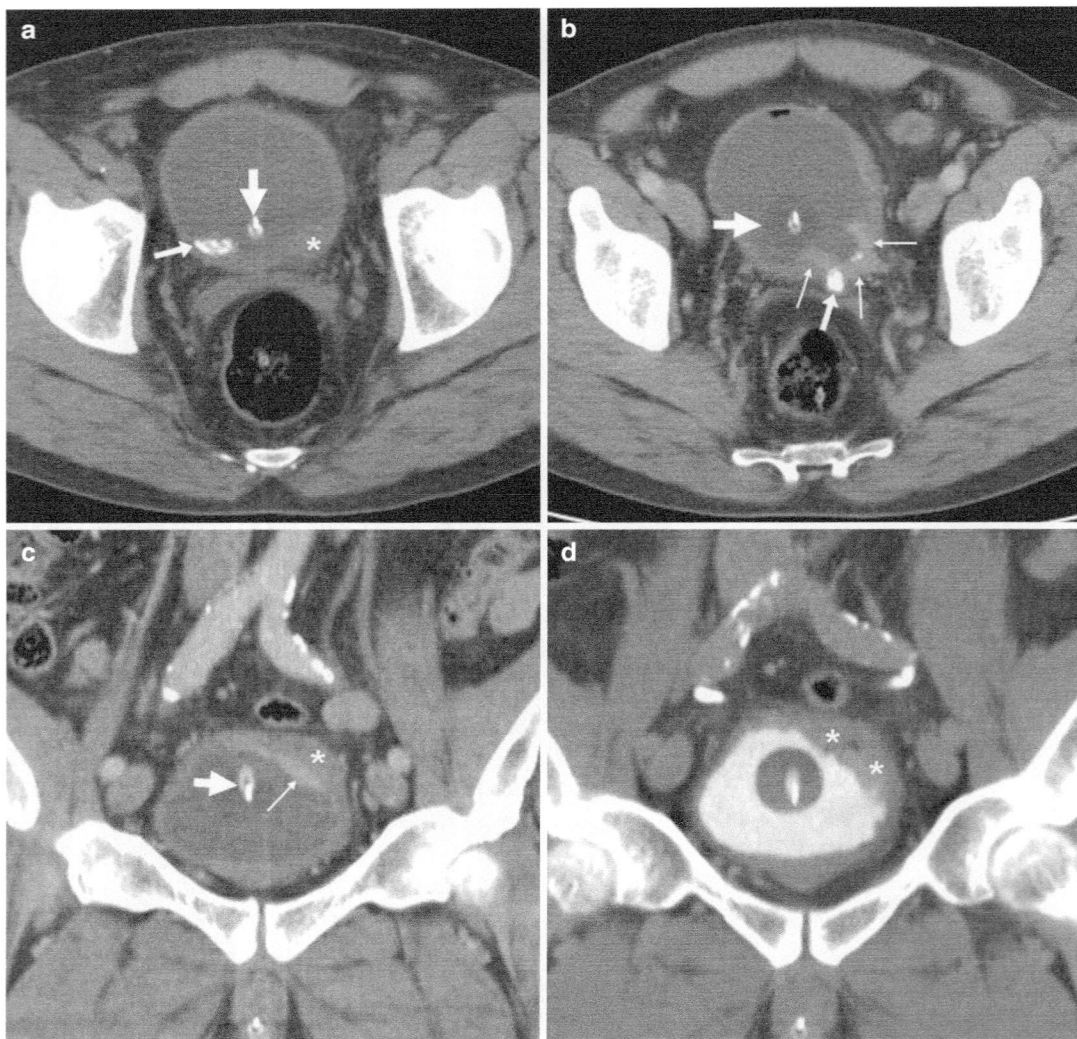

Fig. 15.9 Muscle-invasive bladder carcinoma in a 54-year-old male with urolithiasis (arrows) and long-term bladder catheterisation (thick arrows). Unenhanced (**a**), portal (**b**, **c**) and excretory (**d**) phase CT images showed focal solid mural thickening (*) at the left posterolateral bladder wall, with an irregular configuration and positive contrast enhancement (thin arrows). Radical cystectomy with orthotopic neobladder reconstruction was performed (Partially reproduced from Open Access Ref.no. [4])

15.3.4 Urinary Bladder Fistulas

Fistulisation between the gastrointestinal and the urinary tract may underlie chronic or recurrent UTI, and the diagnosis is generally unsuspected when pathognomonic symptoms such as pneumaturia and faecaluria are absent. Most colovesical fistulas (CVFs) develop secondary to sigmoid colon diverticulitis, occasionally from colorectal carcinomas. Crohn's disease (CD) represents the most frequent cause of enterovesical fistulas (EVFs), particularly in young males, since the presence of the uterus and adnexa protects the bladder from penetration of full-thickness chronic ileal inflammation. However, enterovesical fistulas cause significant morbidity and generally mandate surgical repair to eradicate chronic urinary infection and prevent systemic sepsis [39–42].

Vesical fistulisation may be confirmed via oral administration of indocyanine green dye or other similar agents. Conversely, visualisation of the fistulous track is generally challenging both at cystoscopy (orifice is identified in less than 50% of cases) and imaging [39–42].

Since most patients with colonic diverticulitis, colorectal cancer and CD are commonly investigated with CT or MRI, radiologists should carefully seek for features consistent with vesical fistulisation. The presence of air in the bladder lumen without catheterisation or recent instrumentation is the commonest albeit indirect finding (Fig. 15.10a, b), but no air may be observed in the bladder if the patient has voided prior to the examination. Other suggestive changes include retraction of the bladder wall, focal or diffuse mural thickening, adhesion and tethering of thickened adjacent bowel loops. Fistulas are directly identified only when filled by air, fluid or enteral contrast (Fig. 15.10c, d). The extraluminal findings, such as bowel wall thickening, diverticula or soft-tissue mass, generally hint to the primary cause of the fistula [43–45].

In our experience, CT-cystography proved to be a fast, cheap and highly accurate modality to depict CVFs and EVFs, since retrograde bladder distension opens and opacifies thin yet patent fistulas (Fig. 15.10e, f). CT-cystography is recommended after failed identification during cystoscopy and CT, particularly when surgical treatment is to be planned [16].

15.4 Cross-Sectional Imaging Appearances of Infections of the Prostate and Seminal Vesicles

15.4.1 Prostatic Infections

The widespread use of antibiotics has led to a decline in the occurrence of UTIs involving both the prostate and seminal vesicles. However, acute bacterial prostatitis (ABP) remains a relatively common, potentially serious infection which is generally diagnosed on clinical grounds and requires intensive parenteral antibiotic therapy [8].

Due to the usual heterogeneous enhancement of the prostate gland, CT provides little clue to the presence of ongoing ABP, which may be suggested by rapid enlargement compared to previous studies or coexistent signs of UTI in the bladder or seminal vesicles (Fig. 15.11). Some reports described MRI appearance of ABP as characterised by T2-hypointense "bands" with absent diffusion restriction and progressive or plateau enhancement, compared to the nodular configuration, marked diffusion abnormality and "spike" enhancement of prostatic carcinoma (PCa). Conversely, chronic prostatitis commonly mimics PCa since it generally involves the peripheral zone and shows low T2 signal intensity, mild to moderate diffusion restriction corresponding to increased cellular infiltrate and early and increased enhancement compared with normal prostatic tissue. Despite these overlapping MRI features, diagnosis of chronic inflammation over PCA may be suggested by:

(a) Geographic configuration
(b) Lack of mass effect, contour deformity and capsular alteration
(c) Lower degree of diffusion restriction than in PCa [3, 46]

The key role of cross-sectional imaging is to differentiate ABP from prostatic abscess (PA), which has similar clinical and laboratory features but a different management. The latter generally results from unrecognised or inappropriately treated UTI or develops following recent transrectal ultrasound (TRUS)-guided prostate biopsy and often requires TRUS- or transperineal CT-guided drainage, sometimes surgical incision. Interestingly, in prostatic infections an increased serum prostate-specific antigen (PSA) is common but generally regresses with therapy [5, 8, 47, 48].

TRUS may detect PAs as single or multiple hypoechoic areas with thick walls, floating echogenic speckles in the cavity, and poorly defined periphery with increased colour Doppler signals. Compared to TRUS, multiplanar CT provides a more comprehensive visualisation of PAs. The usual appearance is single, septated or

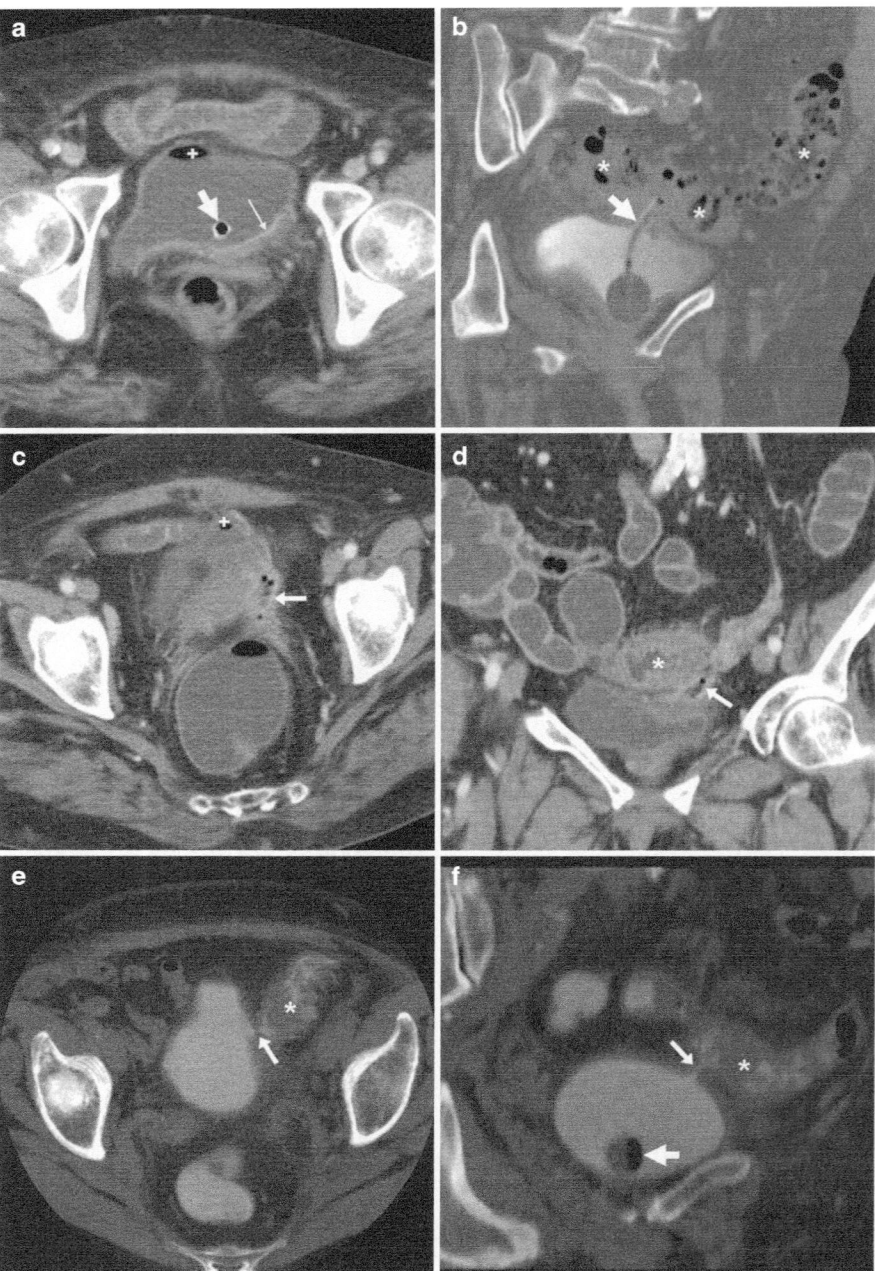

Fig. 15.10 Three different cases of colovesical fistulas (CVFs). In an 88-year-old female with medically treated acute diverticulitis, contrast-enhanced multidetector CT revealed urinary bladder with some intraluminal gas (+ in A) which was attributed to catheterisation (thick arrows) and thin urothelial hyperenhancement (thin arrow in **a**) consistent with active UTI. On excretory phase acquisition (**b**), tip of the Foley catheter (thick arrow) was seen protruding into the thickened diverticular sigmoid colon (*) through a CVF, which required surgical repair including segmental colic resection, colostomy and bladder suture. In a 78-year-old female investigated with water enema CT colonography (**c**,

d) for an endoscopically impassable stricture, a fluid-filled CVF (arrows) containing gas bubbles was directly identifiable communicating with the thickened sigmoid colon (*). Note minimal air in the bladder (+ in **c**) without previous instrumentation. In a 79-year-old woman with chronic UTI and previous CT demonstration of sigmoid colon diverticulosis and intravesical air, cystoscopy failed to detect fistulous orifices. Additional CT-cystography (**e**, **f**) through the Foley catheter (thick arrow) showed leakage of diluted contrast in the sigmoid colon (*) through a short CVF (arrows), which was surgically repaired (Partially reproduced from Open Access Ref.no. [16])

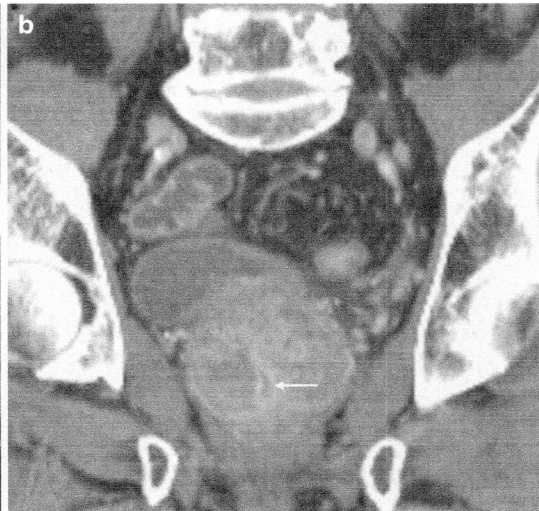

Fig. 15.11 An 80-year-old male was hospitalised because of suspected urosepsis. As the sole acute abnormality, contrast-enhanced multidetector CT showed moderate enlargement of the prostate compared to a previous CT study (not shown), with heterogeneous structure and per-ceptible thin hyperenhancement along the prostatic ure-thra (thin arrows), without appreciable abscess cavities. Consistent clinical and laboratory findings confirmed the diagnosis of acute bacterial prostatitis

multiple fluidlike (−19 to 13 HU attenuation) collections, often with perceptible peripheral or septal enhancement, which cause more or less symmetric prostatic enlargement of variable entity (Fig. 15.12). Furthermore, CT easily shows extraprostatic penetration of PAs in the prevesical space, rectum, perineum or ischiorec-tal fossa and consistently allows monitoring changes after medical or surgical treatment. The usual differential diagnosis is PCa, particularly with regressive changes after treatment (Fig. 15.13) [3–5].

15.4.2 Infections of the Seminal Vesicles

Seminal vesicle abscesses (SVAs) are even more uncommon than PAs and frequently associated with other lower UTIs such as AIC, ABP or epididymo-orchitis. Albeit characteristic, haemo-spermia is not unusually absent [8, 49].

Transabdominal or transrectal ultrasound may detect SVAs (Fig. 15.14) as hypo-anechoic masses. Compared to normal finely septated sem-inal vesicles with fluidlike CT attenuation, low T1- and fluidlike T2-hyperintense MRI signal, cross-sectional CT imaging depicts SVAs as uni- or bilateral gland enlargement with thick irregu-lar enhancing wall, internal hypoattenuating regions and adjacent fat inflammatory changes (Fig. 15.14). In normal conditions, some asym-metry may exist between the seminal vesicles, which reach 3.5 × 2 cm in size when fully dis-tended in young adults, and normally show enhancing walls and septa. Conversely, the semi-nal vesicles tend to shrink with age; therefore any enlargement in elderly patients should be viewed with suspicion [4, 49, 50].

The differential diagnosis of seminal vesicle infections encompasses congenital or acquired cysts, tuberculosis, benign and malignant tumours and particularly metastases from pros-tate, bladder or rectal cancers [49, 51].

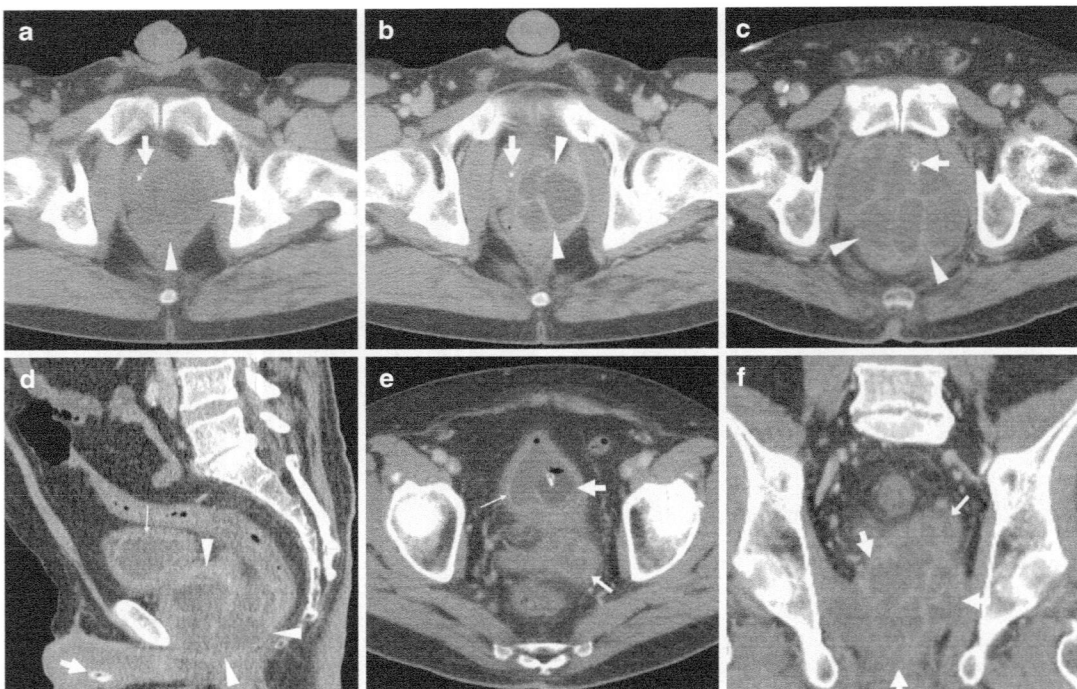

Fig. 15.12 Prostatic abscess in a 48-year-old male with perineal pain and abnormally increased CRP. Axial unenhanced (**a**) and post-contrast (**b**) CT images showed mild asymmetric prostatic enlargement occupied by a 4-cm septated fluidlike collection (arrowheads) with peripheral and septal enhancement. Note displacement of periurethral calcifications (thick arrows) from midline. Ultrasound-guided transperineal drainage confirmed *Escherichia coli* infection. Another case of large prostatic abscess from ESBL-positive *Escherichia coli* infection in a 61-year-old male with previous chemo- and radiotherapy for non-Hodgkin lymphoma, fever (38 °C), dysuria, pelvic pain and enlarged tender prostate at digital rectal examination. Multiplanar CT images (**c–f**) showed marked prostatic enlargement by confluent nonenhancing hypoattenuating (17-19 HU) regions, with peripheral and septal enhancement (arrowheads). The prostatic infection involved also the left seminal vesicle (arrows in **e**, f), displaced upwards the urinary bladder with mild circumferential mural thickening and mucosal hyperenhancement (thin arrows) indicating UTI. The abscess was relieved by transperineal evacuation (Partially reproduced from Open Access Ref.no. [4])

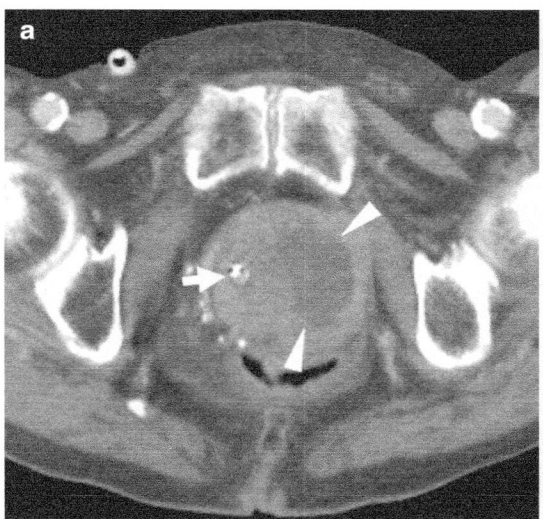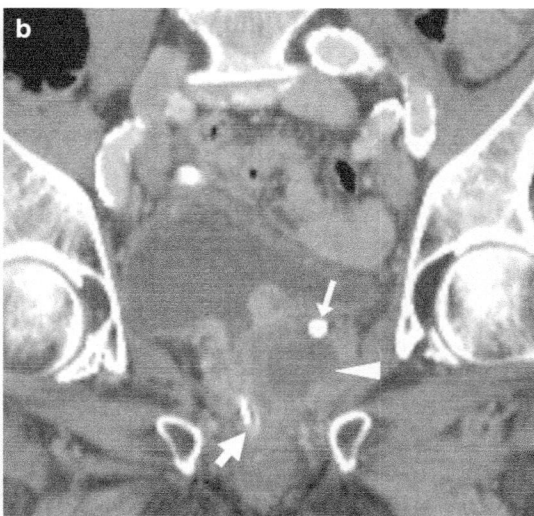

Fig. 15.13 Prostate carcinoma with post-treatment regressive (necrotic) changes in an 86-year-old elderly male with indwelling catheter (thick arrows). Axial (**a**) and coronal (**b**) post-contrast CT images depicted a 3 × 2 cm left-sided hypoenhancing region (arrowheads) causing enlargement of the ipsilateral prostate gland, initially interpreted as an abscess. Note residual brachytherapy seed indicated by arrow in (**b**) (Reproduced from Open Access Ref.no. [4])

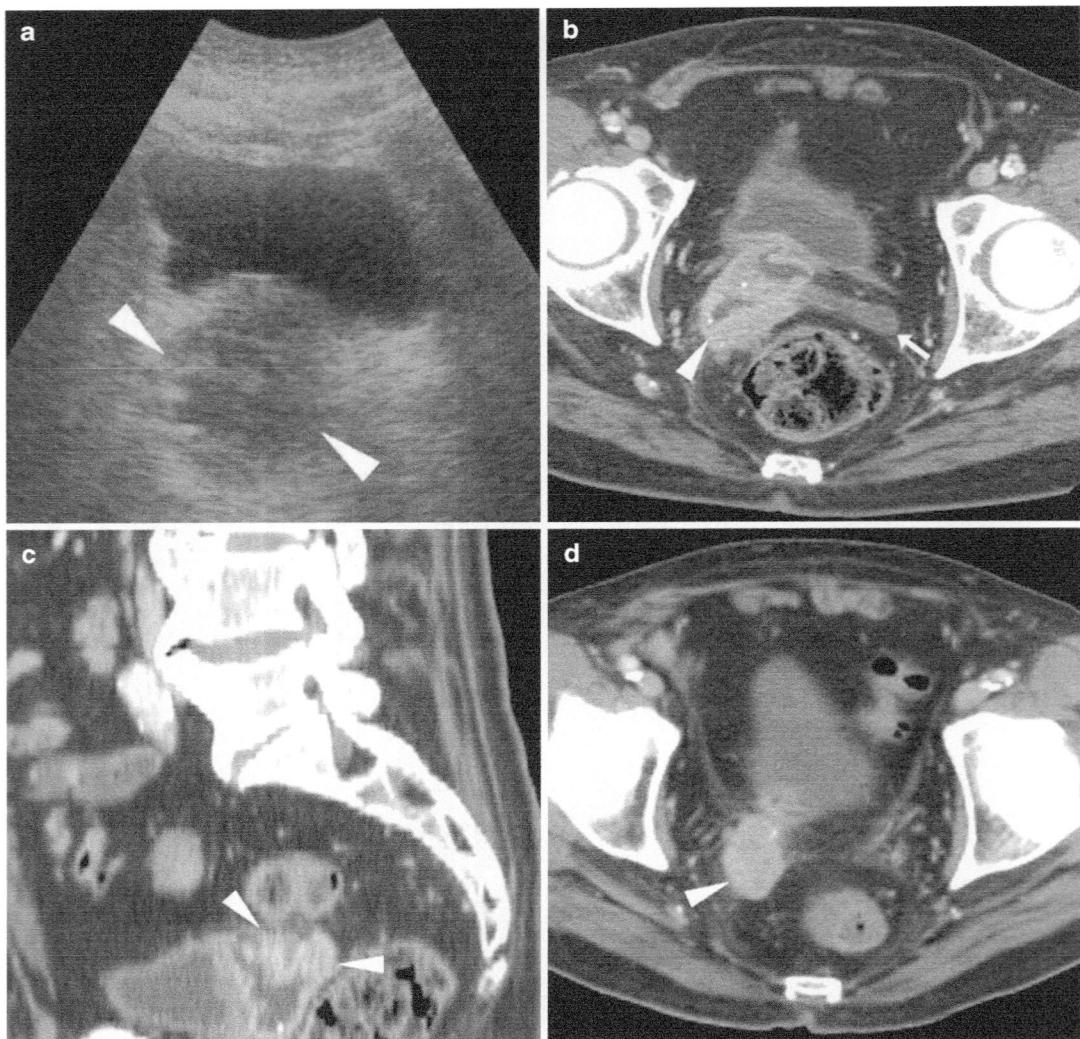

Fig. 15.14 Seminal vesicle abscess in a 74-year-old male with recurrent UTIs, suffering from malaise, persistent fever, pelvic tenderness and dysuria. Transabdominal ultrasound (**a**) revealed a right paramedian inhomogeneous hypo-anechoic multiseptated mass (arrowhead), exerting compression on the urinary bladder. CT (**b, c**) confirmed markedly enlarged right seminal vesicle (arrowheads) with thick, strongly enhancing walls and septa, speckled calcifications and internal liquefied areas. After intensive antibiotic treatment, the abscess partially decreased with disappearance of mass effect and of liquefied portions at follow-up CT (**d**). Serum prostate-specific agent (PSA) normalised from 10 to 5 ng/mL over 2 months (Reproduced from Open Access Ref.no. [4])

References

1. Avery LL, Scheinfeld MH (2013) Imaging of penile and scrotal emergencies. Radiographics 33: 721–740
2. Pavlica P, Barozzi L (2001) Imaging of the acute scrotum. Eur Radiol 11:220–228
3. Schull A, Monzani Q, Bour L et al (2012) Imaging in lower urinary tract infections. Diagn Interv Imaging 93:500–508
4. Tonolini M, Ippolito S (2016) Cross-sectional imaging of complicated urinary infections affecting the lower tract and male genital organs. Insights Imaging 7(5):689–711
5. Yu M, Robinson K, Siegel C et al (2016) Complicated genitourinary tract infections and mimics. Curr Probl Diagn Radiol 46(1):74–83. https://doi.org/10.1067/j.cpradiol.2016.1002.1004
6. Sartelli M, Viale P, Catena F et al (2013) 2013 WSES guidelines for management of intra-abdominal infections. World J Emerg Surg 8:3

7. Browne RF, Zwirewich C, Torreggiani WC (2004) Imaging of urinary tract infection in the adult. Eur Radiol 14(Suppl 3):E168–E183

8. Grabe M, Bartoletti R, Bjerklund-Johansen TE et al (2014) Guidelines on urological infections. European Association of Urology, The Netherlands. Available at: http://uroweb.org/wp-content/uploads/19-Urological-infections_LR2.pdf.

9. Sorensen SM, Schonheyder HC, Nielsen H (2013) The role of imaging of the urinary tract in patients with urosepsis. Int J Infect Dis 17:e299–e303

10. EuropeanSociety, Radiology Oxford University (2016) ESUR Guidelines on Contrast Media 9.0. Available at: www.esur.org/guidelines

11. Stacul F, van der Molen AJ, Reimer P et al (2011) Contrast induced nephropathy: updated ESUR contrast media safety committee guidelines. Eur Radiol 21:2527–2541

12. Cook TS, Hilton S, Papanicolaou N (2013) Perspectives on radiation dose in abdominal imaging. Abdom Imaging 38:1190–1196

13. Van Der Molen AJ, Cowan NC, Mueller-Lisse UG et al (2008) CT urography: definition, indications and techniques. A guideline for clinical practice. Eur Radiol 18:4–17

14. Kekelidze M, Dwarkasing RS, Dijkshoorn ML et al (2010) Kidney and urinary tract imaging: triple-bolus multidetector CT urography as a one-stop shop--protocol design, opacification, and image quality analysis. Radiology 255:508–516

15. Vaccaro JP, Brody JM (2000) CT cystography in the evaluation of major bladder trauma. Radiographics 20:1373–1381

16. Tonolini M, Bianco R (2012) Multidetector CT cystography for imaging colovesical fistulas and iatrogenic bladder leaks. Insights Imaging 3:181–187

17. Chan DP, Abujudeh HH, Cushing GL Jr et al (2006) CT cystography with multiplanar reformation for suspected bladder rupture: experience in 234 cases. AJR Am J Roentgenol 187:1296–1302

18. Singh AK, Desai H, Novelline RA (2009) Emergency MRI of acute pelvic pain: MR protocol with no oral contrast. Emerg Radiol 16:133–141

19. Heverhagen JT, Klose KJ (2009) MR imaging for acute lower abdominal and pelvic pain. Radiographics 29:1781–1796

20. Ditkofsky N, Singh A, Avery LL et al (2014) The role of emergency MRI in the setting of acute abdominal pain. Emerg Radiol 21:615–624

21. Wasnik AP, Elsayes KM, Kaza RK et al (2011) Multimodality imaging in ureteric and periureteric pathologic abnormalities. AJR Am J Roentgenol 197:W1083–W1092

22. Hsu KF, Char DL, Lee YL et al (2009) Extensive bladder wall abscess. J Trauma 67:413

23. Lawrentschuk N, Gani J, Bolton DM et al (2004) Spontaneous bladder wall abscess. J Urol 171:2379

24. Sarkar KK, Philp T, Thurley P (1990) Intramural vesical abscess. Br J Urol 66:665

25. Jia JB, Lall C, Tirkes T et al (2015) Chemotherapy-related complications in the kidneys and collecting system: an imaging perspective. Insights Imaging 6:479–487

26. Wong-You-Cheong JJ, Woodward PJ, Manning MA et al (2006) From the archives of the AFIP: inflammatory and nonneoplastic bladder masses: radiologic-pathologic correlation. Radiographics 26:1847–1868

27. Schieda N, Malone SC, Al Dandan O et al (2014) Multi-modality organ-based approach to expected imaging findings, complications and recurrent tumour in the genitourinary tract after radiotherapy. Insights Imaging 5:25–40

28. Smit SG, Heyns CF (2010) Management of radiation cystitis. Nat Rev Urol 7:206–214

29. Suresh UR, Smith VJ, Lupton EW et al (1993) Radiation disease of the urinary tract: histological features of 18 cases. J Clin Pathol 46:228–231

30. Bluemke DA, Fishman EK, Kuhlman JE et al (1991) Complications of radiation therapy: CT evaluation. Radiographics 11:581–600

31. Gray DJ, Ross AG, Li YS et al (2011) Diagnosis and management of schistosomiasis. BMJ 342:d2651

32. Khalaf I, Shokeir A, Shalaby M (2012) Urologic complications of genitourinary schistosomiasis. World J Urol 30:31–38

33. Zaghloul MS, Gouda I (2012) Schistosomiasis and bladder cancer: similarities and differences from urothelial cancer. Expert Rev Anticancer Ther 12:753–763

34. Zaghloul MS, Nouh A, Moneer M et al (2008) Time-trend in epidemiological and pathological features of schistosoma-associated bladder cancer. J Egypt Natl Canc Inst 20:168–174

35. Mostafa MH, Sheweita SA, O'Connor PJ (1999) Relationship between schistosomiasis and bladder cancer. Clin Microbiol Rev 12:97–111

36. Heyns CF, van der Merwe A (2008) Bladder cancer in Africa. Can J Urol 15:3899–3908

37. Kim JK, Park S-Y, Ahn AJ et al (2004) Bladder cancer: analysis of multi–detector row helical CT enhancement pattern and accuracy in tumor detection and perivesical staging. Radiology 231:725–731

38. Kundra V, Silverman PM (2003) Imaging in oncology from the University of Texas M. D. Anderson cancer Center. Imaging in the diagnosis, staging, and follow-up of cancer of the urinary bladder. AJR Am J Roentgenol 180:1045–1054

39. Melchior S, Cudovic D, Jones J et al (2009) Diagnosis and surgical management of colovesical fistulas due to sigmoid diverticulitis. J Urol 182:978–982

40. Solem CA, Loftus EV Jr, Tremaine WJ et al (2002) Fistulas to the urinary system in Crohn's disease: clinical features and outcomes. Am J Gastroenterol 97:2300–2305

41. Yamamoto T, Keighley MR (2000) Enterovesical fistulas complicating Crohn's disease: clinicopathological features and management. Int J Color Dis 15:211–215. discussion 216–217

42. Ruffolo C, Angriman I, Scarpa M et al (2006) Urologic complications in Crohn's disease: suspicion criteria. Hepato-Gastroenterology 53:357–360

43. Goldman SM, Fishman EK, Gatewood OM et al (1985) CT in the diagnosis of enterovesical fistulae. AJR Am J Roentgenol 144:1229–1233

44. Yu NC, Raman SS, Patel M et al (2004) Fistulas of the genitourinary tract: a radiologic review. Radiographics 24:1331–1352

45. Tonolini M, Villa C, Campari A et al (2013) Common and unusual urogenital Crohn's disease complications: spectrum of cross-sectional imaging findings. Abdom Imaging 38:32–41

46. Kitzing YX, Prando A, Varol C et al (2016) Benign conditions that mimic prostate carcinoma: MR imaging features with histopathologic correlation. Radiographics 36:162–175

47. Saglam M, Ugurel S, Kilciler M et al (2004) Transrectal ultrasound-guided transperineal and tran-srectal management of seminal vesicle abscesses. Eur J Radiol 52:329–334

48. Oliveira P, Andrade JA, Porto HC et al (2003) Diagnosis and treatment of prostatic abscess. Clin Urol 29:30–34

49. Kim B, Kawashima A, Ryu JA et al (2009) Imaging of the seminal vesicle and vas deferens. Radiographics 29:1105–1121

50. Zagoria RJ, Papanicolaou N, Pfister RC et al (1987) Seminal vesicle abscess after vasectomy: evaluation by transrectal sonography and CT. AJR Am J Roentgenol 149:137–138

51. Kubik-Huch RA, Hailemariam S, Hamm B (1999) CT and MRI of the male genital tract: radiologic-pathologic correlation. Eur Radiol 9:16–28

Cross-Sectional Imaging of Urethral, Penile and Scrotal Infections

16

Massimo Tonolini

16.1 Introduction

As discussed in the dedicated chapter of this book, colour Doppler ultrasound represents the mainstay first-line technique to investigate the lower urinary and male genital tract, particularly to differentiate testicular torsion from epididymo-orchitis [1–3].

During the last decade, state-of-the art multi-detector computed tomography (CT) and magnetic resonance imaging (MRI) have been increasingly used to provide a comprehensive multiplanar assessment of genitourinary structures and disorders with high spatial and contrast resolution. In particular, MRI arguably represents the best technique to investigate suspected or known periurethral and penile disorders [1, 4–7], abnormalities affecting the perianal and perineal structures [8, 9] and the scrotum [10–12].

Mostly relying upon our personal experience at a tertiary care hospital focused on treatment of infectious illnesses [13], this chapter complements the preceding one by presenting with examples the CT and MRI appearances and differential diagnoses of urinary tract infections (UTIs) involving the urethra, penis, perineum and scrotum, which may develop from either sexual contact or catheterization and urologic instrumentation [14–16].

Some of these imaging findings, particularly acute funiculitis, may be incidentally encountered in cross-sectional studies performed for other clinical diagnoses, such as unspecific abdominal pain, suspected acute gynaecologic disorder or renal colic. Furthermore, as described in the previous chapter about technical protocols, in patients with UTI or sepsis, the entire pelvis and genital region should be included in the cross-sectional acquisition. The groins, perineum and scrotum should be carefully scrutinized for subtle abnormalities or asymmetry, and familiarity with the usual appearances of such is warranted [3, 13, 17–19].

16.2 Cross-Sectional Imaging Appearances of Infections of the Urethra, Perineum and Scrotum

16.2.1 Acute Urethritis and Perineal Abscess

Acute urethritis is generally diagnosed on the basis of clinical symptoms such as pruritus, mucopurulent discharge, alguria and dysuria, plus consistent laboratory and culture findings. The role of imaging is mostly reserved to look for further complications, particularly in those patients with one or more RENUC risk factors (see Table 1 of the Chap. 1) [13, 14].

In the past, conventional radiographic studies with injection of iodinated contrast medium

M. Tonolini, M.D.
Radiology Department, "Luigi Sacco" University Hospital, Via G.B. Grassi 74, Milan 20157, Italy
e-mail: mtonolini@sirm.org

© Springer International Publishing AG 2018
M. Tonolini (ed.), *Imaging and Intervention in Urinary Tract Infections and Urosepsis*,
https://doi.org/10.1007/978-3-319-68276-1_16

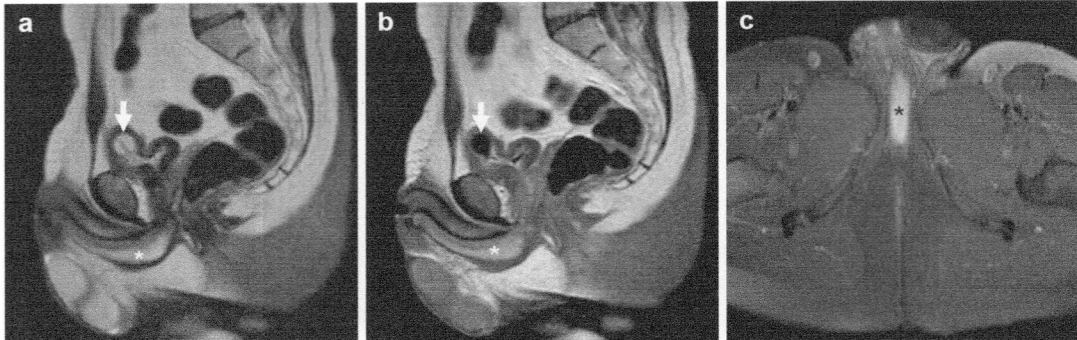

Fig. 16.1 Uncomplicated acute urethritis in a 30-year-old male with neurogenic bladder treated by intermittent self-catheterization, manifesting with purulent urethral secretions and physical finding of induration and tenderness of the corpus spongiosum. MRI images revealed T2-weighted (**a**) diffuse, uniform hypersignal in the corpus spongiosum (*) with corresponding intense homogeneous enhancement on post-gadolinium T1-weighted sequences (**b, c**). The infection did not interrupt the dartos tunica and Buck's fascia and did not involve the corpora cavernosa, scrotum and ischioanal spaces. Note Foley catheter in place (thick arrows). The patient successfully recovered with temporary suprapubic catheter and intravenous and topical antibiotics [Reproduced with permission from Open Access Ref.no [13]]

(CM) were the mainstay techniques for imaging the male urethra, particularly to assess traumatic injuries and strictures: however, retrograde urethrography and voiding cystourethrography could not assess the periurethral structures [4, 20, 21].

Conversely, nowadays the use of MRI can effectively visualize periurethral abnormalities [6, 13]. In our experience, uncomplicated acute urethritis may be seen as diffuse thickening of the penile urethra and surrounding corpus spongiosum with intermediate-to-high signal intensity on T2-weighted images and corresponding intense contrast enhancement (Fig. 16.1) [13, 17].

If untreated, urethritis may be complicated by a periurethral abscess through infection of Littrè glands. Since the penile tunica albuginea prevents the dorsal spread of infection, abscesses tends to track ventrally along the corpus spongiosum [14].

Periurethral abscesses may be also demonstrated sonographically, but ultrasound is generally cumbersome due to inflammatory swelling and tenderness of the penile and perineal structures. MRI consistently visualizes penile abscesses as fluid- or pus-filled cavities with enhancing periphery, typically located ventrally and in communication with the urethra (Fig. 16.2), and may clearly depict the involvement of corpora cavernosa and fibrous tunicae. The key differential diagnosis is a urethral diverticulum, which is most commonly located in the distal urethra and may closely resemble an abscess. Moreover, periurethral abscesses may further progress inferiorly breaching through the Buck fascia, thus leading to fasciitis and gangrenous necrosis of the subcutaneous tissue of the perineum and scrotum (Fournier's gangrene) [7, 12, 13, 17].

In our experience, in patients with previous radical prostatectomy, persistent UTI may be complicated by pubic osteomyelitis through contiguous spread of infection; therefore, in these cases scrutinizing CT images with a bone window setting and comparison with previous studies may be useful to appreciate irregularities and erosions of the bony surfaces, cortical discontinuity or frank osteolysis (Fig. 16.3).

16.2.2 Funiculitis and Epididymitis

As mentioned above and extensively discussed in the appropriate chapter, ultrasound with colour Doppler rapidly supports a clinical and laboratory diagnosis of epididymo-orchitis. However, in our experience CT may occasionally reveal signs of a clinically unsuspected

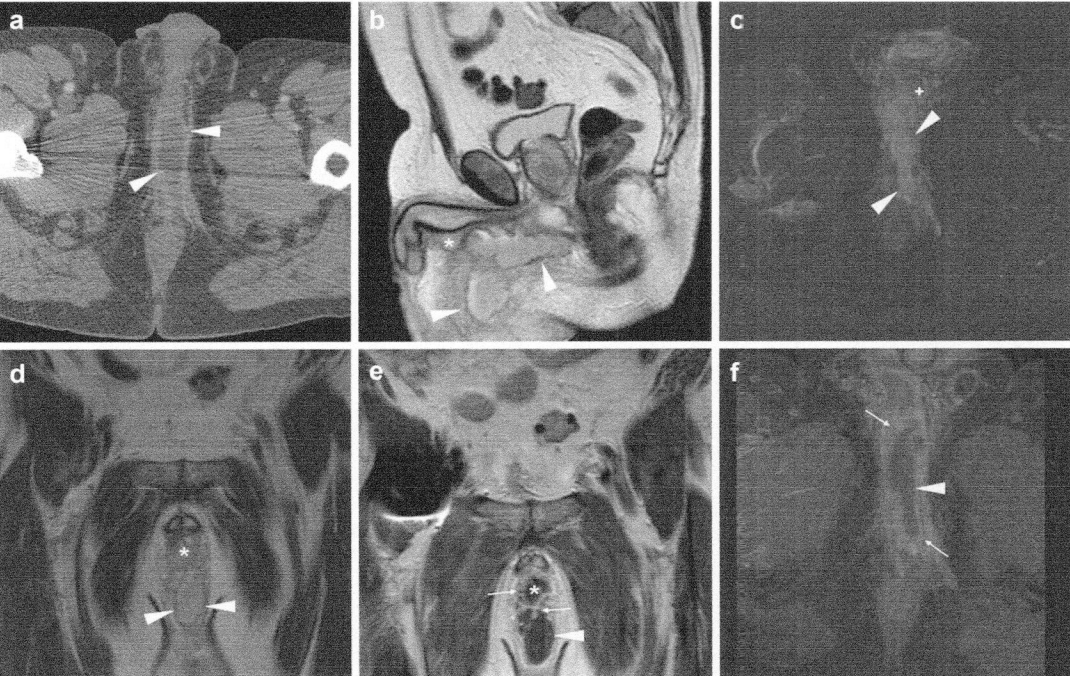

Fig. 16.2 Penile and perineal abscess from progression of urethral infection in a 53-year-old male with tender, inflamed swelling despite antibiotic therapy. Perineal infection was initially detected at contrast-enhanced CT (**a**) as an elongated midline abscess with peripheral enhancement (arrowheads) and internal fluid. MRI showed corresponding inhomogeneous fluid-like content on T2-weighted sequences (**b–d**) with surrounding inflammatory stranding (+), strong contrast enhancement in the abscess walls (arrowheads in **e, f**). The infected corpus spongiosum (*) showed similar signal features. Surgical evacuation was required to relieve the abscess [Reproduced with permission from Open Access Ref. no [13]]

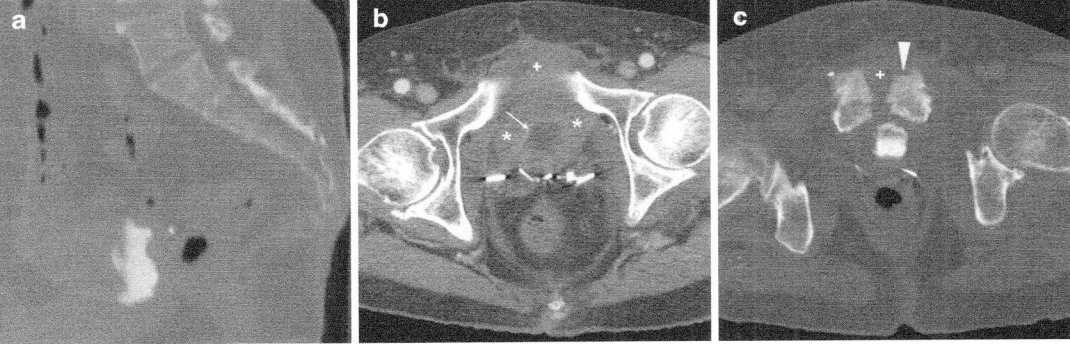

Fig. 16.3 Pubic osteomyelitis in a 78-year-old male with history of radical prostatectomy and pelvic radiotherapy, suffering from recurrent urinary tract infections (UTIs). CT urography showed a wide vertical opacified cavity corresponding to the contracted urinary bladder, vesico-urethral anastomosis and proximal urethra (**a**). The contracted bladder showed circumferential mural thickening (*) and thin urothelial hyperenhancement (thin arrow) consistent with ongoing UTI in the venous phase (**b**), plus a soft-tissue attenuation inflammatory tissue (+) extending ventrally to surround the pubic symphysis. Note metallic clips in (**b**). As seen with bone window settings (**c**), the latter showed irregular erosions more pronounced on the left side (arrowhead) consistent with development of osteomyelitis, which was not present in a previous MRI (not shown) and required intensive antibiotic therapy

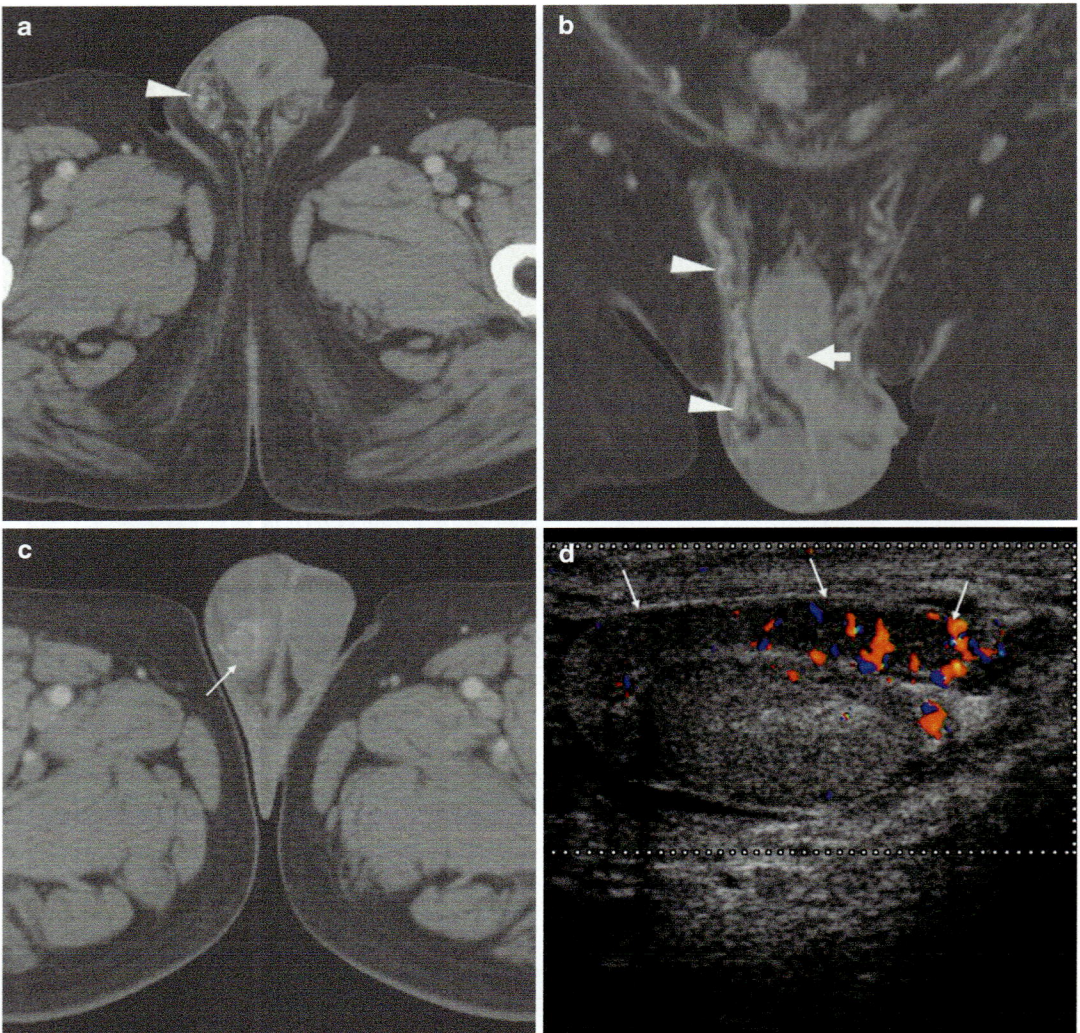

Fig. 16.4 Unsuspected funiculitis and acute epididymitis in a 75-year-old male with persistent fever, acute urinary retention, pyuria, markedly increased leukocyte count and acute phase reactants. Contrast-enhanced CT (**a–c**) revealed asymmetric thickening and vascular engorgement of the right spermatic cord (arrowheads), enlarged and hyperenhancing epididymis (thin arrow in **c**) com-pared to contralateral structure. Note Foley catheter (thick arrow in **b**). Subsequent colour Doppler ultrasound (**d**) confirmed thickened hypoechoic ipsilateral epididymis (thin arrows), particularly at the tail with increased flow signals consistent with acute inflammation. Despite nega-tive cultures after empiric antibiotic therapy, levofloxacin effectively treated the infection

genital infection, including unilateral spermatic cord thickening of variable entity, with inflammatory "fat stranding" and engorged enhancing blood vessels on the affected side. These features reflect infectious hyperaemia, should be reported as consistent with acute funiculitis and are strongly associated with ipsilateral infectious epididymitis and/or orchitis (Figs. 16.4, 16.5). Hypervascularity of the epididymis may be also observed at CT (Figs. 16.5, 16.6). Similarly to CT, MRI may also depict engorged vessels along the spermatic cord, plus epididymal enlargement with increased or heterogeneous T2 signal intensity and hypervascularity. Anyway, in these instances, scrotal colour Doppler ultrasound is warranted to confirm abnormal CT or MRI findings (Figs. 16.4, 16.5) [10, 12, 13, 17].

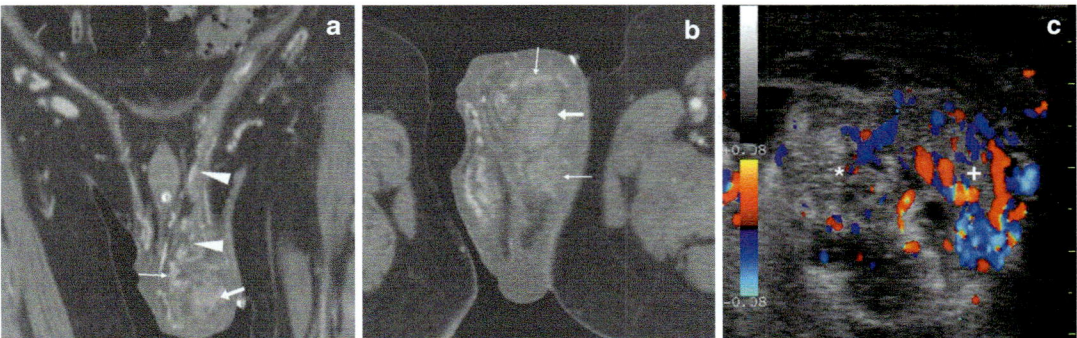

Fig. 16.5 Acute epididymo-orchitis in a 47-year-old Sri Lankan male with multiple myeloma on bortezomib therapy, suffering from fever and acute scrotal pain, tenderness and induration. Contrast-enhanced CT (**a**, **b**) performed to investigate impending urosepsis depicted a thickened engorged left spermatic cord, with inhomogeneous vascularization of the ipsilateral epididymis (thin arrows) and testis (arrows). Note catheter (in **a**) and thickened and increased oedematous attenuation of the scrotal skin and external tunicae. Colour Doppler (**c**) revealed hypervascularization of the epididymis (**+**). Unresponsive to antibiotics, this infection caused by *Klebsiella pneumoniae* ultimately required orchiectomy [Reproduced with permission from Open Access Ref.no [13]]

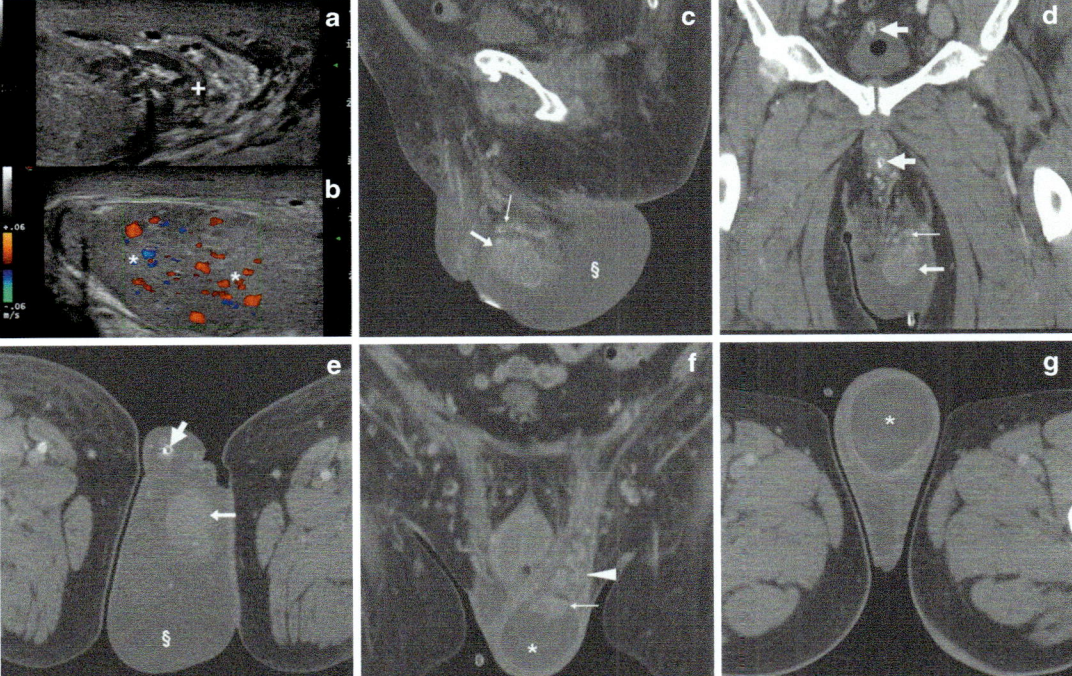

Fig. 16.6 Surgically confirmed epididymo-orchitis with pyocele in a 72-year-old diabetic male with haematuria and enlarged left scrotum, history of transurethral resection of bladder carcinoma and bladder neck stricture treated by long-term catheterization (thick arrows). Colour Doppler ultrasound revealed ipsilateral enlarged inhomogeneous epididymal head (**+** in **a**) and hypervascularized testis (* in **b**). After ineffective antibiotic therapy, contrast-enhanced CT (**c–e**) showed hypervascularized left epididymis (thin arrows) and testis (arrows) compared to contralateral structures and development of a large posterior scrotal collection (§). Another surgically proven case of testicular abscess and necrosis in a 59-year-old male with epididymo-orchitis unresponsive to medical therapy: post-contrast CT (**f**, **g**) revealed vascular engorgement along the left spermatic cord (arrowhead), faintly enhanced epididymal head (thin arrow in **e**) and ipsilateral scrotum occupied by fluidlike collection (*) with thin peripheral enhancing rim [Partially reproduced with permission from Open Access Ref.no [13]]

The commonest differential diagnosis of inflammatory cord enlargement is left-sided untreated or recurrent varicocele. Alternatively, spermatic vascular engorgement may be secondary to the presence of a testicular tumour. Furthermore, radiologists should be aware of the early postoperative spermatic cord thickening secondary to surgical manipulation during inguinal hernia repair: this condition typically appears tubular shaped, generally does not exceed 1 cm in diameter and regresses at follow-up. Albeit with regression of hypervascularity, some asymmetry in thickness of the pelvic extra-inguinal spermatic cord between the operated side and the contralateral one may be sometimes encountered months to years after surgery. Finally, epididymal abnormalities found on cross-sectional imaging may correspond to tubercular involvement, spermatocele (sperm granuloma), sometimes metastases or rare primary neoplasms [13, 22, 23].

16.2.3 Orchitis and Scrotal Abscesses

Compared to epididymitis, infectious involvement of the adjacent testis is less common and generally has similar or more severe clinical and laboratory manifestations [14, 16].

Since the scrotum should be included in a comprehensive abdomino-pelvic CT scan obtained for UTI or sepsis, familiarity with its normal appearance is warranted. Some fluid hydrocele is often present and should be reported, although often without pathologic significance. The normal testes are symmetric ovoid-shaped hypoattenuating structures, which are poorly differentiated by the scrotal tunicae and from hydrocele. At MRI the normal testes appear homogeneous, T1 isointense to muscle and T2 hyperintense, and the albuginea and mediastinum testis are identifiable as low-signal bands [10, 12, 13, 17].

On cross-sectional imaging studies, acute orchitis is suggested by testicular asymmetry with unilateral enlargement and increased contrast enhancement of the affected testis compared to the contralateral one; signs of funiculitis and epididymitis are generally associated (Fig. 16.6). Compared to CT, MRI better shows testicular inflammation as decreased T1 and increased T2 signal intensity in respect to the normal testis, with either intense homogeneous enhancement or the characteristic "tiger skin" post-contrast pattern corresponding to preserved septa. Focal or diffuse orchitis may be challenging to differentiate from testicular tumours, which generally show mass effect, solid-type CT attenuation and MRI signal features and are not associated with clinical and biochemical signs of infection [10–12, 17].

Untreated epididymo-orchitis may be further complicated by necrosis and/or development of a scrotal abscess or pyocele, which require surgical treatment [14, 16]. Loss of contrast enhancement is the hallmark of testicular necrosis, which is most easily demonstrated by avascularity at colour Doppler ultrasound [1–3]. CT and MRI features of pyocele include complex, heterogeneous fluidlike collections, surrounded by an enhancing periphery (Fig. 16.6) or by hyperaemic inflamed surrounding parenchyma [10–13].

16.2.4 Differential Diagnosis of Perineal and Genital Infections

Fournier's gangrene (FG) is an uncommon necrotizing polymicrobial infection of the genital, perineal and perianal regions that involves both superficial and deep fascial planes. The clinical presentation includes local pain, swollen oedematous or gangrenous overlying skin, sometimes with appreciable crepitus, and fever. FG constitutes a surgical emergency that must be recognized early because it is rapidly progressive; aggressive surgical debridement and broad-spectrum antibiotics are required to prevent a fatal outcome. The origin of infection is occult in

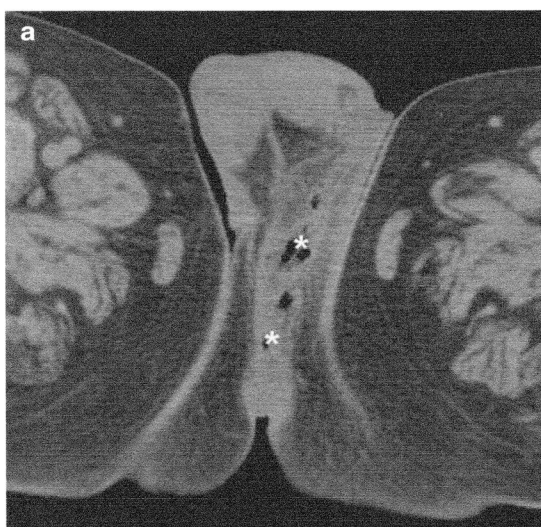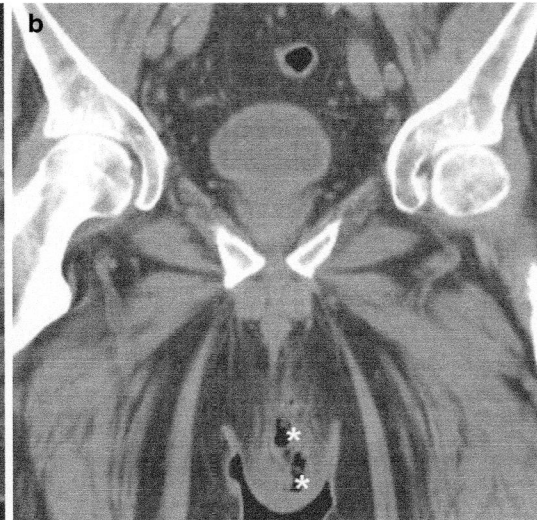

Fig. 16.7 Surgically treated Fournier's gangrene in a 63-year-old diabetic male with recurrent UTIs and perineal painful swelling. Unenhanced CT (**a**, **b**) revealed asymmetric left-sided thickening of the skin and subcutaneous fat infiltration with presence of gas collections (*) at the perineum and dorsal aspect of the scrotum

6–45% of patients and may be colorectal (such as tumour, diverticulitis, inflammatory bowel disease, perirectal abscess), urologic (lower UTI) or cutaneous (e.g. pressure ulceration) in descending order of frequency [24, 25].

Multidetector CT is by far the preferred modality since it has higher specificity for the diagnosis of FG and provides superior evaluation of disease extent. CT features include asymmetric fascial thickening, subcutaneous fat stranding at the involved areas, superficial or deep fluid and air-attenuation collections. Subcutaneous emphysema produced by anaerobic bacteria is the hallmark of FG (Fig. 16.7); however, air is absent in up to 10% of cases. Furthermore, CT can define the starting point of the infectious process, thereby allowing differentiation of complicated perineal infections from urinary versus an alternative source, particularly cryptogenetic perianal sepsis (Fig. 16.8) [13, 24–26].

Another uncommon differential diagnosis of perineal and scrotal infections is hidradenitis suppurativa (HS), a rare inflammatory disease of the genital, perineal and gluteal regions with unclear pathogenesis and chronic progressive course, which is mostly encountered in black people and males in association with poor hygiene [27–29].

In our experience, MRI offers two key advantages in this uncommon disorder: it accurately describes the affected regions, thus allowing optimal planning of wide excision and ultimately a decreased recurrence rate, which is proportional to the radicality of surgery [27, 28]. On the other hand, since skin inflammation, abscesses and fistulous tract are nonspecific physical manifestations, MRI may support a diagnosis of HS over epididymo-orchitis and scrotal abscess by demonstrating that tissue inflammation and abscesses are confined to the skin and subcutaneous tissues, with a characteristic symmetric distribution and lacking communication with pelvic organ. Inflamed tissue and abscesses are easily identified with MRI sequences acquired with fat suppression and after intravenous contrast (Fig. 16.9) [30].

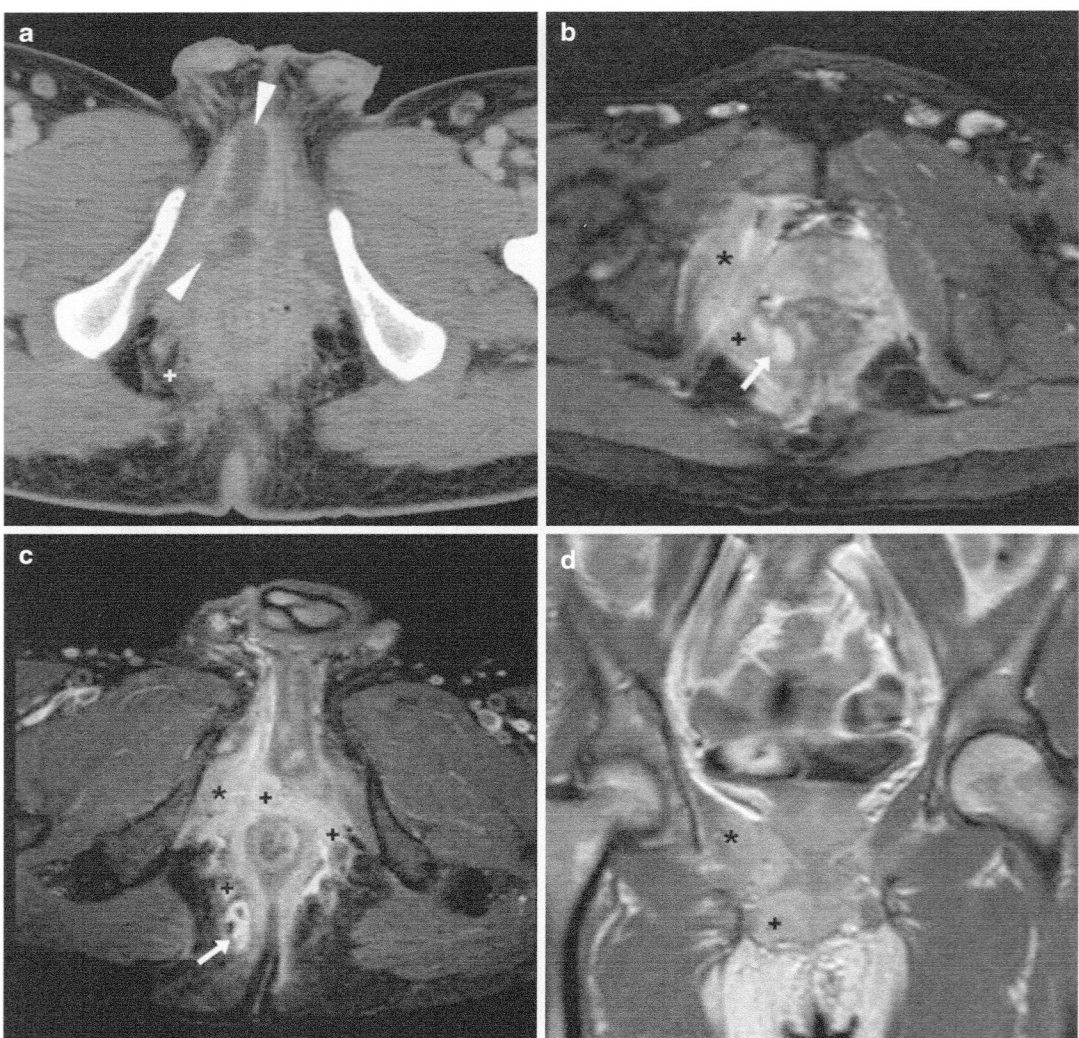

Fig. 16.8 Extensive cryptogenetic perianal inflammation in a 56-year old diabetic male with fever. Axial post-contrast CT image (**a**) revealed perineal abscess (arrowheads) closely similar to that depicted in Fig. 16.2. Additional MRI including axial STIR (**b**), post-gadolinium axial fat-suppressed (**c**) and coronal (**d**) T1-weighted images showed extensive inflammatory signal abnormalities and hyperenhancement (+) surrounding the anus, involving the right sphincter complex and obturator internus (*) muscles and extending to the ischioanal fossa. Tiny abscess collections (arrows in **b** and **c**) were present. Topography of infection, sparing of prostate and corpora cavernosa and clinical examination were inconsistent with complicated UTI [Reproduced with permission from Open Access Ref.no [13]]

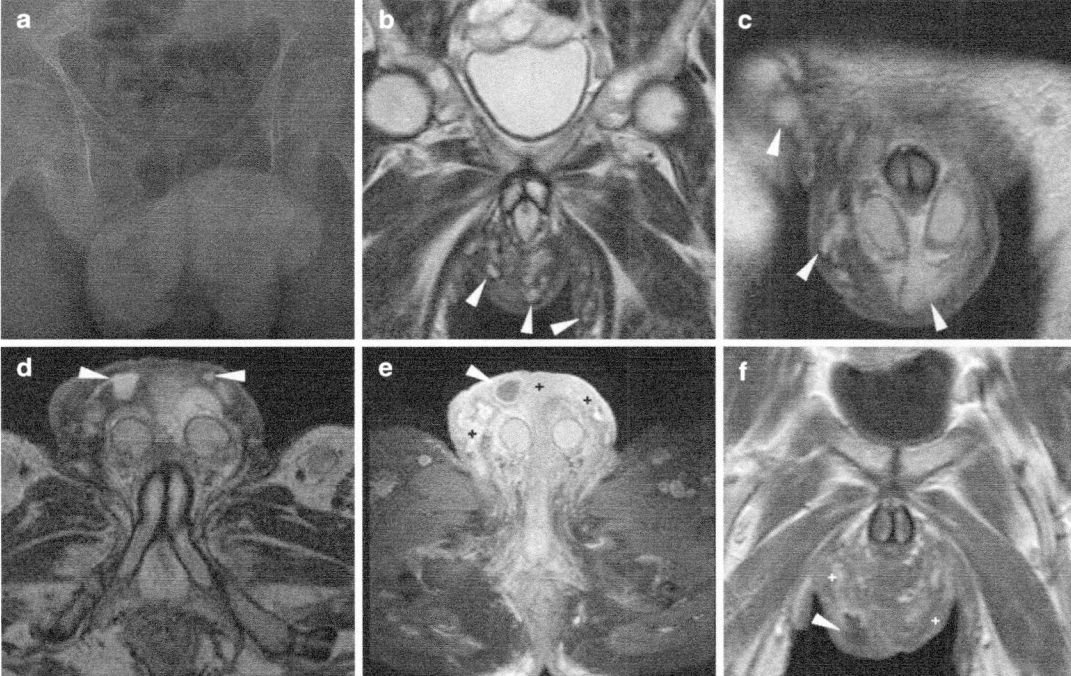

Fig. 16.9 Surgically confirmed hidradenitis suppurativa in a 51-year-old male with hepatitis C, complaining of progressive, painful swelling of perineum, scrotum and penis, with thickened skin and fistulous orifices. Plain radiographs (**a**) excluded air collections in the swollen scrotum. MRI including multiplanar T2-weighted (**b–d**), post-gadolinium axial fat-suppressed (**e**) and coronal (**f**) T1-weighted images depicted marked symmetrical thick-ening of the skin and subcutaneous planes with abnormal inflammatory signal intensity and hyperenhancement (+ in **e**, **f**) involving the medial aspect of the thighs, perineal region and scrotum. Small purulent collections with peripheral enhancement (arrowheads) and inflamed inguinal lymph nodes were present. The testes (not shown) did not show appreciable abnormalities [Reproduced with permission from Open Access Ref.no [13]]

References

1. Avery LL, Scheinfeld MH (2013) Imaging of penile and scrotal emergencies. Radiographics 33:721–740
2. Pavlica P, Barozzi L (2001) Imaging of the acute scrotum. Eur Radiol 11:220–228
3. Schull A, Monzani Q, Bour L et al (2012) Imaging in lower urinary tract infections. Diagn Interv Imaging 93:500–508
4. Ryu J, Kim B (2001) MR imaging of the male and female urethra. Radiographics 21:1169–1185
5. Kirkham AP, Illing RO, Minhas S et al (2008) MR imaging of nonmalignant penile lesions. Radiographics 28:837–853
6. Del Gaizo A, Silva AC, Lam-Himlin DM et al (2013) Magnetic resonance imaging of solid urethral and peri-urethral lesions. Insights Imaging 4:461–469
7. Pretorius ES, Siegelman ES, Ramchandani P et al (2001) MR imaging of the penis. Radiographics 21(Supp 1):S283–S298. discussion S298-289
8. Tonolini M, Villa C, Campari A et al (2013) Common and unusual urogenital Crohn's disease complications: spectrum of cross-sectional imaging findings. Abdom Imaging 38:32–41
9. Torkzad MR, Karlbom U (2011) MRI for assessment of anal fistula. Insights Imaging 1:62–71
10. Cassidy FH, Ishioka KM, McMahon CJ et al (2010) MR imaging of scrotal tumors and pseudotumors. Radiographics 30:665–683
11. Mohrs OK, Thoms H, Egner T et al (2012) MRI of patients with suspected scrotal or testicular lesions: diagnostic value in daily practice. AJR Am J Roentgenol 199:609–615
12. Parenti GC, Feletti F, Brandini F et al (2009) Imaging of the scrotum: role of MRI. Radiol Med 114:414–424
13. Tonolini M, Ippolito S (2016) Cross-sectional imaging of complicated urinary infections affecting the lower tract and male genital organs. Insights Imaging 7(5):689–711

14. Grabe M, Bartoletti R, Bjerklund-Johansen TE et al (2014) Guidelines on urological infections. European Association of Urology, The Netherlands. Available at: http://uroweb.org/wp-content/uploads/19-Urological-infections_LR2.pdf.

15. Barozzi L, Valentino M, Menchi I et al (2010) Clinical uroradiology: the standardisation of terminology for lower urinary tract function and dysfunction. Radiol Med 115:272–286

16. Trojian TH, Lishnak TS, Heiman D (2009) Epididymitis and orchitis: an overview. Am Fam Physician 79:583–587

17. Kubik-Huch RA, Hailemariam S, Hamm B (1999) CT and MRI of the male genital tract: radiologic-pathologic correlation. Eur Radiol 9:16–28

18. Browne RF, Zwirewich C, Torreggiani WC (2004) Imaging of urinary tract infection in the adult. Eur Radiol 14(Suppl 3):E168–E183

19. Yu M, Robinson K, Siegel C et al (2016) Complicated genitourinary tract infections and mimics. Curr Probl Diagn Radiol 46(1):74–83. https://doi.org/10.1067/j.cpradiol.2016.1002.1004

20. Kawashima A, Sandler CM, Wasserman NF et al (2004) Imaging of urethral disease: a pictorial review. Radiographics 24(Suppl 1):S195–S216

21. Pavlica P, Barozzi L, Menchi I (2003) Imaging of male urethra. Eur Radiol 13:1583–1596

22. Gupta SA, Horowitz JM, Bhalani SM et al (2014) Asymmetric spermatic cord vessel enhancement on CT: a sign of epididymitis or testicular neoplasm. Abdom Imaging 39:1014–1020

23. Tonolini M (2016) Multidetector CT of expected findings and complications after contemporary inguinal hernia repair surgery. Diagn Interv Radiol 22(5):422–429

24. Levenson RB, Singh AK, Novelline RA (2008) Fournier gangrene: role of imaging. Radiographics 28:519–528

25. Piedra T, Ruiz E, Gonzalez FJ et al (2006) Fournier's gangrene: a radiologic emergency. Abdom Imaging 31:500–502

26. Khati NJ, Sondel Lewis N, Frazier AA et al (2015) CT of acute perianal abscesses and infected fistulae: a pictorial essay. Emerg Radiol 22(3):329–335

27. Alikhan A, Lynch PJ, Eisen DB (2009) Hidradenitis suppurativa: a comprehensive review. J Am Acad Dermatol 60:539–561. quiz 562–533

28. Anderson BB, Cadogan CA, Gangadharam D (1982) Hidradenitis suppurativa of the perineum, scrotum, and gluteal area: presentation, complications, and treatment. J Natl Med Assoc 74:999–1003

29. Buimer MG, Wobbes T, Klinkenbijl JH (2009) Hidradenitis suppurativa. Br J Surg 96:350–360

30. Kelly AM, Cronin P (2005) MRI features of hidradenitis suppurativa and review of the literature. AJR Am J Roentgenol 185:1201–1204

Part IV

Miscellaneous Topics

Cross-Sectional Imaging of Urosepsis

17

Massimo Tonolini

17.1 Introduction

Although extremely common, urinary tract infections (UTI) encompass a wide range of conditions which range from asymptomatic bacteriuria and simple cystitis causing local symptoms to potentially life-threatening conditions. Generally, urinary sepsis or urosepsis is defined by the presence of bacteraemia with a urinary tract infectious focus [1].

The incidence of sepsis is reportedly increasing, in both community-acquired and healthcare-associated (nosocomial) UTIs. Patients with the RENUC risk factors (as listed in Table 1.1 in the introductory chapter of this book) are much more likely to develop urosepsis, such as diabetics, immunosuppressed and transplant recipients, those treated with corticosteroid or chemotherapy, those with urolithiasis, obstructed urinary tract, neurogenic bladder and congenital abnormalities, or following recent instrumentation. Although associated with a better prognosis compared to other systemic infections, urosepsis remains a critical situation, particularly in the elderly and immunocompromised. The associated mortality is estimated to fall in the range between 20 and 40% and is probably declining due to improvements in patient care. However, mortality remains considerable in severe sepsis (defined by the development of organ dysfunction) and in septic shock with persistent hypotension despite fluid resuscitation [1, 2].

17.2 Role of Imaging in Urosepsis

Suspected urosepsis requires early diagnosis and timely treatment, particularly in those patients with risk factors for complicated UTI. The role of imaging includes:

(a) To detect urological complications requiring directed treatment, such as abscess and pyonephrosis
(b) To document congenital, acquired or postsurgical anatomical situations which predispose to infection
(c) To confirm urological cause of sepsis while excluding other potential sources in the body

The ultimate aim is to prevent renal function deterioration and to decrease morbidity and mortality [1, 3].

As well known, first-line ultrasound readily allows detecting urinary obstruction and pyonephrosis requiring prompt drainage without use of ionizing radiation and intravenous contrast medium. However, as extensively discussed in other chapters of this book, multidetector CT (including intravenous contrast enhancement unless contraindicated) is superior to ultrasound in the detection of infection and abscesses and by

M. Tonolini, M.D.
Radiology Department, "Luigi Sacco" University Hospital, Via G.B. Grassi 74, Milan 20157, Italy
e-mail: mtonolini@sirm.org

© Springer International Publishing AG 2018
M. Tonolini (ed.), *Imaging and Intervention in Urinary Tract Infections and Urosepsis*,
https://doi.org/10.1007/978-3-319-68276-1_17

far represents the ideal modality to comprehensively investigate severe UTI and possible complications [4–10].

Figures 17.1, 17.2, and 17.3 present three clinical examples of cross-sectional imaging investigation of urinary sepsis. In our experience, the use of CT is particularly useful in the postoperative setting after urological instrumentation and surgery [9, 11–13].

In a large study including 221 adult patients experiencing first-time urosepsis, the use of CT discovered major findings in almost one-third

(32%) of patients, particularly hydro- or pyonephrosis (17%) and urolithiasis (7.6%). Other findings in descending order or frequency included tumours, renal abscesses, ureteral dilatation, calyceal dilatation, duplex kidney, ureteral structure, infected polycystic kidney, emphysematous pyelonephritis and displaced nephrostomy. Clinical predictors of major abnormalities include increased serum creatinine, type 2 diabetes, diabetic complications, known renal disease or urological abnormality. Interestingly, abnormal CT findings led to urological intervention in approximately one-half

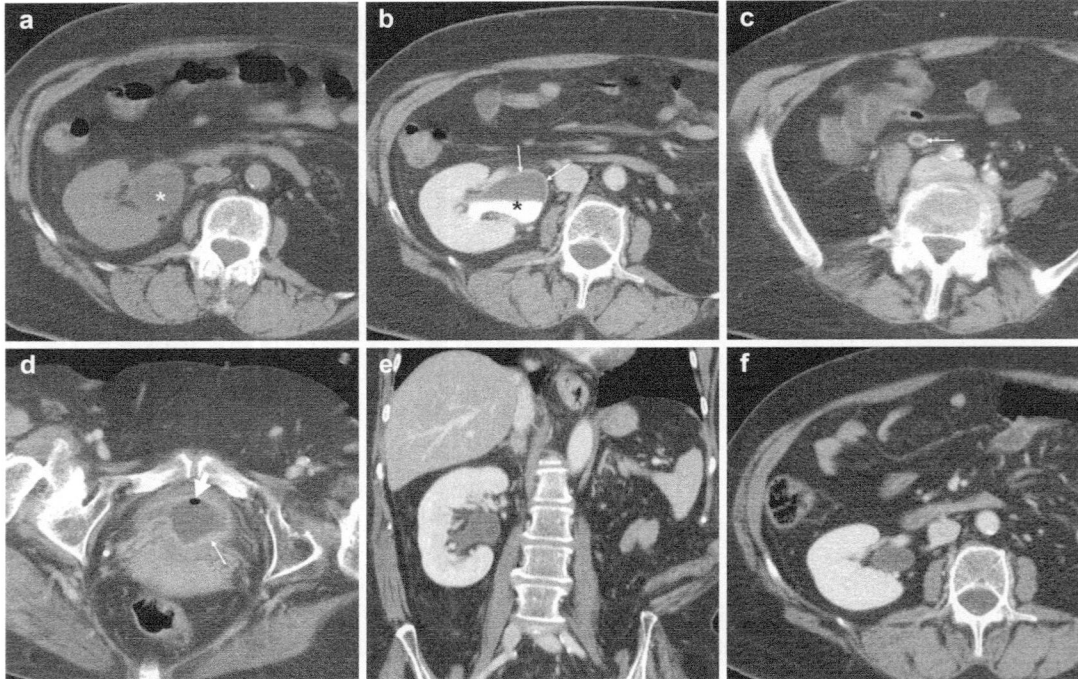

Fig. 17.1 A 71-year-old female with a congenital solitary kidney was hospitalized for voiding difficulty and high fever unresponsive to empirical antibiotics. Urgent unenhanced (**a**) and post-contrast (**b–d**) multidetector CT revealed mild hydronephrosis with preserved renal function. The dilated renal pelvis (*) showed minimal, enhancing mural thickening (thin arrows in **b**) which was even more pronounced along the ureter (thin arrow in **c**) and in the bladder (thin arrow in **d**; note Foley catheter indicated by thick arrow). Findings were consistent with diagnosis of urosepsis which required prolonged in-hospital treatment. Four months after discharge, repeated CT (**e**, **f**) showed decreased hydronephrosis, normalized mural thickening and disappearance of urothelial hyperenhancement. Note absent left kidney

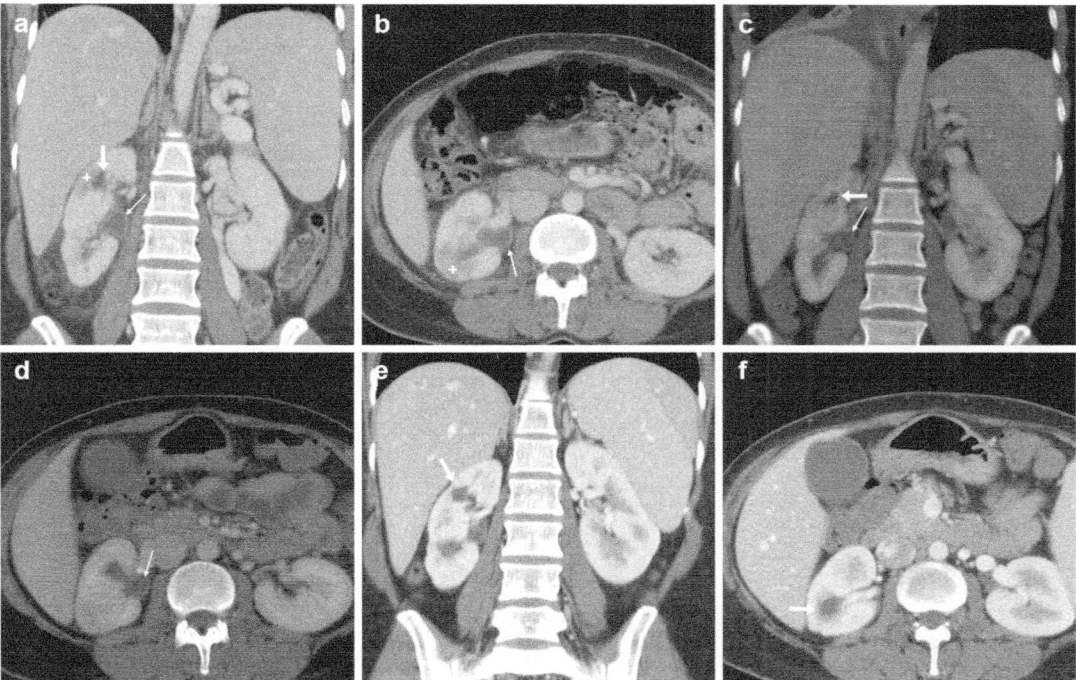

Fig. 17.2 A 41-year-old female immigrant from the Middle East had history of renal colic 2 years ago. Currently attended at emergency department for abdominal and right flank pain associated with shivers, high fever and dysuria. Laboratory tests revealed leukocytosis and increased acute phase reactants. Urgent contrast-enhanced CT (**a, b**) showed mild, hyperenhancing thickening of the renal pelvis (thin arrows), calyceal dilatation (arrow) at the upper renal third, two wedge-shaped hypoperfused parenchymal areas (*), consistent with right acute pyelitis and pyelonephritis. Transferred to intensive care unit, she progressively improved with medical therapy. Urine cultures diagnosed *Escherichia coli* infection. Before discharge, repeated CT (**c, d**) showed resolution of parenchymal changes and persistence of calyceal dilatation (arrow) and of pelvic urothelial enhancement (thin arrows). Distant follow-up CT (**e, f**) showed resolved hydronephrosis and urothelial enhancement and persistent upper calyceal dilatation (arrows) with focal thinning of the overlying parenchyma consistent with chronic "scarring"

of cases, such as positioning or replacement of nephrostomy or ureteral stent, sometimes cyst drainage, catheter replacement, stone removal and occasionally even nephrectomy [3].

Furthermore, multidetector CT provides panoramic body exploration, thus allowing to detect infectious changes resulting from haematogenous dissemination in other anatomical regions, which are most usually found in the lungs, the brain, the liver and spleen and the iliopsoas muscles [14]. Finally, as exemplified in Figs. 17.1, 17.2, and 17.3, cross-sectional CT imaging is highly valuable to provide consistent follow-up of severe or complicated UTIs during medical or interventional therapy, in order to document resolution of infectious changes or long-term sequelae [5–8].

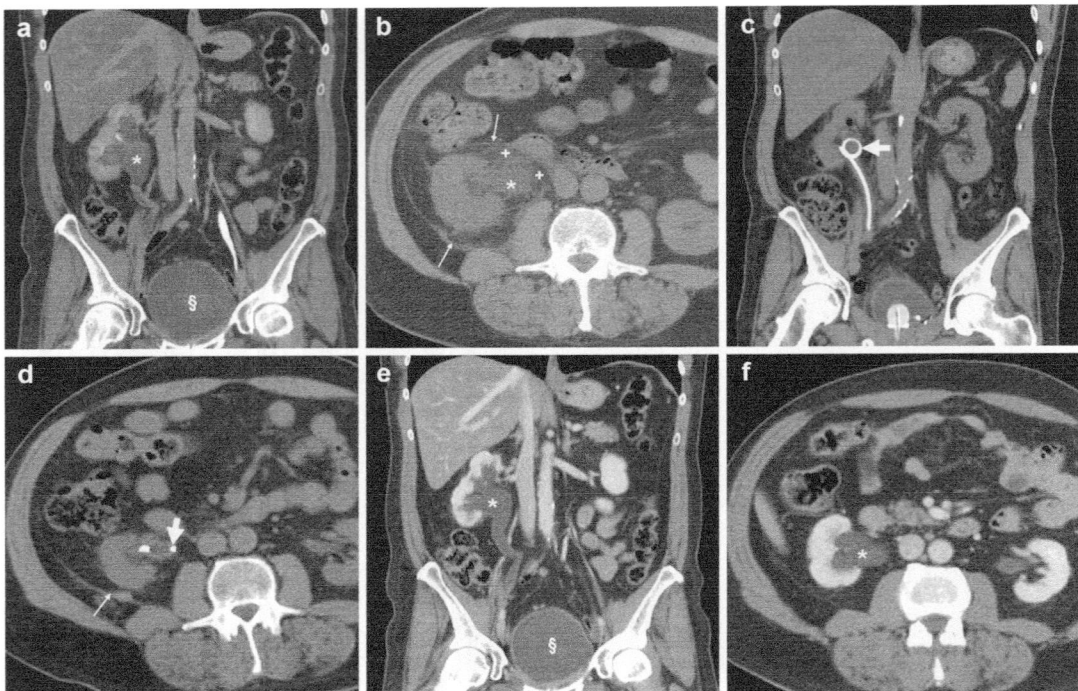

Fig. 17.3 A 61-year-old male with recent radical cystectomy for bladder carcinoma and orthotopic neobladder (*§*) reconstruction, as documented by postoperative multidetector CT urography. Note right-sided hydronephrosis (*) with delayed contrast excretion. A year later, he was hospitalized for sepsis and acute renal failure. Unenhanced CT (**b**) showed stable dilatation of the right renal pelvis (*) with appearance of peripelvic and perirenal "fat stranding" (+) and of ipsilateral fascial thickening (thin arrows). Pyonephrosis was relieved by ureteral stenting (thick arrows) as seen on repeated unenhanced CT (**c, d**) with resolution of perirenal inflammation and persistently thickened posterior renal fascia (thin arrow in **d**). With resolution of urosepsis and improved renal function, follow-up contrast-enhanced CT (**e, f**) showed resolution of infectious changes, preserved nephrographic effect, stable hydronephrosis (*) compared to (**a**) and well-distended neobladder (*§*)

References

1. Grabe M, Bartoletti R, Bjerklund-Johansen TE et al (2014) Guidelines on urological infections. European Association of Urology, The Netherlands. Available at: http://uroweb.org/wp-content/uploads/19-Urological-infections_LR2.pdf
2. Foxman B (2003) Epidemiology of urinary tract infections: incidence, morbidity, and economic costs. Dis Mon 49:53–70
3. Sorensen SM, Schonheyder HC, Nielsen H (2013) The role of imaging of the urinary tract in patients with urosepsis. Int J Infect Dis 17:e299–e303
4. van Nieuwkoop C, Hoppe BP, Bonten TN et al (2010) Predicting the need for radiologic imaging in adults with febrile urinary tract infection. Clin Infect Dis 51:1266–1272
5. Ifergan J, Pommier R, Brion MC et al (2012) Imaging in upper urinary tract infections. Diagn Interv Imaging 93:509–519
6. Craig WD, Wagner BJ, Travis MD (2008) Pyelonephritis: radiologic-pathologic review. Radiographics 28:255–277. quiz 327–258
7. Demertzis J, Menias CO (2007) State of the art: imaging of renal infections. Emerg Radiol 14:13–22
8. Browne RF, Zwirewich C, Torreggiani WC (2004) Imaging of urinary tract infection in the adult. Eur Radiol 14(Suppl 3):E168–E183
9. Tonolini M, Ippolito S (2016) Cross-sectional imaging of complicated urinary infections affecting the lower tract and male genital organs. Insights Imaging 7(5):689–711
10. Lee MJ (2002) Non-traumatic abdominal emergencies: imaging and intervention in sepsis. Eur Radiol 12:2172–2179

11. Tonolini M, Ierardi AM, Varca V et al (2015) Multidetector CT imaging of complications after laparoscopic nephron-sparing surgery. Insights Imaging 6:465–478

12. Tonolini M, Villa F, Ippolito S et al (2014) Cross-sectional imaging of iatrogenic complications after extracorporeal and endourological treatment of urolithiasis. Insights Imaging 5:677–689

13. Tonolini M, Villa F, Bianco R (2013) Multidetector CT imaging of post-robot-assisted laparoscopic radical prostatectomy complications. Insights Imaging 4:711–721

14. Tonolini M, Campari A, Bianco R (2012) Common and unusual diseases involving the iliopsoas muscle compartment: spectrum of cross-sectional imaging findings. Abdom Imaging 37:118–139

Modern Imaging of Urogenital Tuberculosis

18

Massimo Tonolini

18.1 Urogenital Tuberculosis: Pathogenesis and Clinical Features

Nowadays, tuberculosis still represents a major public health problem worldwide, with a high prevalence in those regions where population concentrates with poor sanitation and unfavourable social and economic status. Despite the availability of effective therapies, in recent years, tuberculosis experienced a recrudescence, particularly in Eastern Europe, in parts of Africa and Asia, and also in nonendemic Western populations: this phenomenon results from a combination of factors such as the appearance of drug-resistant mycobacteria, increased population migrations and the human immunodeficiency virus (HIV) epidemic [1–3].

Compared to lung tuberculosis, extrapulmonary disease accounts for a minority of cases but is increasingly encountered, particularly in individuals with HIV or medication-related immunosuppression. After the lymph nodes, urogenital tuberculosis (UG-TB) is the second most common (27–35% of cases) form of extrapulmonary disease and generally occurs in adults, since the interval between the primary pulmonary infection and UG-TB presentation varies from 5 to 40 years (over 20 years on average); conversely UG-TB is rare in children [1–5].

The pathogenetic mechanisms are closely related to the clinical manifestations and imaging patterns. UG-TB primarily develops through haematogenous spread of *Mycobacterium tuberculosis* from the lungs to the kidneys. At this point, the acquired cellular immunity blocks bacterial multiplication and contains the infection by forming inactive microscopic granulomas. Subsequently, when the host's immunity decreases, reactivation occurs into the kidney medulla. The renal involvement is initially bilateral and cortical, reflecting its origin from dissemination in the bloodstream. Later on, when the mycobacteria are shed into the urine, the disease spreads downward to involve the calyces, renal pelvis, ureter and ultimately bladder, causing urothelial inflammation and mucosal thickening [1, 4–6].

The presentation of UG-TB varies according to the disease stage and is often subtle, in approximately half of patients in the absence of active lung infection. History and radiographic evidence of previous lung tuberculosis are often

M. Tonolini, M.D.
Radiology Department, "Luigi Sacco" University
Hospital, Via G.B. Grassi 74, Milan 20157, Italy
e-mail: mtonolini@sirm.org

© Springer International Publishing AG 2018
M. Tonolini (ed.), *Imaging and Intervention in Urinary Tract Infections and Urosepsis*,
https://doi.org/10.1007/978-3-319-68276-1_18

lacking. Renal tuberculosis, collecting system and unilateral ureteral involvement are generally asymptomatic. Chronic inflammation causes reduced compliance and capacity of the urinary bladder, which manifests with increased frequency of micturition, dysuria and ultimately urgency. Since more than 50% of all patients complain of irritative voiding symptoms, UG-TB is frequently discovered when the lower urinary tract is already involved. One of the most common manifestations is recurrent or resistant urinary tract infection with microscopic or macroscopic haematuria. Unspecific back or flank pain and constitutional symptoms such as fever, malaise and weight loss are commonly present. Further progression of UG-TB causes ureteral stricture, upstream hydronephrosis and ultimately renal function loss: according to the development of healthcare, the prevalence of nonfunctioning kidneys at diagnosis varies from 58 to 71% in developing countries to 8% in the United States. Generally, in low-income countries, patients are more symptomatic at presentation, with frequent irreversible destruction of the urinary tract [1, 4, 6, 7].

Tuberculosis also commonly affects the prostate, epididymis, seminal vesicles and fallopian tubes. Prostatic tuberculosis has coexistent renal involvement in 85% of cases and is often poorly symptomatic but sometimes characteristically manifests as haemospermia. Nearly half of male patients have scrotal complaints or abnormal physical findings, and in developing countries UG-TB is a common cause of infertility in both sexes [1, 4, 6, 7].

Alternatively, imaging signs of genitourinary involvement are detected in patients with lung or disseminated tuberculosis which may affect the neck and mediastinal lymph nodes, liver and spleen, peritoneum, abdominal nodes and digestive tract, central nervous system and spine [8–12].

However, the diagnosis of UG-TB is frequently delayed and probably underestimated; therefore a high degree of suspicion should be exercised. Confirmation requires the demonstra-

tion of *Mycobacterium tuberculosis* in urine or other body sample, coupled with consistent imaging findings. Recently nuclei acid amplification tests have become the method of choice [1, 4, 6, 7, 13].

The prolonged combination drug therapies used in respiratory tuberculosis effectively cure UG-TB too. However, surgical treatment is often performed in complicated cases, which may require ablative procedures (partial or total nephrectomy, ureterectomy, cystectomy, transurethral resection of prostate, epididymectomy and salpingectomy) or reconstructive ones such as ureteral stricture repair, ureteral stenting or nephrostomy, urinary diversion or bladder augmentation cystoplasty [4, 5, 14].

18.2 Cross-Sectional Imaging of Urogenital Tuberculosis

The most experienced radiologists are often familiar with the classical radiographic signs of UG-TB, as demonstrated by intravenous urography (IVU). Until a decade ago, IVU allowed detecting subtle changes reflecting early renal and collecting system damage such as the "moth-eaten" calyx, papillary necrosis and calyceal dilatation. The diagnosis of UG-TB was relatively straightforward when faced with collecting system and ureteral distortion by multiple strictures and partial or complete replacement of the kidney by calcifications [8, 10, 15–20].

In the current era of multidetector CT, IVU has been abandoned. CT offers several advantages over IVU because it provides combined morphologic and functional information and visualizes parenchymal abnormalities even in nonfunctioning kidneys and the possible extrarenal extension of tubercular changes. Furthermore, CT is most sensitive to detect calcifications, renal cavities, mural thickening and ureteral strictures [8, 10, 15–21].

18.2.1 Renal and Collecting System Involvement

The earliest CT renal features of UG-TB reflect localized tissue oedema from active inflammation and include focal hypoperfused parenchymal areas and sometimes small-sized cortical abscess-like collections; therefore, the appearance closely mimics that of bacterial acute pyelonephritis. Occasionally, tuberculosis may masquerade as a solid renal mass with minimal enhancement which may be misinterpreted as tumour. The involvement of the collecting system generally begins with calyceal deformity and loss of sharpness, focal or uneven caliectasis from infundibular strictures at different sites; diffuse caliectasis without dilatation of the renal pelvis represents a characteristic pattern. The fluid contained in dilated cavities sometimes shows higher-than-water attenuation (10–30 HU) corresponding to debris and caseation. A mild, uniform and enhancing urothelial thickening (Fig. 18.1) is commonly

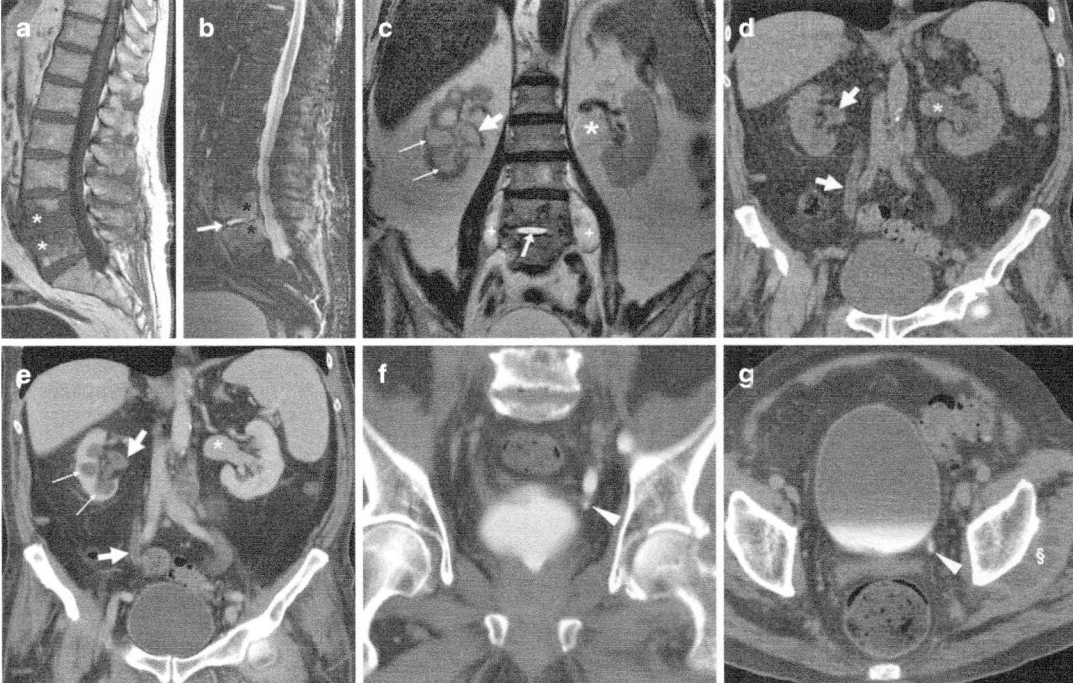

Fig. 18.1 An 82-year-old male was diagnosed with lumbar spondylodiscitis on the basis of characteristic inflammatory-type MR signal changes affecting the L4 and L5 vertebral bodies (T1-weighted **a**, short-tau inversion recovery **b**, T2-weighted **c**) and abscessualized intervertebral disc (*arrows* in **b**, **c**). The hypothesis of spinal tuberculosis was suggested by the presence of bilateral paravertebral abscesses (+ in **c**). Incidental findings included moderate left-sided hydronephrosis (*), right kidney with parenchymal thinning, dilated and distorted calyces (*thin arrows*) and non-dilated pelvis with some mural thickening (*thick arrow*). Unenhanced CT acquisition (**d**) did not reveal urinary tract calcifications. The mild urothelial thickening along the right renal pelvis and ureter (*thick arrows*) showed positive contrast enhancement (**e**). The atrophied right kidney had uneven calyceal dilatation (*thin arrows* in **e**). The left-sided hydronephrosis (* in **e**) was confirmed, with preserved nephrographic phase and contrast excretion, and secondary to a short stricture of the distal ureter (*arrowheads* in delayed phase images **f** and **g**). Tuberculosis was confirmed by positive QuantiFERON assay and vertebral biopsy and improved after specific combined therapy (Adapted from Open Access Ref.no [21])

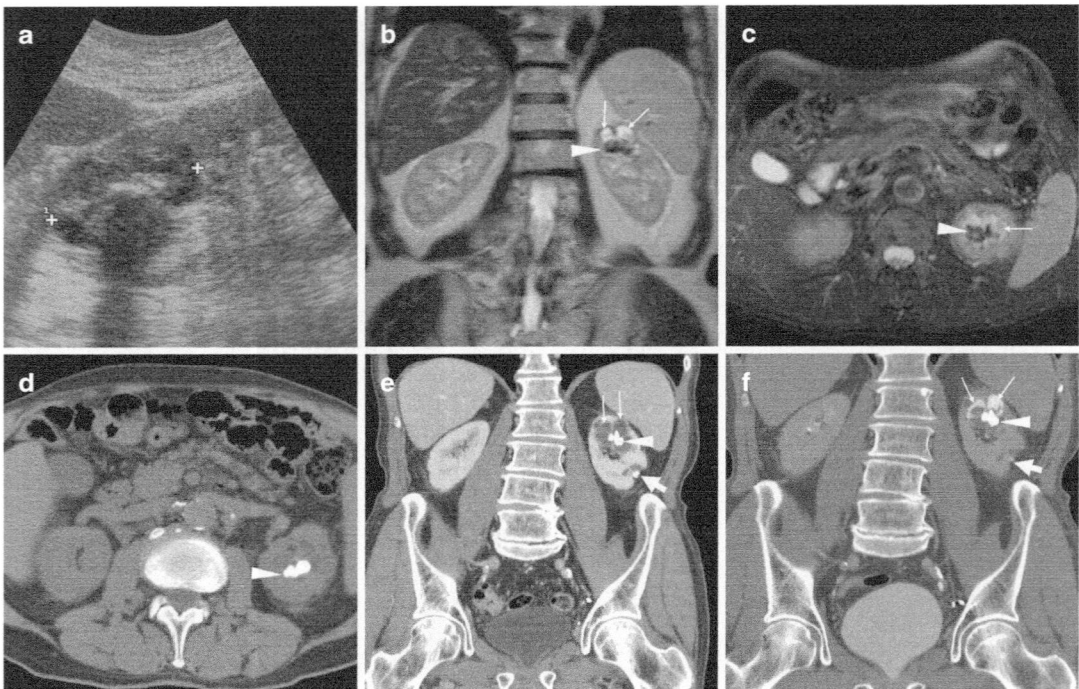

Fig. 18.2 An 80-year-old male being investigated for reasons unrelated to the urinary tract had sonographic detection of a hypo-anechoic upper pole lesion (calipres) of the left kidney, mostly occupied by a large calcification causing posterior acoustic shadowing. Coronal (**b**) and fat-saturated axial (**c**) T2-weighted images from MR cholangiopancreatography depicted very low-signal structures (arrowheads) suggestive of calcifications, located within dilated calyces (thin arrows). Calcifications (arrowheads) were well visible on CT including preliminary unenhanced scan (**d**). After intravenous contrast, nephrographic (**e**) acquisition confirmed left upper renal pole with thinned parenchyma and dilated and distorted calyces opacified by urine in the delayed excretory (**f**) phase. An additional focal renal scarring with calcification was noted (thick arrow). Findings were consistent with chronic tubercular infection, without appreciable abnormalities of the excretory tract and bladder

appreciable and similar to that observed in other active urinary infections [8, 10, 15–21].

Late renal changes consistent with advanced disease include a multiloculated cystic appearance from progression and confluence of caliectasis, and presence of calcifications (Fig. 18.2). The latter are seen in over half of patients and may take several forms such as amorphous, granular or curvilinear. Chronic UG-TB is indicated by the pathognomonic lobar distribution of calcifications or even by complete replacement of the kidney (tuberculous autonephrectomy) [8, 10, 15–21].

18.2.2 Ureteral and Bladder Involvement

The ureter is involved in almost 50% of patients with UG-TB. Chronic infection causes intramural fibrosis and ultimately leads to stricture formation with upstream hydronephrosis. CT visualizes the thickened ureteral wall and strictures, which have a predilection for sites of normal anatomic narrowing and therefore occur in descending order of frequency at the distal third of the ureter (Fig. 18.1), ureteropelvic junction and mid-ureter. Sometimes multiple, tuberculous strictures are

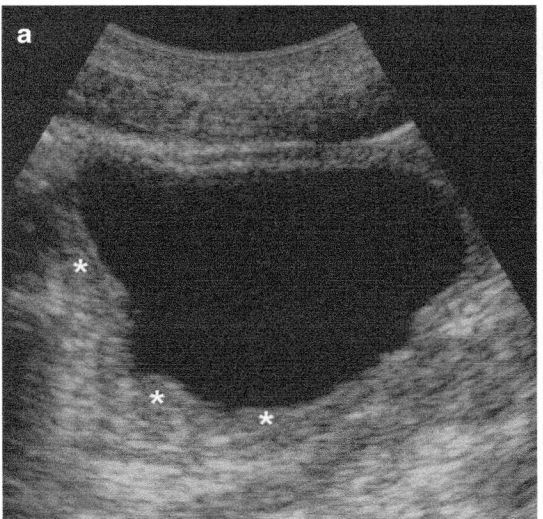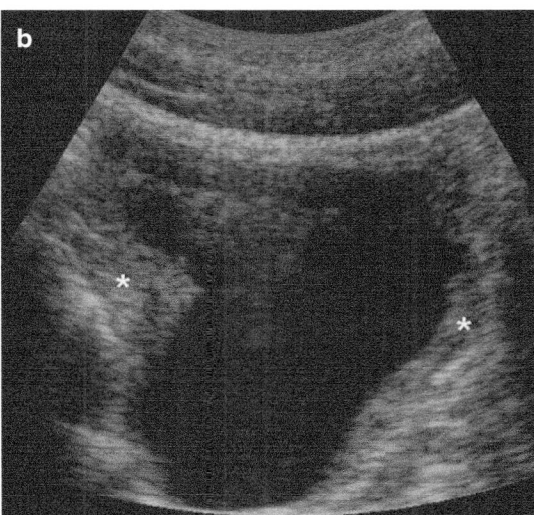

Fig. 18.3 A 14-year-old adolescent boy immigrated from Eastern Europe suffered from persistent dysuria and macroscopic haematuria. Transverse (**a**) and longitudinal (**b**) ultrasound images showed normally distended urinary bladder with circumferential mural thickening (*), particularly severe on the right posterolateral and upper aspects. The kidneys and collecting system did not show significant abnormalities; the ureters were not dilated. Cystoscopy confirmed extensive, severe inflammatory changes of the bladder wall. Diagnosis of urinary tuberculosis was ultimately made, after negative urinary tests and cultures

nowadays frequently misinterpreted as urotheliomas (Fig. 18.1) unless suggestive clinical features or other imaging signs suggest the diagnosis. Long-standing hydronephrosis ultimately leads to parenchymal atrophy with thinned, poorly functioning parenchyma [8, 10, 15–21].

The earliest bladder change is represented by decreased capacity. Disease progression leads to formation of mural thickening, irregularities from ulceration and filling defects representing granulomas (Fig. 18.3). Advanced disease causes extensive fibrotic wall scarring which appears as low-volume, severely thickened "thimble" bladder [8, 10, 15–22].

18.2.3 Genital Tuberculosis

In both sexes, tubercular involvement of the genital organs may occur through haematogenous spread, lymphatic spread or contiguous extension from the lower urinary tract. CT appearances of UG-TB affecting the prostate and seminal vesicles include characteristic calcifications and hypoattenuating changes from inflammation and caseous necrosis, which are indistinguishable from pyogenic abscesses. The epididymis may show focal or diffuse swelling with hypoechoic sonographic appearance and low T2 MRI signal intensity consistent with chronic inflammation and fibrosis. Granulomatous prostatitis may mimic cancer at multiparametric MRI, as it manifests as focal or extensive T2 hypointensity within the peripheral zone, with moderate or marked diffusion restriction and contrast enhancement, and occasionally demonstrates extraprostatic extension too; when caseating necrosis develops, both the T2-weighted signal intensity and diffusion restriction increase, but dynamic enhancement disappears [8, 10, 15–20, 23].

The majority of affected females have fallopian tubes involvement in the form of uni- or bilateral hydrosalpinx or complex adnexal masses

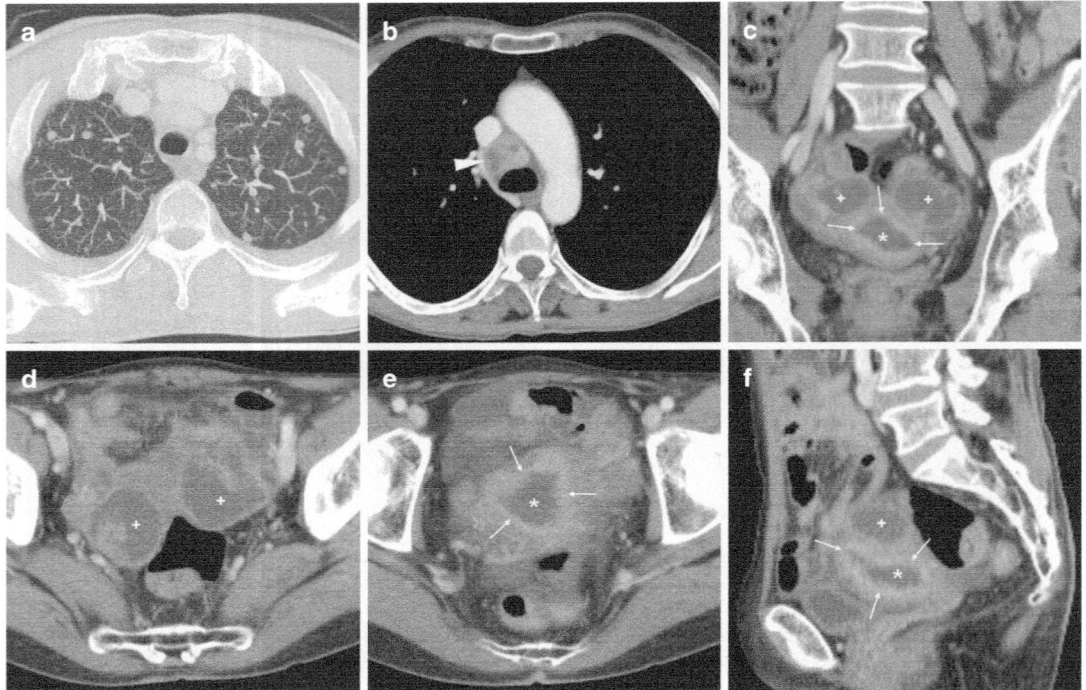

Fig. 18.4 A 58-year-old woman was transferred from Albania under presumptive diagnosis of ovarian carcinoma including increased serum CA125 tumour marker. A year earlier, her husband was diagnosed affected with lung tuberculosis. Contrast-enhanced body CT revealed several centimetric non-calcified and non-cavitary pulmonary nodules (**a**), particularly at both apical regions; necrotic mediastinal adenopathies (arrowhead in **b**); bilateral adnexal enlargement from pear-shaped fluid collections (+) with thin, minimally irregular enhancing periphery; dilatation of the uterine cavity (*) lined by thick, strongly enhancing endometrium (thin arrows). Consultation with attending gynaecologist diagnosed bilateral tubo-ovarian abscesses and pyometra. After inconclusive microbiological assays, endometrial washing and biopsy yielded purulent necrotic material with epithelioid giant cell granulomas, without microorganisms at microscopy and culture. Genital tuberculosis was confirmed by positive QuantiFERON test and polymerase chain reaction for mycobacterial DNA (Adapted from Open Access Ref.no [25])

(Fig. 18.4) which are easily confused with pyogenic tubo-ovarian abscesses and even ovarian tumours [13, 24, 25].

Conclusion

Recognition of UG-TB is important since if left untreated, it leads to shrunken, non-functioning kidneys. However, it is usually a challenging clinical diagnosis due to subtle, unspecific symptoms and time-consuming, difficult cultures. Albeit the majority of cases occur in the Third World, UG-TB is occasionally but increasingly encountered in Western countries and should be suspected in patients with unexplained haematuria, resistant urinary tract infection ("sterile pyuria") and prostatic, epididymal or adnexal lesions, particularly in immigrants from endemic areas or immunosuppressed such as HIV-positive patients [2, 4].

Cross-sectional imaging, particularly with multidetector CT, comprehensively evaluates the entire urogenital tract and consistently supports the diagnosis of UG-TB particularly when a combination of multiple findings is observed. Table 18.1 summarizes the early and late urinary changes which should alert the radiologist to the possibility of tuberculosis, particularly if multiple and bilateral [11, 12, 20].

Table 18.1 Early and advanced cross-sectional imaging features suggesting urinary tuberculosis, particularly if multiple and bilateral (Reproduced from Open Access Ref.no [21])

Early changes	• Renal low-attenuation, hypoperfused parenchymal regions with or without abscess-like collections
	• Uneven pelvicalyceal dilatation and/or distortion, particularly caliectasis without pelvic dilatation
Advanced changes	• Variably distributed renal calcifications
	• Diffuse renal scarring and atrophy
	• Replacement of kidney by cavities communicating with the collecting systems
	• Multiple pyelo-ureteral strictures, particularly including deformed ureterovesical junction
	• Hydronephrosis and/or poorly functioning kidney without obstructing calculi
	• Contracted thickened urinary bladder

References

1. Figueiredo AA, Lucon AM, Gomes CM et al (2008) Urogenital tuberculosis: patient classification in seven different groups according to clinical and radiological presentation. Int Braz J Urol 34:422–432. discussion 432

2. Figueiredo AA, Lucon AM, Junior RF et al (2008) Epidemiology of urogenital tuberculosis worldwide. Int J Urol 15:827–832

3. Daher Ede F, da Silva GB Jr, Barros EJ (2013) Renal tuberculosis in the modern era. Am J Trop Med Hyg 88:54–64

4. Zajaczkowski T (2012) Genitourinary tuberculosis: historical and basic science review: past and present. Cen Eur J Urol 65:182–187

5. Abbara A, Davidson RN (2011) Etiology and management of genitourinary tuberculosis. Nat Rev Urol 8:678–688

6. Kapoor R, Ansari MS, Mandhani A et al (2008) Clinical presentation and diagnostic approach in cases of genitourinary tuberculosis. Indian J Urol 24:401–405

7. Altiparmak MR, Trabulus S, Balkan II et al (2015) Urinary tuberculosis: a cohort of 79 adult cases. Ren Fail 37:1157–1163

8. Burrill J, Williams CJ, Bain G et al (2007) Tuberculosis: a radiologic review. Radiographics 27:1255–1273

9. Vanhoenacker FM, De Backer AI, Op de BB et al (2004) Imaging of gastrointestinal and abdominal tuberculosis. Eur Radiol 14(Suppl 3):E103–E115

10. Harisinghani MG, McLoud TC, Shepard JA et al (2000) Tuberculosis from head to toe. Radiographics 20:449–470. quiz 528-449, 532

11. Zissin R, Gayer G, Chowers M et al (2001) Computerized tomography findings of abdominal tuberculosis: report of 19 cases. Isr Med Assoc J 3:414–418

12. Engin G, Acunas B, Acunas G et al (2000) Imaging of extrapulmonary tuberculosis. Radiographics 20: 471–488. quiz 529-430, 532

13. Turkmen IC, Bassullu N, Comunoglu C et al (2012) Female genital system tuberculosis: a retrospective clinicopathological study of 1,548 cases in Turkish women. Arch Gynecol Obstet 286:379–384

14. Lee JY, Park HY, Park SY et al (2011) Clinical characteristics of genitourinary tuberculosis during a recent 10-year period in one center. Korean J Urol 52:200–205

15. Sallami S, Ghariani R, Hichri A et al (2014) Imaging findings of urinary tuberculosis on computerized tomography versus excretory urography: through 46 confirmed cases. Tunis Med 92:743–747

16. Merchant S, Bharati A, Merchant N (2013) Tuberculosis of the genitourinary system-urinary tract tuberculosis: renal tuberculosis-part II. Indian J Radiol Imaging 23:64–77

17. Merchant S, Bharati A, Merchant N (2013) Tuberculosis of the genitourinary system-urinary tract tuberculosis: renal tuberculosis-part I. Indian J Radiol Imaging 23:46–63

18. Kulchavenya E, Zhukova I, Kholtobin D (2013) Spectrum of urogenital tuberculosis. J Infect Chemother 19:880–883

19. Wang LJ, Wong YC, Chen CJ et al (1997) CT features of genitourinary tuberculosis. J Comput Assist Tomogr 21:254–258

20. Jung YY, Kim JK, Cho KS (2005) Genitourinary tuberculosis: comprehensive cross-sectional imaging. AJR Am J Roentgenol 184:143–150

21. Tonolini M, Bonzini M (2016) Case 14115. Urinary tuberculosis: multidetector CT findings {Online}. EuroRAD Available at: URL: http://www.eurorad.org/case.php?id=14115

22. Wong-You-Cheong JJ, Woodward PJ, Manning MA et al (2006) From the archives of the AFIP: inflammatory and nonneoplastic bladder masses: radiologic-pathologic correlation. Radiographics 26:1847–1868

23. Kitzing YX, Prando A, Varol C et al (2016) Benign conditions that mimic prostate carcinoma: MR imaging features with Histopathologic correlation. Radiographics 36:162–175

24. Sharma JB, Karmakar D, Hari S et al (2011) Magnetic resonance imaging findings among women with tubercular tubo-ovarian masses. Int J Gynaecol Obstet 113:76–80

25. Tonolini M, Bonzini M (2016) Case 14163. Female genital tuberculosis {Online}. EuroRAD Available at: URL: http://www.eurorad.org/case.php?id=14163

Imaging Infections in Transplanted Kidneys

19

Stefano Palmucci, Pietro Valerio Foti,
and Massimiliano Veroux

19.1 Imaging Infections in Transplanted Kidneys

Infections are common in renal transplant recipients, with more than 80% of infections developing in the first year after transplantation [1]. They still represent a cause of rejection in transplant patients, even if technical advances in surgery and immunosuppressive treatment have reduced the failure rate of renal grafts. The optimization of immunosuppressive therapy has diminished the percentage of rejection but at the same time has increased the risk of renal infection [2, 3].

Infections may be reported in renal and extra-renal locations [1]; in addition, as reported by Akbar et al., they may be distinguished on the basis of the timing of their appearances:

1. Infections that occur in the first week
2. Infections that develop from the 1st month to 6th months after transplantation
3. Infections from 6 months onward

These infections are schematically classified as *early*, *intermediate*, and *late* infections [4, 5].

In the first week, early infections are usually represented by pneumonia, surgical wound infections, urinary tract infections, vascular access infection, and *Clostridium difficile* colitis. From the 1st to 6th month, intermediate infections are caused by opportunistic agents or *Cytomegalovirus*: in this period, surgical site infections or *reactivations of dormant host infections* [6] may be observed.

19.1.1 Imaging Techniques

In the evaluation of infective diseases in transplanted kidneys, two main topics need to be addressed in more detail:

1. Firstly, kidney transplant recipients are often represented by immunocompromised subjects. This means that infections develop with a different clinical course from healthy people.
2. Secondly, transplanted kidneys should be investigated avoiding the use of contrast-enhancing techniques, because iodinate contrasts or gadolinium agents are nephrotoxic; kidney transplant recipients, particularly when involved with

S. Palmucci (✉) • P.V. Foti
Department of Medical and Surgical Sciences and
Advanced Technologies "G.F Ingrassia"—
Radiodiagnostic and Radiotherapy Unit, University
Hospital "Policlinico-Vittorio Emanuele", Via Santa
Sofia 78, Catania 95123, Italy
e-mail: spalmucci@sirm.org; pietrofoti@hotmail.com

M. Veroux
Department of Medical and Surgical Sciences and
Advanced Technologies "G.F. Ingrassia"—
Vascular Surgery and Organ Transplant Unit,
University Hospital "Policlinico-Vittorio Emanuele",
Via Santa Sofia 78, Catania 95123, Italy
e-mail: veroux@unict.it

© Springer International Publishing AG 2018
M. Tonolini (ed.), *Imaging and Intervention in Urinary Tract Infections and Urosepsis*,
https://doi.org/10.1007/978-3-319-68276-1_19

infections, may have impaired renal function and reduced creatinine clearance. Therefore, radiologists should carefully evaluate the risk of contrast-associated nephropathy.

Based on previous considerations, UltraSonography (US) is routinely performed as first imaging modality [7]: it can safely investigate patients avoiding ionizing radiation exposure. It provides also functional information—thanks to different Doppler sonographic indexes. Multidetector Computed Tomography (MDCT) could be used as second-step imaging modality: it has excellent spatial resolution, even if performed without contrast agent. However, unenhanced scans have some limitations, mainly represented by poor contrast resolution for the detection and characterization of focal lesions in transplanted kidneys.

Magnetic Resonance (MR), thanks to its great contrast resolution, shows high accuracy in the characterization of renal and extrarenal lesions, providing information about the content (blood, serous, proteinaceous material). In the past, it has been considered a very important diagnostic tool in the assessment of transplanted renal complications: indeed, gadolinium agents were considered safe, without risk of nephrotoxicity. MR was considered as the gold standard for the evaluation of vascular and nonvascular complications in kidney transplant recipients.

Since 2006, several articles have reported in literature that the risk of Nephrogenic Systemic Fibrosis (NSF) in subjects with impaired renal function [8] and contrast-enhanced MR has been discounted.

Recently, functional evaluation has been gradually introduced into the MR protocol for characterization of focal renal lesions: Diffusion-Weighted Imaging (DWI) and Diffusion Tensor Imaging (DTI) have been used in several studies to assess renal function and characterize renal lesions [9–11].

An MR protocol should include not only morphological sequences but also functional acquisitions for the evaluation of transplanted kidneys. On the basis of previous studies published in literature [9, 11], the following sequences are generally acquired:

- Conventional T2-weighted single-shot Fast Spin-Echo (FSE) sequence, acquired with large Field Of View (FOV), covering from L2 to the perineum.
- Axial and coronal T2-weighted fast recovery FSE sequences, with FOV limited to pelvis, acquired from the upper portion of transplanted kidney to the perineum; sequences may be repeated with spatial fat saturation.
- Axial T1-weighted FSE sequence, acquired with the same space orientation and extension of axial T2-weighted sequences.
- Diffusion-weighted sequences, using multiple b-values (from 0 to 800); if a b multi-fitting is not allowed, a couple of b-values (0 and 800 and/or 0 and 500) are used.

Functional sequences need to be positioned with the same orientation of morphological axial T1 and T2 sequences, in order to provide high correlation of altered signal areas; diffusion sequences may be also performed on a coronal plane.

19.1.2 Urinary Tract Infections

Urinary Tract Infection (UTI) occurs in >75% in kidney transplant recipients [12]. It has been described as the most common infective complication after kidney transplantation [13].

UTIs represent the most common bacterial infections that require hospitalization in kidney transplant recipients: they occur more frequently than pneumonia, postoperative infections, and septicemia [14].

In the management of renal transplant recipients, several critical problems may be associated with UTI: the interaction between antibiotic treatments and immunosuppression agents, the development of resistant bacteria, and the high tendency for recurrence in transplanted kidneys [12].

Several causes and risk factors have been identified in the pathogenesis of UTI: pretransplant UTI, prolonged period of hemodialysis before hospitalization, polycystic kidney disease, diabetes mellitus, urinary catheterization, immunosuppression, allograft trauma, and technical complications related to ureteral anastomosis

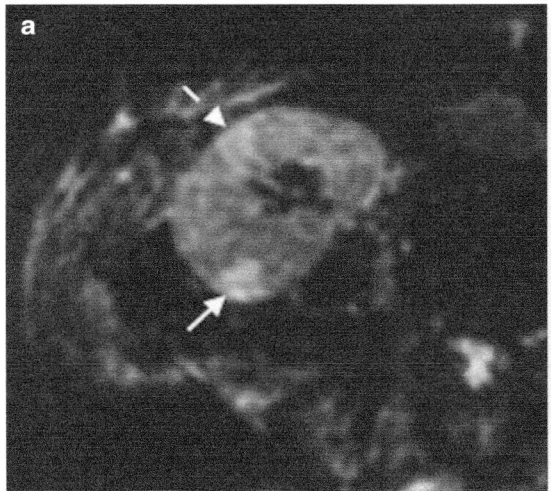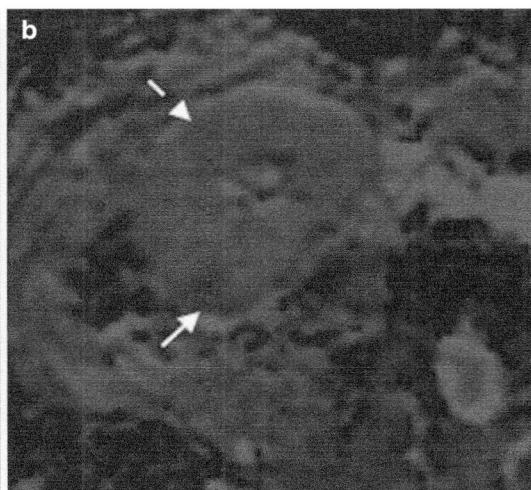

Fig. 19.1 A 55-year-old woman with pyelonephritis affecting transplanted kidney. On diffusion sequences (**a**), PN areas appear as triangle-shaped hyperintense lesions (white arrow posteriorly and dashed arrow anteriorly); on ADC map (**b**), lesions show mild to moderate signal restriction. The clinical features—fever and right iliac pain—and the MR reports suggested the diagnosis of urinary infection

[15]; in addition, predisposing factors include female gender, age, urinary tract abnormalities, and organ from deceased donor [12].

The impact of UTI on allograft function has been investigated with several parameters— such as iothalamate Glomerular Filtration Rate (iGFR), estimated Glomerular Filtration Rate (eGFR), and creatinine value [16]. However, variations of these parameters are controversial; in one study published by Giessing et al., measurements of creatinine values and eGFR were not statistically different between transplanted kidneys with and without UTI [12]; the iGFR values were different between the two groups.

Clinically, UTIs are associated with bacteremia and fever, which is reported in approximately half of patients [6]. Patients may also present not only with classic UTI symptoms but also with gastrointestinal alterations or asymptomatic bacteriuria [14].

In most cases, UTIs are represented by *pyelonephritis*, *renal abscesses*, and *peritransplant abscesses*.

On ultrasonography, *pyelonephritis* (PN) may involve renal parenchyma in a focal or diffuse pattern. Focal PN is depicted as a small area of increased or decreased echogenicity. This sonographic pattern is not specific, mostly when multiple focal areas of pyelonephritis are present in the renal parenchyma. A differential diagnosis includes acute rejection [17], which is characterized by organ enlargement, swelling of the medullar pyramids, loss of cortico-medullary differentiation, and edema in the renal sinus fat [18].

MR examinations are very helpful in the assessment of renal infection in kidney transplant recipients. PNs may be demonstrated as areas with hypointense signal on T1-weighted acquisitions and hyperintense signal on T2-weighted acquisitions. Currently, morphological T1-weighted and/ or T2-weighted sequences are combined with DWI [19, 20], providing a more accurate diagnosis of infection in renal parenchyma (Fig. 19.1). It may also help radiologists in the differential diagnosis between acute and chronic processes in the renal parenchyma.

In a recent paper by Henninger et al., DWI has been investigated for the assessment of nephritis [19]. In this study, T1-weighted and T2-weighted sequences were compared to DWI for the presence of regions with altered signal in renal parenchyma. DWI sequences demonstrated with high accuracy pathological areas in all 21 patients with infection, whereas conventional T2-weighted acquisitions were able to demonstrate "obvious"

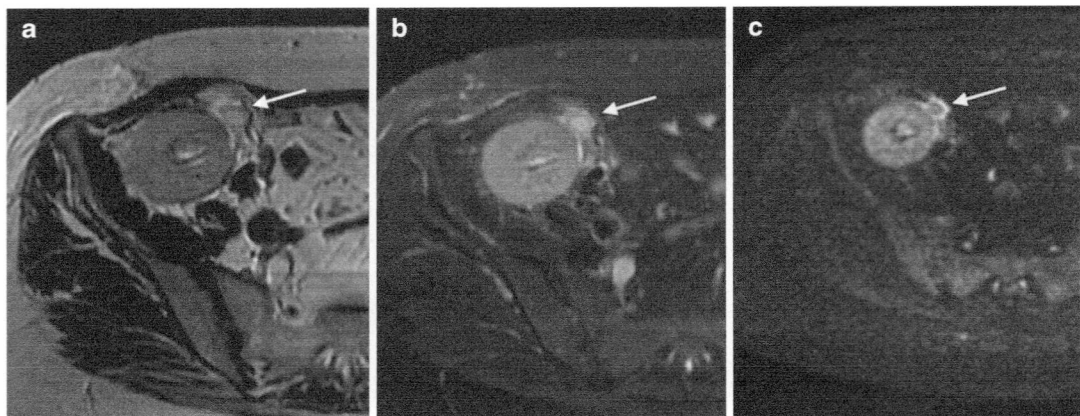

Fig. 19.2 Axial T2-weighted images (without and with spatial fat saturation, respectively, on **a** and **b**) and DWI sequence (**c**) show ureter inflammation signs in right iliac fossa, occurring in a 54-year-old woman. Figures clearly show increased thickness of ureteral wall; moderate hyperintensity is also depicted along the course of the ureter, due to inflammation (white arrows)

abnormal signal in 3 out of 21 patients and "slightly pathological signal" in 17 out of 21 subjects [19]. In one patient, T2-weighted sequences did not reveal abnormal signal on renal parenchyma. Based on these results, authors declared that "DWI of the kidneys seems to be highly sensitive for the detection of infections within the kidney" [19].

PNs—in a focal or diffuse pattern—should be differentiated from renal infarction, which appears as wedge-shaped triangular area with no perfusion on color Doppler. The identification of other extrarenal imaging features may be helpful in obtaining a differential diagnosis. Indeed, the ureteral wall thickening may be another feature commonly detected on US or MR examinations, suggesting an infective disease (Fig. 19.2).

The presence of a variable echogenicity inside a dilated pyelocaliceal system is clinically significant for pyonephrosis [17]; the presence of gas in the renal parenchyma is typical of emphysematous pyelonephritis [17], which could be also found as complication of a normal renal infection.

CT may be limited in the diagnosis of UTI: unenhanced scans, very often acquired to prevent renal damage from iodinate contrast, are able to provide nonspecific signs, represented by renal enlargement and perivisceral fluid collections. In some cases, small hypo-attenuated areas may be detected in the renal parenchyma, but they may overlap with renal infarction or cortical cyst. Thickened borders are usually associated with infections or abscesses and no with infarcted areas.

Peritransplant abscesses are uncommon and occur after the first week (Fig. 19.3). These abscesses could be due to extrarenal extension of pyelonephritis; they may be also caused by colonization of bacterial in fluid collections as urinoma, lymphocele, and hematoma.

A *peritransplant abscess* should be differentiated from lymphocele, which is a fluid collection without epithelial border; on US, typical imaging features of lymphocele are represented by a variable in size anechoic area, often with lobulated shape, without borders (Fig. 19.4). Lymphocele is clearly depicted as a fluid water-density collection on CT images (Fig. 19.5); on MR sequences, it appears as a fluid collection with homogeneous high signal on T2-weighted acquisitions and hypointense signal on T1-weighted images (Fig. 19.5). No restriction signal is observed on functional imaging.

Hematomas may also occur as peritransplant fluid collection: an intralesional fluid-fluid level—depicted on sonographic images—may

Fig. 19.3 A 69-year-old transplanted kidney recipient from cadaveric donor, with a perirenal abscess and a surgical wound infection. Coronal T2-weighted acquisitions (**a** and **c**) show a small fluid collection, located adjacent to the lower portion of transplanted kidney: the fluid collection is hyperintense on T2-weighted image, peripherally bordered by thickened wall. On DWI sequence (**b**), obtained at the level of the fluid collection described, homogeneous high signal intensity is depicted (white arrow). On T2-weighted acquisition repeated with spatial fat saturation (**d**), obtained at the level of perirenal abscess described, another fluid collection (white arrow) is evident in the subcutaneous fat near the surgical site

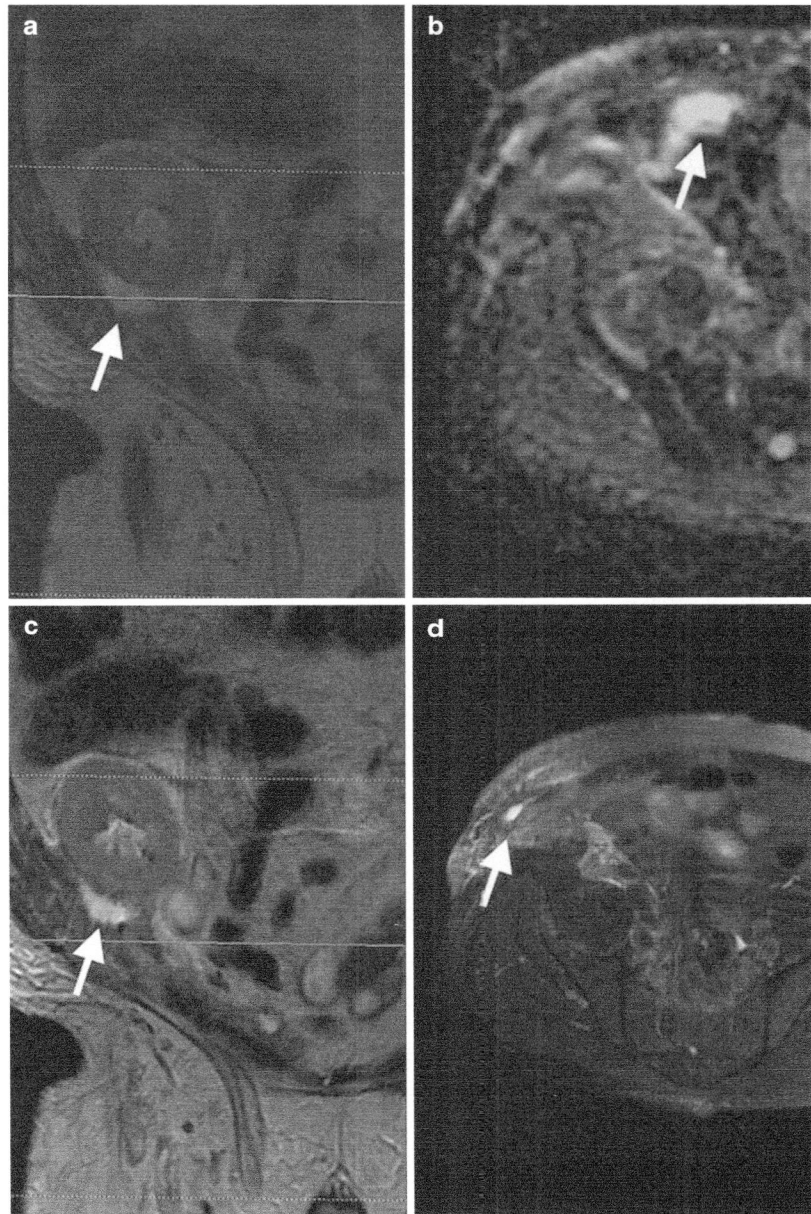

be a helpful sign to provide a differential diagnosis. MR is able to demonstrate hematomas as fluid collection with high signal on T1-weighted sequences, due to the presence of intralesional blood degradation products (Fig. 19.6).

However, the differential diagnosis for peritransplant fluid collections—abscesses, lymphoceles, and hematomas—may be very difficult considering only imaging features; very often, imaging features overlap and do not allow a diagnosis. Some perirenal abscesses may have a complex appearance on US, showing, occasionally, an internal fluid-fluid level. In addition, a lymphocele may be colonized, developing thickened border due to the infection.

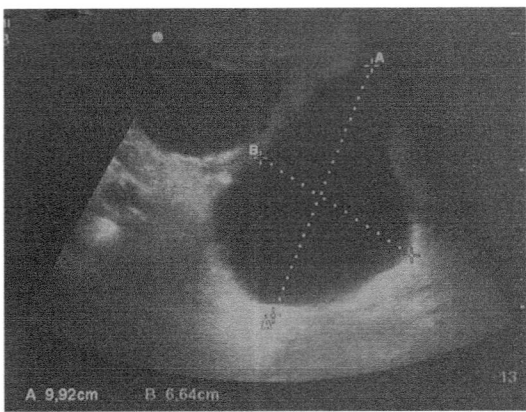

Fig. 19.4 A 38-year-old transplanted kidney recipient. A large fluid collection is clearly appreciable in left iliac region. On US image, this fluid collection seems to have no border, without complex signs inside; these imaging findings suggest a simple fluid content and the diagnosis of lymphocele, which is clearly depicted as a fluid water-density collection on US, CT, or MR exams

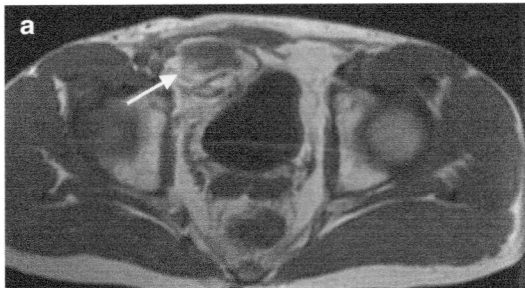

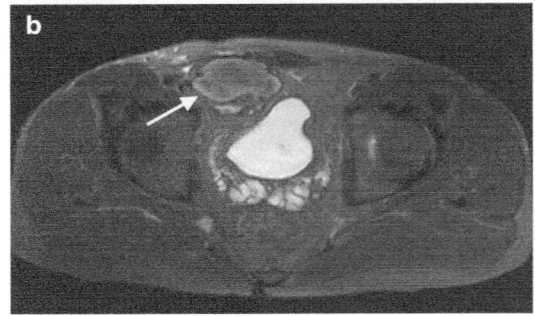

Fig. 19.6 A 50-year-old man with right transplanted kidney from cadaveric donor. MR acquisition demonstrates a fluid collection located in the right iliac-inguinal region, behind the rectum muscle. On T1-weighted sequences (**a**), this fluid collection shows peripherally high signal, due to the presence of intralesional blood degradation products; the high signal is well appreciated on T1-weighted acquisition obtained after fat saturation (**b**)

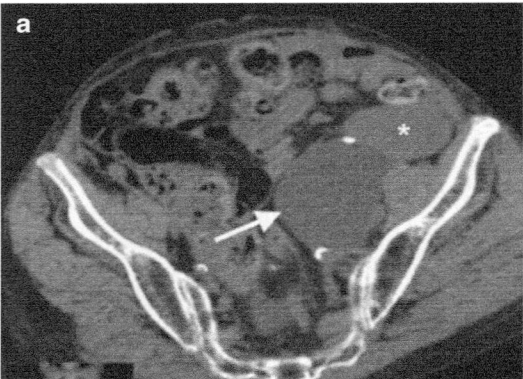

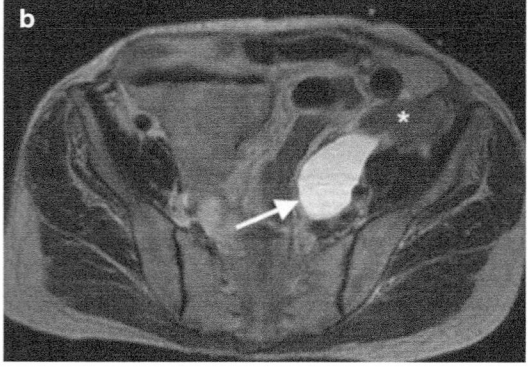

Fig. 19.5 A 61-year-old woman with transplanted kidney in left iliac region (white asterisk). A large fluid collection is demonstrated on CT and MR images (**a** and **b**, respectively); the lesion is homogeneous hypodense on CT (white arrow in **a**) and hyperintense on MR (white arrow in **b**)

Conclusion

Infections of transplant renal recipients are commonly detected in the posttransplant period. Imaging plays a crucial role in the detection of renal and extrarenal infections; very often, it has to provide a correct diagnosis in infected organs with impaired renal function, which limits the utilization of contrast agent.

References

1. Akbar SA, Jafri SZ, Amendola MA, Madrazo BL, Salem R, Bis KG (2005) Complications of renal transplantation. Radiographics 25(5):1335–1356
2. Fishman JA, Rubin RH (1998) Medical progress: infection in organ transplant recipients. N Engl J Med 338:1741–1751
3. Sia IG, Paya CV (1998) Infectious complications following renal transplantation. Surg Clin North Am 78:95–112

4. Fishman JA (2007) Infection in solid-organ transplant recipients. N Engl J Med 357:2601–2614
5. Tanphaichitr NT, Brennan DC (2000) Infectious complications in renal transplant recipients. Adv Ren Replace Ther 7:131–146
6. http://www.emdocs.net/transplant-emergencies-part-i-infection-rejection-and-medication-effects/
7. Sharfuddin A (2014) Renal relevant radiology: imaging in kidney transplantation. Clin J Am Soc Nephrol 9:416–429
8. Thomsen HS, Morcos SK, Dawson P (2006) Is there a causal relation between the administration of gadolinium based contrast media and the development of nephrogenic systemic fibrosis (NSF)? Clin Radiol 61:905–906
9. Palmucci S, Mauro LA, Failla G, Foti PV, Milone P, Sinagra N, Zerbo D, Veroux P, Ettorre GC, Veroux M (2015) Magnetic resonance with diffusion-weighted imaging in the evaluation of transplanted kidneys: updating results in 35 patients. Transplant Proc 44:1884–1888. https://doi.org/10.1016/j.transproceed.2012.06.045
10. Erbay G, Koc Z, Karadeli E, Kuzgunbay B, Goren MR, Bal N (2012) Evaluation of malignant and benign renal lesions using diffusion-weighted MRI with multiple b values. Acta Radiol 53:359–365. https://doi.org/10.1258/ar.2011.110601
11. Palmucci S, Cappello G, Attinà G, Foti PV, Siverino RO, Roccasalva F, Piccoli M, Sinagra N, Milone P, Veroux M, Ettorre GC (2015) Diffusion weighted imaging and diffusion tensor imaging in the evaluation of transplanted kidneys. Eur J Radiol Open 16:71–80. https://doi.org/10.1016/j.ejro.2015.05.001
12. Giessing M (2012) Urinary tract infection in renal transplantation. Arab J Urol 10:162–168. https://doi.org/10.1016/j.aju.2012.01.005
13. Castañeda DA, León K, Martín R, López L, Pérez H, Lozano E (2013) Urinary tract infection and kidney transplantation: a review of diagnosis, causes, and current clinical approach. Transplant Proc 45:1590–1592. https://doi.org/10.1016/j.transproceed.2013.01.014
14. Karuthu S, Blumberg EA (2012) Common infections in kidney transplant recipients. Clin J Am Soc Nephrol 7:2058–2070
15. Muñoz P (2001) Management of Urinary Tract Infections and Lymphocele in renal transplant recipients. Clin Infect Dis 33(Suppl 1):S53–S57. Review
16. Ariza-Heredia EJ, Beam EN, Lesnick TG, Cosio FG, Kremers WK, Razonable RR (2014) Impact of urinary tract infection on allograft function after kidney transplantation. Clin Transpl 28:683–690. https://doi.org/10.1111/ctr.12366
17. Kolofousi C, Stefanidis K, Cokkinos DD, Karakitsos D, Antypa E, Piperopoulos P (2012) Ultrasonographic features of kidney transplants and their complications: an imaging review. ISRN Radiol 2013:480862. https://doi.org/10 5402/2013/480862. eCollection 2013
18. Al-Khulaifat S (2008) Evaluation of a transplanted kidney by Doppler ultrasound. Saudi J Kidney Dis Transpl 19:730–736
19. Henninger B, Reichert M, Haneder S, Schoenberg SO, Michaely HJ (2013) Value of diffusion-weighted MR imaging for the detection of nephritis. Sci World J 2013:348105. https://doi.org/10.1155/2013/348105
20. Verswijvel G, Vandecaveye V, Gelin G, Vandevenne J, Grieten M, Horvath M, Oyen R, Palmers Y (2002) Diffusion-weighted MR imaging in the evaluation of renal infection: preliminary results. JBR-BTR 85:100–103

Interventional Radiology for Drainage of Urine

20

Anna Maria Ierardi, Salvatore Alessio Angileri,
Enrico Maria Fumarola, and Gianpaolo Carrafiello

20.1 Indications

Ureteral obstruction is a heterogeneous clinical entity, and it is often challenging for the clinician to determine the optimal method of decompression [1].

Urinary obstruction can affect the urinary tract at any level, and it can be caused by a variety of pathologic processes, intrinsic and extrinsic to the urinary system.

Patients with urinary tract obstruction can have a wide range of clinical presentations, varying from urosepsis to asymptomatic dilated urinary systems found incidentally on imaging [2].

The approach to each patient will differ significantly depending on infection of urinary obstruction or not. Pyonephrosis can rapidly deteriorate into life-threatening sepsis as infection gains access to the vascular system.

Urosepsis mandates emergent urinary drainage and can significantly reduce mortality, whereas obstructive uropathy can be managed on an urgent or elective basis.

Therefore, the keys in determining the optimal drainage strategy and how likely it is to achieve

the desired outcome are the review of anatomical and functional imaging, laboratory, and clinical data [3].

Simple percutaneous nephrostomy (PCN) catheter placement is the primary method of draining an obstructed, infected urinary system. Because these patients are at high risk for sepsis, it is critical to confirm they receive an appropriate antibiotic within 60 min of starting the procedure [4].

The most common reason for benign obstruction is stone disease [5]. In this situation, PCN serves to preserve renal function, relief colic pain caused by repeated muscular contractions of the ureter against the obstructing calculus, and access for definitive stone therapy once the acute episode has resolved [6].

PCN permits access to the collecting system for percutaneous stone removal or for temporary decompression until the stone has migrated or has been disintegrated with extracorporeal shockwave lithotripsy [7].

Noninfected urinary obstruction caused by malignancy is another common indication for drainage. The clinical goal for such patients is to preserve or to recover renal function [3]. The most common reason for malignant upper urinary obstruction is advanced pelvic disease. The majority of these patients have a poor prognosis. Sometimes, it is difficult to decide whether aggressive decompression of the upper urinary tract should be performed or whether

A.M. Ierardi (✉) • S.A. Angileri
E.M. Fumarola • G. Carrafiello
Diagnostic and Interventional Radiology Department,
ASST Santi Paolo e Carlo, Via A di Rudinì 8, Milan
20142, Italy
e-mail: amierardi@yahoo.it; alessioangileri@gmail.com;
em.fumarola@gmail.com; gcarraf@gmail.com

© Springer International Publishing AG 2018
M. Tonolini (ed.), *Imaging and Intervention in Urinary Tract Infections and Urosepsis*,
https://doi.org/10.1007/978-3-319-68276-1_20

only palliative noninvasive treatment should be offered [8].

Following ureteral reimplantation into the bladder or after cystectomy and creation of an ileal conduit or neo-bladder, ureteral obstruction may occur because of ureteral ischemia and stenosis, surgical mishap, or recurrent urothelial tumor.

Ureteral injuries represent known risk of some non-urologic surgical procedures; the consequences may be a complete transection of the ureter or a leak of urine or a stricture scar.

Initial management of a urine leak includes drainage of the urinoma or urinary ascites and is often followed by nephrostomy or ureteral stent placement for urinary diversion. Careful review of prior imaging and presentation data of the patient and cooperation with colleagues who proposed for radiologic procedure are extremely important to obtain the desired endpoint [3].

20.2   Patient Preparation

Given the high risk of pyonephrosis, defined as the infection of urine within the collecting system, routine intravenous (IV) antibiotic prophylaxis is recommended [4].

In the periprocedural management of coagulation status and hemostasis risk, urinary drainage interventions in interventional radiology must be considered from moderate- to high-risk procedures.

For moderate-risk procedures, INR should be <1.5 and platelet > 50,000/μL with transfusion recommended under this threshold; patients undergoing anticoagulant and/or anti-aggregating therapy should be interrupted at least 7 days before the procedure, with the introduction of fractionated heparin when necessary. Low molecular weight heparin (LMWH) needs to be stopped one dose before the procedure with no need to withhold aspirin [9].

For high-risk procedures, INR should be <1.5 and platelet > 50,000/μL with necessary transfusion under this threshold; anticoagulant and/or anti-aggregating therapy have to be withhold 7 days before the procedure. Heparin has to be stopped 24 h or up to two doses before the procedure [10].

20.3   Percutaneous Renal Access

Knowing the orientation of the kidney upon the psoas and being familiar with basic renal anatomy is essential to the optimum percutaneous approach. In particular, knowledge of the principal renal vascular structures and their relationships to the renal collecting system can decrease the risk of hemorrhagic events [11]. The main renal artery typically divides into an anterior and a posterior division. The avascular field between the anterior and posterior divisions, known as Brodel's bloodless line, is the ideal point of renal entry. Because of the orientation of the kidney in the body, entry through a posterior calix usually traverses this line [12].

But, for example, in a nearly horizontal kidney, a puncture of an inferior pole calyx will mean to approach the kidney from the "deepest" part of it, resulting in an increased risk of bleeding. In general, the most effective approach in these cases is through a superior pole calyx, between the 11th and 12th ribs, as close as possible to the 12th rib so as to avoid injury to the subcostal artery.

Preprocedural evaluation of prior imaging (CT, intravenous pyelogram, or ultrasound) is essential. CT is far preferable, as it will help assess the kidney's angle, determine the presence of renal cysts, and alert the operator to unusual positions of the colon, spleen, or liver. Procedures are done with the patient in the prone or semi-prone position. It is essential to be aware that with the patient prone, the kidney's position is often more superior than it appears on a supine CT. So a planned superior pole approach must sometimes be aborted, as it would require entering superior to the 11th rib and significantly increase the risk of lung injury. Before making the puncture, it is beneficial to mark the spot on the skin and check it fluoroscopically; the C-arm can be rotated into a lateral position to see the inferior tip of the lung in relation to the proposed puncture site. The same information can now be gained with add-on software that gives C-arms CT-type imaging capabilities, but rotating the C-arm is quicker with less radiation exposure [11].

20.3.1 Fluoroscopic Guidance

Fluoroscopically guided percutaneous access requires opacification of the renal collecting system. Most commonly radiographic contrast medium is instilled via cystoscopically placed ureteral catheters. The side which needs to be treated is slightly elevated on a foam pad, a maneuver that brings the posterior calices into a more vertical position. The neck of the patient is placed in a neutral position with a chest roll positioned to facilitate ventilation. The upper extremity ipsilateral to the affected kidney is placed at 90-degree flexion, and the contralateral upper extremity is tucked at the side to allow the C-arm to be positioned as close to the patient as possible. Biplanar fluoroscopy is the most commonly used imaging method. Radiographic guidance of needle puncture into the collecting system for anterograde percutaneous access is routinely performed using one of two techniques, including eye of the needle and triangulation.

With the C-arm in the 30-degree position, an 18-gauge diamond tip access needle is positioned, so that the targeted calix, needle tip, and needle hub are in line with the image intensifier, giving a bull's-eye effect on the monitor.

Continuous fluoroscopic monitoring is performed to ensure that the needle maintains the proper trajectory. Needle depth is ascertained by rotating the C-arm to a vertical orientation. If the needle is aligned with the calix in this view, the operator should be able to aspirate urine from the collecting system, confirming proper positioning [12].

20.3.2 Ultrasound Guidance

In recent years, ultrasonography has emerged as an adjunct imaging modality to reduce time and radiation exposure, without compromising the success of the procedure [13].

Doppler technology represents another advantage and can help to visualize and to avoid renal blood vessels during percutaneous puncture [14].

A direct approach to the kidney, likewise to vascular procedures, can be obtained with the Seldinger technique. The Seldinger technique involves an ultrasound-guided puncture of the collecting system with a sheathed 18-gauge needle. US guidance permits visualization of the needle from the skin entrance site to the target renal calyx (Fig. 20.1). After injection of a small amount of iodinated contrast medium to opacify the cavity, under fluoroscopy, an hydrophilic guidewire can be inserted and, upon this wire, advanced the needle sheath. Lastly, the hydrophilic wire is replaced with a super-stiff guidewire to insert, usually, a pigtail catheter (Fig. 20.2) [15].

Constraining the access trajectory to the posterolateral aspect of the kidney can create an undesirable geometry resulting in the catheter

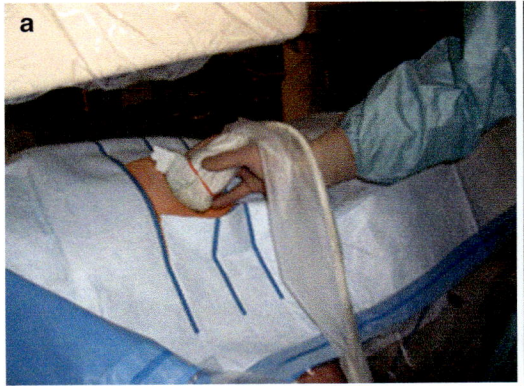
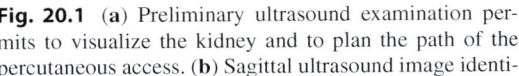
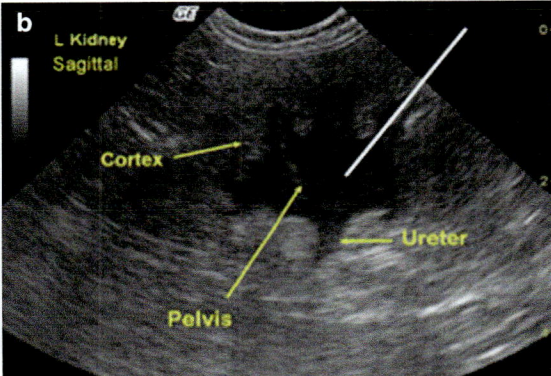

Fig. 20.1 (**a**) Preliminary ultrasound examination permits to visualize the kidney and to plan the path of the percutaneous access. (**b**) Sagittal ultrasound image identifies the kidney (cortex, pelvis, and ureter): the white line indicates the path of percutaneous access

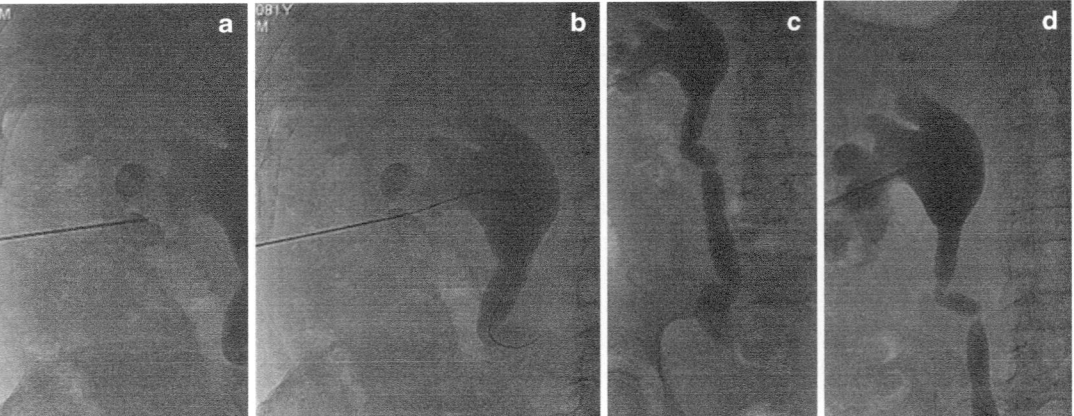

Fig. 20.2 (**a**) Through the needle, an injection of a small amount of iodinated contrast medium permits to opacify the cavity. (**b**) Under fluoroscopy, a hydrophilic guidewire can be inserted. (**c**) The hydrophilic wire is replaced with a super-stiff guidewire. (**d**) A pigtail catheter is correctly deployed

exiting posteriorly. Instead, for patient comfort, a more lateral approach that allows the patient to rest comfortably in a supine position is preferred.

Collection of a sample for urine culture may be obtained when access to the collecting system has been established.

A sample of urine for culture may be useful when [3]:

1. There is clinical suspicion of urinary tract infection.
2. If there is an indwelling or recently removed stent or hardware.
3. Patients have an ureteroenteric anastomosis.

20.3.3 Percutaneous Access of Nondilated Renal Collecting System

These procedures are often relatively difficult to perform for two reasons: first, the renal collecting systems are typically completely decompressed due to the leak; second, many of these patients have recently undergone a significant operation via a ventral approach, making patient positioning difficult [10].

Different techniques may be used [16].

The first choice should always be ultrasound (US), given its low risk and ready accessibility,

even because, although the collecting system may be completely decompressed, many of these patients will have chronically dilated renal collecting systems due to prior ureteral obstruction [17].

Sometimes, a central puncture may be performed more easily, but a drainage can't be deployed; therefore, once the collecting system is opacified, a second needle can be guided under fluoroscopy into a more suitably peripheral calyx. It is important to remember that in the prone position, contrast material pools dependently in anterior calices. Once needle position within the collecting system is confirmed, visualization of posterior (antidependent) calices can be accomplished by injection of several milliliter room air into the collecting system [17].

Another option for accessing a nondilated collecting system is to use a 21-gauge needle to access the renal pelvis under US guidance; this needle can then be used to opacify the collecting system, and a second needle (e.g., greater than 18G) can be advanced into a target calyx under fluoroscopy [10].

CT-guided access may also be described, particularly when selection of a specific calyx is critical [18].

Another technique to access to a nondilated collecting system is similar to the way a nondilated biliary tree is accessed: a small needle is advanced into the kidney under US or fluoro-scopic observation, and then during slow retraction with gentle aspiration, the operator observes the needle hub for the appearance of urine. Contrast material is then injected to evaluate the position. Alternately, following needle placement, gentle injection of contrast can be performed as the needle is retracted, taking care not to create large contrast stains in the parenchyma by alternating gentle injection and aspiration [19].

If these techniques are not successful and there is no contraindication, the intravenous (IV) administration of approximately 50–80 mL of iodinated contrast can be helpful to visualize the renal collecting system [17].

Once acceptable needle access to the urinary system has been established, a wire is advanced through the needle into the collecting system. It is unimportant whether the wire passes down the ureter or loops within an upper pole calyx, so long as there is a portion of stiff wire in the collecting system adequate to support exchange for a coaxial introducer. When advancing the coaxial dilator, care should be taken not to traumatize the urothelium with the guidewire or to injure it by advancing stiffened components beyond the parenchyma. Seldinger exchange concludes with placement of a 0.035-in. guidewire into the collecting system. Over this wire, a nephrostomy tube can be inserted; or, a sheath can be placed to facilitate access to the ureter and urinary bladder [16].

If all the above procedures are unsuccessful, a combined approach with urologist may be most appropriate. By performing a combined approach, contrast can be injected retrograde into the ureter of interest through a cystoscope, providing a direct fluoroscopic target of the calyces. This approach also allows distension of the renal calyces if enough contrast is injected [16].

20.4 Urinary Drainage Devices

Urinary drainage can be external (nephrostomy): internal-external (nephroureteral stent) or internal (double-J stent, metallic stents) without an externalized catheter. These are the devices most commonly used by interventional radiologists for urinary drainage.

20.4.1 External Devices: Nephrostomy

Pigtail catheter positioned in the renal pelvis provide obligatory external drainage for ipsilateral obstruction and for external diversion of urine for patients with ureteral or bladder injury or leak. Patients with neurogenic bladder or chronic bladder outlet obstruction may be managed with a transurethral Foley catheter or a suprapubic cystostomy locking loop catheter placed percutaneously into the urinary bladder from the anterior abdominal wall [20].

After placement, routine exchange of nephrostomy catheters is required to prevent encrustation and subsequent infections. Patients are typically scheduled for exchange at 8–10-week intervals; replacement should be anticipated if signs or symptoms of tube obstruction or malposition occur. Signs of obstruction include any combination of fever, flank pain, any malfunctions of the drainage, or pericatheter leakage.

20.4.2 Internal-External Devices: Nephroureteral Stents

Percutaneous nephroureteral stent (NUS) is a more stable urinary drainage device than a simple nephrostomy. It has a ureteral limb with a pigtail in the bladder. The external portion of the catheter is indistinguishable from a simple nephrostomy.

It is important to match the length of the ureteral limb of the catheter to the length of the ureter. The length of the NUS depends on the patient's height. Patients shorter than 178 cm typically receive a 22-cm ureteral limb. Between heights of 178 and 193 cm, a 24-cm NUS typically suffices. More than 193 cm, a 26-cm tube is usually required [21].

It is important to make allowance for extra length when hydroureteronephrosis causes substantial ureteral dilation and tortuosity or if there is marked deviation of the ureter.

20.4.3 Internal Devices: Plastic Double-J Stents and Metallic Stents

Placement of a plastic double-J ureteral stent restores physiologic urinary drainage without need for an externalized catheter [22] (Fig. 20.3).

Most often, stents are placed in retrograde fashion by urologists using a cystoscope. Cystoscopic placement requires the operator to be able to visualize and catheterize the ureteral orifice from the urinary bladder.

Most patients who undergo anterograde percutaneous stenting are proposed by urologists when transurethral retrograde positioning of the stent was not possible (due to obstruction of the ureterovesical junction, stricture at the ureteropelvic junction in an ileal diversion, or tumoral stricture of the ureteral papillae) or for failure of stent positioning, which occurs in 14% of cases (27% of cases with malignant obstructions, 6% of cases with benign obstructions) [17].

While self-expandable stents are among the most common metal stents (Fig. 20.4), there is a growing interest in covered stents in an attempt to reduce complications such as ingrowth and stent obstruction. Biodegradable stents are made with high molecular weight polymers such as polyglucolide, poly-lactide, Uriprene, etc. These stents absorb over time, obviating the need for cystoscopic removal and, thus, mitigating procedure-related complications, cost, and patient discomfort [22].

Heparin-coated stents have been shown to be effective at reducing stent encrustation. In vivo studies showed no encrustation at 10–12 months dwell time, compared to the 76% encrustation rate of polymer stents at 12 months [23].

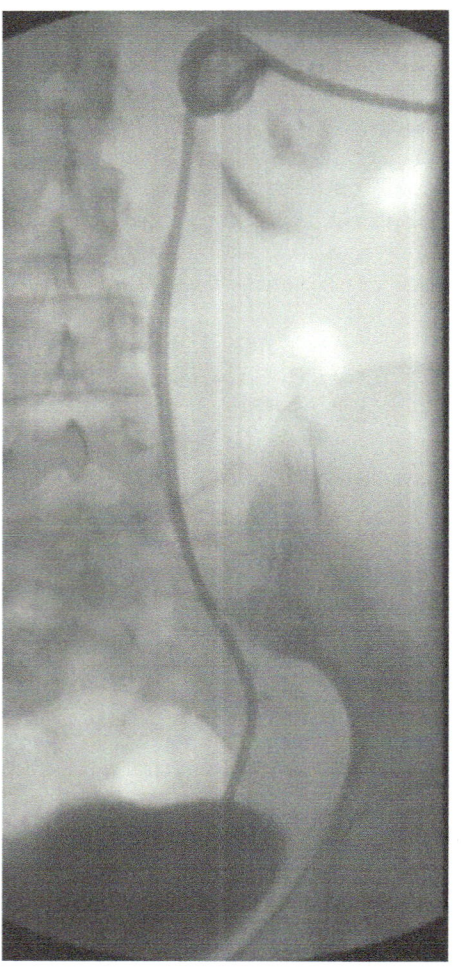

Fig. 20.3 Plastic double-J ureteral stent correctly placed

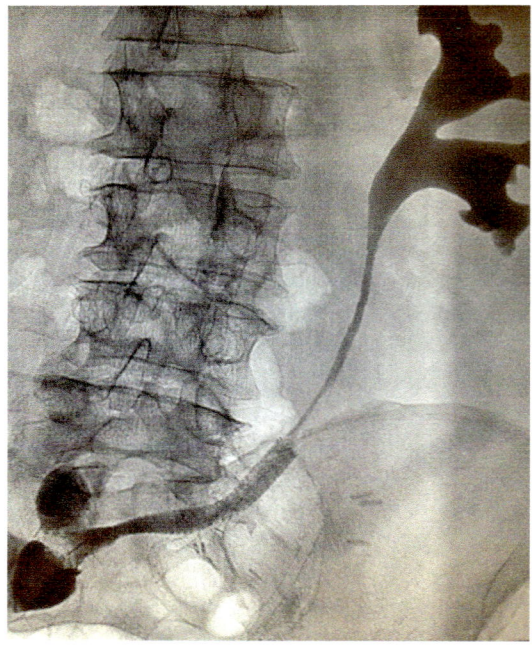

Fig. 20.4 Self-expandable metallic stent correctly deployed

Polytetrafluoroethylene has been applied as coating for metallic stents in animal studies and is effective against urothelial hyperplasia [24].

The clinical evidence for paclitaxel- and chlorhexidine-eluting stents is still pending [25].

In conclusion, metallic stents or resonance metallic stents have been introduced to maintain prolonged patency of ureters compromised by encasing neoplasm ([26, 27], but they are associated with epithelial hyperplasia and have not been helpful, even in malignant cases with short survival expectancy [28].

20.5 Stent Placement

Following successful access to the collecting system, anterograde pyelography demonstrates the location of ureteral obstruction. Maneuvers to cross the obstruction are facilitated and secured by use of a safety wire and a side-arm sheath. A true safety wire in this context is placed alongside the working sheath to secure access. A safety wire can be obtained by placing a second wire through the sheath already in place and removing and reinserting the sheath over one of the two wires [3].

An angled catheter is then placed in the ureter proximal to the point of obstruction, and a guidewire is placed through it. Guidewires with either straight, shapeable, or gently curved tips to try to cross the obstruction can be used. With the angled catheter 1–2 cm above the obstruction, the wire's tip can fully assume its shape in the ureter. The wire is then gently advanced during continuous rotation and retracted iteratively until it engages the obstructed lumen, at which point gentle rotation and advancement of the wire typically delivers it into the distal unobstructed lumen. This technique of careful "twiddling" allows for interrogation of the ureteral surfaces at the level of obstruction, and its success relies heavily on operator responsiveness to tactile and visual stimuli that signal engagement of the luminal opening followed by controlled, atraumatic passage through the obstruction [22].

When the obstruction is difficult to cross, different guidewires in combination with several catheters may be used; alternatively, a long sheath may be placed as near as possible to the obstruction to ensure more stability, and a microcatheter may be tried [22]. Usually a combination of these maneuvers is required to cross the obstruction, and occasionally none of them are successful. When even after a reasonable effort it's impossible to accomplish the procedure, a nephrostomy catheter is placed, and the patient may be reschedule for a second attempt after few weeks of external drainage. The rationale of a second attempt is to not have inflammation associated with organic obstruction after a period of external drainage [3].

After crossing the obstruction, contrast media is injected to visualize ureteral anatomy not seen by anterograde pyelography. The catheter can then be advanced over the wire into the urinary bladder where contrast injection is performed to document the correct intravesical position. Wire passage into the urinary bladder often produces irritative bladder symptoms that can be minimized by placing only as much wire as needed into the viscus. Injection of several cc lidocaine into the urinary bladder can also reduce symptoms of bladder spasm related to catheter placement [3].

20.5.1 Ureteroplasty and Cutting Balloon

In case of severe ureteral stenosis, to allow a correct insertion of the stent, a predilation of the ureter stenosis with a 4–7-mm conventional angioplasty balloon catheter can be necessary (Fig. 20.5). In exceptional cases, it can be difficult to advance a 7–8-Fr JJ-catheter over a tight resistant ureter stenosis following unsuccessful high-pressure balloon dilation [29–31].

Cutting-balloon angioplasty (CBA) represents an alternative system of balloon angioplasty, which combines the features of conventional balloon angioplasty with advanced microsurgical capabilities. This newly developed device has the potential to better dilate also ischemic and fibrotic lesions resistant to conventional ureteroplasty, with a very low and controlled pressure (<8 atm.), potentially reducing the procedural risk [32].

Fig. 20.5 (**a**)
Ureteroplasty of a severe
stenosis of the distal
ureter. (**b**) The guidewire
has crossed the stenosis

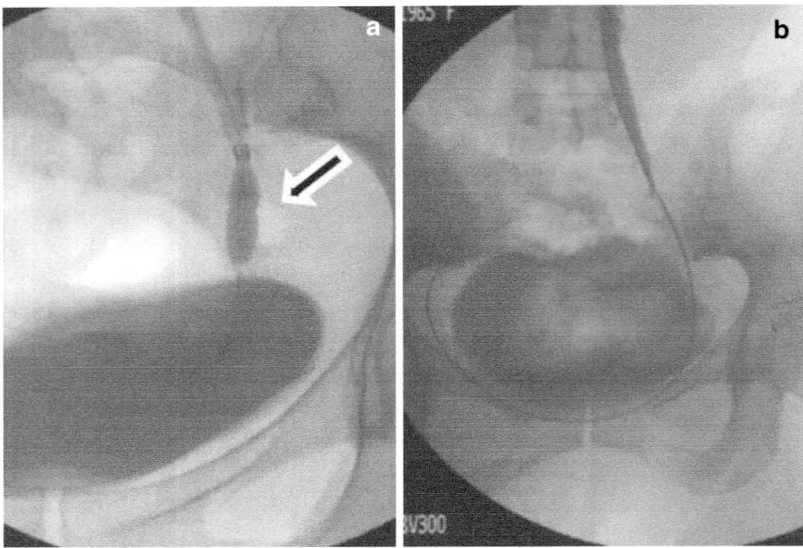

20.5.2 Placement of Double-J Plastic Ureteral Stents

After distention of the bladder with a 3:1 solution of iodinated contrast material and saline to reduce pain and facilitate intravescical maneuvers, the dilution is chosen to obtain sufficient bladder opacification to provide a landmark for the fluoroscopic maneuvers without affecting visualization of the devices [33].

Under fluoroscopic guidance, plastic ureteral stent is advanced up to the bladder; the wire is retracted to the proximal ureter. Under continuous fluoroscopic guidance, the proximal end of the stent may be allocated in renal pelvis, and the wire is pulled completely out of the stent. When the operator considers necessary, the wire may be redirected into the renal pelvis where a nephrostomy tube may be ultimately positioned to ensure an immediate future percutaneous approach if the stent does not work. Placement of NUS: with a wire positioned in the urinary bladder from a percutaneous renal puncture, an 8.5-Fr NUS with a soft stiffener can usually be advanced into the bladder without the need for serial dilations. Larger catheters may require serial dilation of the tract or use of a peel-away sheath to facilitate insertion. Occasionally there is resistance to catheter advancement at the point of ureteral obstruction. This may be

accompanied by prolapse of the proximal catheter and guidewire into the upper pole of the collecting system. Exchange for a stiffer guidewire, use of a long peel-away sheath, and occasionally balloon dilation of the stenosis may be required to allow catheter placement [3].

Alternatively, a double-J plastic ureteral stent and a nephrostomy may be deployed: the first one to ensure a correct course of the urine through the obstructed ureter and the second one to ensure an external diversion of the urine, when necessary [34].

Metallic stents may be deployed both through anterograde and retrograde approaches: the technique is the same of that used for vascular stenting; post-dilation of the stent may be performed when necessary [22].

20.5.3 Retrograde Ureteral Stent Replacement

Ureteral stent replacement was typically performed with cystoscopy; retrograde replacement with cystoscopy imposes the use of stents with calibers no greater than 6 F owing to the diameter of the operational portion of the cystoscope. These stents therefore are more prone to occlusion compared with those positioned in an anterograde manner [33].

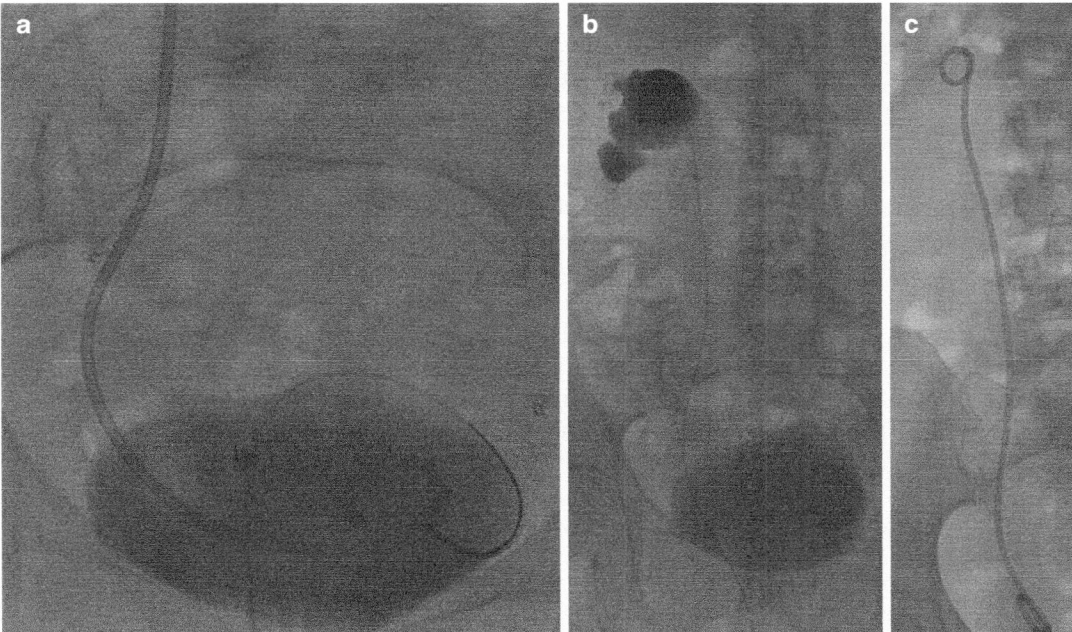

Fig. 20.6 (**a**) Capture of the distal extremity of the ureteral stent using a gooseneck catheter through a transureteral approach. (**b**) Guidewire was inserted in the lumen of the removed stent with the distal tip in the renal pelvis. (**c**) Through the guidewire, a NUS stent was correctly deployed

Fluoroscopically guided retrograde removal and replacement with snare catheters may be used when the cystoscopic approach is unfeasible or fails (patients with "frozen pelvis" or bladder-neck sclerosis in whom cystoscope manipulation may be difficult; malignant obstructions involving the ureteral papilla; patients with ankyloses who are unable to assume the lithotomy position for cystoscope insertion; patients with bleeding-prone bladder tumors because the introduction of cystoscopy instruments that are larger in caliber than those used in fluoroscopic removal carries a higher risk of bleeding; patients with a urostomy). In such cases, the advantage of fluoroscopically guided replacement lies in the smaller caliber of the devices (6–8 F), which are easier to manipulate inside the bladder and consequently involve a lower risk of bleeding in neoplastic disease. In addition, fluoroscopically guided recanalization of the stent being removed allows maintenance of ureteral-tract patency and the possibility to check that the distal extremity of the new stent has reached the renal pelvis. This maneuver is fundamental, especially in patients with severe stenosis due to malignancy ([33, 35] (Fig. 20.6).

Other advantages of the retrograde approach include the avoidance of a general anesthesia and the possibility to perform the procedure in the angiographic suite in outpatients. Technically, the bladder needs to be sufficiently full to allow the snare to grasp the distal end of the ureter more easily. Because the male urethra is longer and grasping and withdrawing of the stent may be more difficult, special care must be taken when performing these maneuvers in men [33].

The use of commercial gooseneck snare catheters or homemade snares consisting of a catheter and a hydrophilic guidewire (which, albeit more difficult to manipulate) was described. Forceps-type devices have seldom been used and appear to be poorly suited to this type of procedure owing to the small caliber of the arms [35].

In the setting of bilateral ureteral stents, after the first stent has been exchanged for a wire, the second stent may be captured before replacing the first to minimize the risk of stent entanglement in the bladder [3].

A cause of failure to replace the stent may occur in the presence of a urinary diversion (ureteroileal conduit). This were hypothesized to be related to intestinal secretions or recurrent urinary tract infections that cause the stent to adhere to the ureteral walls and prevent its withdrawal [36].

Some shrewdness may be considered, for example, the use of stiff guidewires or micro-wires to try to cross encrustation. Retrograde replacement may also prove unfeasible in the case of proximal stent migration into the renal pelvis with distal end at ureteral level. A further advantage is that pyelographic intraprocedural monitoring with intracavitary injection of contrast material can be performed in addition to fluoroscopic control to ensure more precise and safer positioning of the cranial extremity of the stent and easier negotiation of possible ureteral kinks or bends [33].

20.5.4 Anterograde Retrieval of Ureteral Stents

The technique of anterograde removal of double-J stent has also been described, but this approach requires a large percutaneous tract and potentially traumatizes the renal parenchyma. As such, this should be reserved for failed retrograde attempts [37].

Early occlusion of cystoscopically placed ureteral stents is an indication for percutaneous renal drainage. In stable patients, the occluded ureteral stent may be removed at the same time of the anterograde drainage [38, 39].

After percutaneous access to the collecting system is established, a side-arm sheath is placed into the collecting system. Through the sheath, either a loop snare or forceps is used to capture the proximal pigtail of the stent, which is then pulled out through the sheath. Once the stent is pulled out of the sheath, a wire is introduced through the stent and advanced back down the ureter to preserve access for anterograde catheter placement. When efforts to capture the proximal pigtail are unsuccessful, repositioning of the stent pigtail into a position more optimal for capture may be helpful. This can be accomplished by inflating a balloon alongside the ureteral portion of the stent and pushing down or pulling up the entire stent.

Other strategies to remove an occluded stent are transureteral introduction of the loop snare into the bladder for capture of the distal pigtail that is then pulled up by the ureter and out the sheath or transurethral placement of a sheath and loop snare for retrograde retrieval of the stent through the urethra [3].

It is important to keep in mind that retrograde stent retrieval by cystoscopy may be performed by urologist if all these attempts fail [39].

20.6 Follow-Up Care

Nephrostomy catheters and NUS were routinely recommended to be changed at 3-month intervals and ureteral stents at 3–6-month intervals [3].

Encrusted catheters can be challenging for both patients and IR physicians alike. This usually occurs when catheters are not changed as frequently as recommended but is also a function of the catheter material, hydration status, and the chemistry of the patient's urine [34, 41].

A stiff hydrophilic wire is sometimes all that is needed in this situation [3].

20.7 Particular Clinical Conditions: Ureteroileal Anastomotic Stricture

Ureteroileal anastomotic stricture and nonvascular renal transplant complications (urinary tract obstruction or leakage and the development of peritransplant fluid collections) are conditions that may present to the attention of the interventional radiologist.

Ureteroileal anastomotic obstruction is a possible complication after radical cystectomy, with urinary diversion to an ileal conduit occurring in up to 15.5% of patients [40].

Given associated comorbid factors, many patients are not suitable candidates for surgical revision of the anastomosis; minimally invasive alternatives including nephroureteral stenting, balloon dilation, ureteroscopic incision, and insertion of metallic stents were applied ([40, 41].

Placement of transileal retrograde nephroureteral stents is an attractive method of managing postoperative ureteroileal obstruction because it reduces the need for externalized flank catheters in patients who are already saddled with having to maintain the ileal stoma, thereby increasing patient comfort. Moreover, they are associated with minimal morbidity, easy of exchange, and durability [40].

20.8   Interventions in Transplanted Kidney

Interventions on the urinary collecting systems of transplanted kidneys and on peritransplant fluid collections can be complex and require an understanding of current surgical techniques, image-guided interventional techniques, and multidisciplinary management strategies.

Key surgical considerations include the donor renal anatomy (pediatric vs. adult), the location and orientation of the kidney within the recipient pelvis, and the type of surgical ureteral anastomosis employed (donor ureter to the recipient bladder or ureter).

Complications such as urinary obstruction or leak can be identified by anterograde pyelography and managed by percutaneous nephrostomy and ureteral stenting. Peritransplant fluid collections, including urinomas or lymphoceles, can be treated by percutaneous image-guided drainage with or without adjunctive sclerosis.

Renal transplants are most commonly placed in a heterotopic extraperitoneal position in the right or left iliac fossa.

Urinary tract complications occur in 3–10% of renal transplant recipients, with urinary obstruction occurring in 2–10% and urinary leak in 1–5%.

Urinary tract obstruction most commonly occurs at the distal ureter or at the ureterovesical anastomosis, often because of ureteral ischemia due to its limited vascular supply, which originates only from the renal hilum. Other potential etiologies include kinking or extrinsic compression of the ureter, urinary calculi, periureteral fibrosis, malignancy, and polyomavirus infection [42].

Urine leak is a potentially life-threatening complication, because of the risk of infection in these patients, who are in an immunosuppressed state, requiring prompt intervention [43]. Most leaks occur at the distal ureter, possibly as a result of necrosis due to ischemia or rejection, or at the ureteroneocystostomy site, stemming from problems at the time of surgery. Leaks occur less frequently in the proximal ureter or pelvicaliceal system secondary to distal ureteral obstruction [44].

Patients with urine leaks may present with pain, swelling, discharge from the wound, or urinoma [45].

20.8.1 Access and Anterograde Pyelography

Planning an adequate access is the key to successful access to the transplanted kidney. So the first step in intervention on the urinary collecting system is a careful sonographic examination of the renal transplant by the operator, noting the position of the kidney relative to other abdominopelvic organs and the lie of the kidney. Usually, a lateral calix is ideal for entry, in order to avoid a more painful and hazardous transperitoneal approach [45].

This calix also provides optimal lines of force if subsequent placement of a nephroureteral drainage tube or anterograde placement of an internal ureteral stent is necessary. It is better to avoid superior calyxes to prevent inadvertent puncture of bowel or solid organs [30].

Local anesthesia is administered along the planned needle trajectory. Real-time sonographic guidance with a high-resolution linear probe, or in larger patients with a vector or small curved probe, is used to guide the needle into the targeted calyx. A small amount of contrast media is then injected to visualize the urinary collecting system.

In cases of suspected or established urinary leak, calyxes and pelvis may be not dilated: considerations and techniques of percutaneous access are the same described above for native kidneys.

When an obstruction is diagnosed (pyonephrosis or ureteral obstruction caused by a calculus or a clot or by extrinsic compression), a nephrostomy tube alone can be deployed or an internal double-J ureteral stent in addition to a "safety" nephrostomy tube (focal ureteral stricture or urinary leak) [45] (Fig. 20.7).

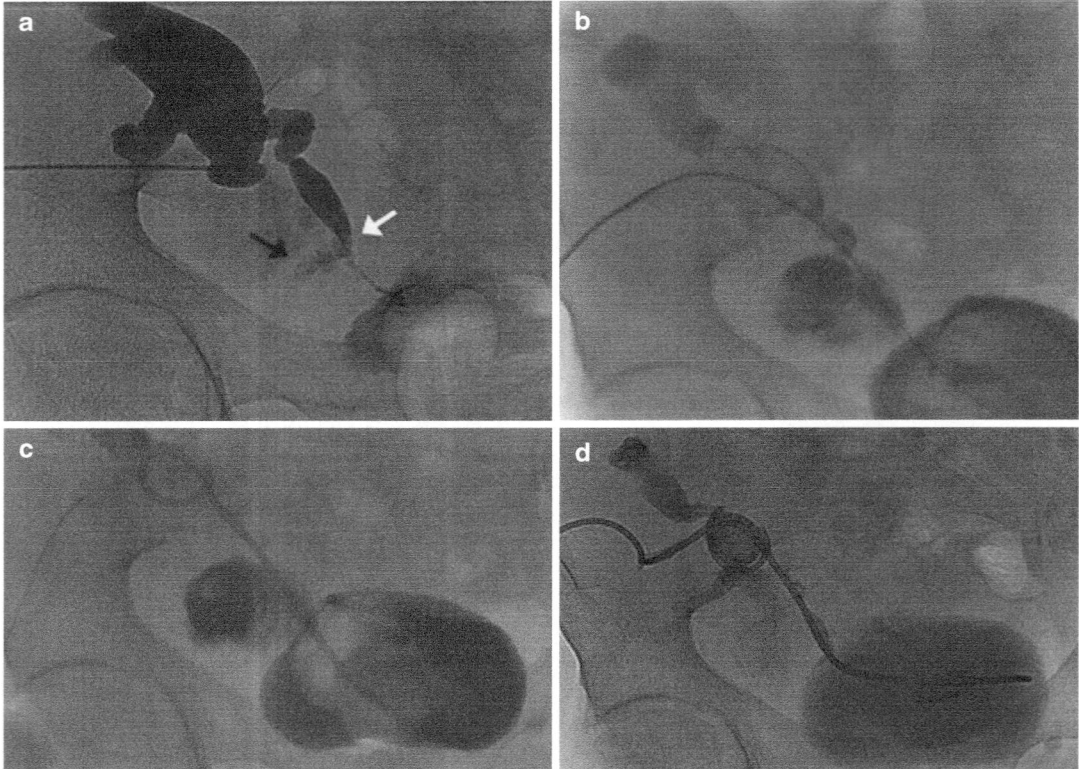

Fig. 20.7 (a) Anterograde pyelography of a transplanted kidney revealed a stricture (white arrow) of the ureter and a leak (black arrow). (b) Leak and stricture were correctly crossed with a guidewire. (c) A double-J ureteral stent was deployed. (d) A nephrostomy was placed

In this last case, like for the leak in native kidneys, the ureteral stent serves to maintain the continuity of the ureter and the nephrostomy drain of the urine outside to maintain the ureter "off."

20.9   Complications

All complications are recorded and classified as minor and major [46].

Major complications were defined as complications that, if untreated, might threaten the patient's life, lead to substantial morbidity and disability, result in hospital admission, or substantially lengthen hospital stay.

Minor complications included situations (like pain or mild hematuria) that do not lead to consequences, requiring no more than symptomatic therapy and include overnight admission for observation only.

Published rates for different types of complications are highly dependent on patient selection and are, in some cases, based on series comprising several hundred patients, which is a larger volume than most individual practitioners are likely to treat.

Complications may be distinguished in hemorrhagic and septic. Moreover, inadvertent bowel or lung transgression represent other rare but possible complications [46].

After a PCN, hemorrhagic complications range from mild to severe hematuria with the need to perform a percutaneous embolization or even a total nephrectomy.

Mild hematuria is also common after ureteral stenting as a result of urothelial irritation [10].

Significant hematuria after ureteral stenting can be caused by arterio-ureteral fistula between the ureter and the common or internal iliac arteries. This rare phenomenon has been reported in the setting of pelvic malignancies treated with surgery and radiation. Inadvertent bowel transgression is a rare complication of PCN when the colon lies in a retro-renal position. Pleural complications including pneumothorax, hemothorax, empyema, and hydrothorax are rare. Inflammatory systemic complications such as sepsis, febrile urinary tract infections, and pyelonephritis may develop as a consequence of drainage and manipulation of potentially infected, obstructed urinary systems, which are further compounded by the immunosuppressive state of advanced malignancy and subsequent systemic treatments [15].

There was no statistically significant difference in the overall stent-related or nephrostomy-related complications as well as the accumulated incidence of inflammatory systemic complications between the two groups. Similarly, no significant difference was observed in the incidence of urinary tract infections between the two treatment modalities [1].

Conclusions

A wide range of clinical situations including preservation of renal function, treatment of infection, urinary diversion, and access for urologic intervention require urinary drainage.

Nowadays several techniques and devices are available. External drainage (nephrostomy) catheters or completely internalized (double-J) stents with NUS and retrograde nephrostomy catheters in between are those most frequently used. Routine maintenance is required for all these devices, and most are associated with some limitation of the patient's lifestyle.

On the other side, the procedures described are permitted to manage clinical and surgical situations unsolved until a few years ago. From this point of view, interventional radiologic techniques improved the quality of life of these patients.

References

1. Hsu L, Li H, Pucheril D et al (2016) Use of percutaneous nephrostomy and ureteral stenting in management of ureteral obstruction. World J Nephrol 5(2):172–181
2. Heyns CF (2012) Urinary tract infection associated with conditions causing urinary tract obstruction and stasis, excluding urolithiasis and neuropathic bladder. World J Urol 30(1):77–83
3. Thornton RH, Covey AM (2016) Urinary drainage procedures in interventional radiology. Tech Vasc Interv Radiol 19(3):170–181
4. Venkatesan AM, Kundu S, Sacks D et al (2010) Practice guidelines for adult antibiotic prophylaxis during vascular and interventional radiology procedures. Written by the Standards of Practice Committee for the Society of Interventional Radiology and Endorsed by the Cardiovascular Interventional Radiological Society of Europe and Canadian Interventional Radiology Association [corrected]. J Vasc Interv Radiol 21(11):1611–1630
5. Bultitude M, Rees J (2012) Management of renal colic. BMJ 345:e5499
6. Mokhmalji H, Braun PM, Martinez Portillo FJ, Siegsmund M, Alken P, Köhrmann KU (2001) Percutaneous nephrostomy versus ureteral stents for diversion of hydronephrosis caused by stones: a prospective, randomized clinical trial. J Urol 165(4):1088–1092
7. Dagli M, Ramchandani P (2011) Percutaneous nephrostomy: technical aspects and indications. Semin Intervent Radiol 28(4):424–437
8. Chitale SV, Scott-barrett S, Ho ET, Burgess NA (2002) The management of ureteric obstruction secondary to malignant pelvic disease. Clin Radiol 57(12):1118–1121
9. Malloy PC, Grassi CJ, Kundu S et al (2009) Consensus guidelines for periprocedural management of coagulation status and hemostasis risk in percutaneous image-guided interventions. J Vasc Interv Radiol 20(7 Suppl):S240–S249
10. Pabon-ramos WM, Dariushnia SR, Walker TG et al (2016) Quality improvement guidelines for percutaneous nephrostomy. J Vasc Interv Radiol 27(3):410–414
11. Springer RM (2015) Planning and execution of access for percutaneous renal stone removal in a community hospital setting. Semin Intervent Radiol. 32(3):311–322
12. Miller NL, Matlaga BR, Lingeman JE (2007) Techniques for fluoroscopic percutaneous renal access. J Urol 178(1):15–23
13. Osman M, Wendt-nordahl G, Heger K, Michel MS, Alken P, Knoll T (2005) Percutaneous nephrolithotomy with ultrasonography-guided renal access: experience from over 300 cases. BJU Int 96(6):875–878
14. Ristau BT, Averch TD, Tomaszewski JJ (2011) Percutaneous renal access by urologist or radiologist: a review of the literature. Nephro-Urol Mon 3(4):252–257
15. Carrafiello G, Laganà D, Mangini M et al (2006) Complications of percutaneous nephrostomy in the treatment of malignant ureteral obstructions: single-centre review. Radiol Med 111(4):562–571
16. Ray CE, Brown AC, Smith MT, Rochon PJ (2014) Percutaneous access of nondilated renal collecting systems. Semin Intervent Radiol. 31(1):98–100
17. Patel U, Abubacker MZ (2004) Ureteral stent placement without postprocedural nephrostomy tube: experience in 41 patients. Radiology 230(2):435–442

18. Sommer CM, Huber J, Radeleff BA et al (2011) Combined CT- and fluoroscopy-guided nephrostomy in patients with non-obstructive uropathy due to urine leaks in cases of failed ultrasound-guided procedures. Eur J Radiol 80(3):686–691

19. Chien GW, Bellman GC (2002) Blind percutaneous renal access. J Endourol 16(2):93–96

20. Lee MJ, Papanicolaou N, Nocks BN, Valdez JA, Yoder IC (1993) Fluoroscopically guided percutaneous suprapubic cystostomy for long-term bladder drainage: an alternative to surgical cystostomy. Radiology 188(3):787–789

21. Pilcher JM, Patel U (2002) Choosing the correct length of ureteric stent: a formula based on the patient's height compared with direct ureteric measurement. Clin Radiol 57(1):59–62

22. Fiuk J, Bao Y, Calleary JG, Schwartz BF, Denstedt JD (2015) The use of internal stents in chronic ureteral obstruction. J Urol 193(4):1092–1100

23. Cauda F, Cauda V, Fiori C, Onida B, Garrone E (2008) Heparin coating on ureteral double J stents prevents encrustations: an in vivo case study. J Endourol 22(3):465–472

24. Chung HH, Lee SH, Cho SB et al (2008) Comparison of a new polytetrafluoroethylene-covered metallic stent to a noncovered stent in canine ureters. Cardiovasc Intervent Radiol 31(3):619–628

25. Krambeck AE, Walsh RS, Denstedt JD et al (2010) A novel drug eluting ureteral stent: a prospective, randomized, multicenter clinical trial to evaluate the safety and effectiveness of a ketorolac loaded ureteral stent. J Urol 183(3):1037–1042

26. Lang EK, Winer AG, Abbey-mensah G et al (2013) Long-term results of metallic stents for malignant ureteral obstruction in advanced cervical carcinoma. J Endourol 27(5):646–651

27. Wang HJ, Lee TY, Luo HL et al (2011) Application of resonance metallic stents for ureteral obstruction. BJU Int 108(3):428–432

28. Hekimoğlu B, Men S, Pinar A et al (1996) Urothelial hyperplasia complicating use of metal stents in malignant ureteral obstruction. Eur Radiol 6(5):675–681

29. Atar E, Bachar GN, Bartal G et al (2005) Use of peripheral cutting balloon in the management of resistant benign ureteral and biliary strictures. J Vasc Interv Radiol 16(2 Pt 1):241–245

30. Fonio P, Appendino E, Calandri M, Faletti R, Righi D, Gandini G (2015) Treatment of urological complications in more than 1,000 kidney transplantations: the role of interventional radiology. Radiol Med 120(2):206–212

31. Kumar S, Jeon JH, Hakim A, Shrivastava S, Banerjee D, Patel U (2016) Long-term graft and patient survival after balloon dilation of ureteric stenosis after renal transplant: a 23-year retrospective matched cohort study. Radiology 281(1):301–310

32. Atar E, Bachar GN, Eitan M, Graif F, Neyman H, Belenky A (2007) Peripheral cutting balloon in the management of resistant benign ureteral and biliary strictures: long-term results. Diagn Interv Radiol 13(1):39–41

33. Carrafiello G, Laganà D, Mangini M et al (2007) Fluoroscopically guided retrograde replacement of ureteral stents. Radiol Med 112(6):821–825

34. Vanderbrink BA, Rastinehad AR, Ost MC, Smith AD (2008) Encrusted urinary stents: evaluation and endourologic management. J Endourol 22(5):905–912

35. De baere T, Denys A, Pappas P, Challier E, Roche A (1994) Ureteral stents: exchange under fluoroscopic control as an effective alternative to cystoscopy. Radiology 190(3):887–889

36. Lang EK, Allaei A, Robinson L, Reid J, Zinn H (2015) Minimally invasive radiologic techniques in the treatment of uretero-enteric fistulas. Diagn Interv Imaging 96(11):1153–1160

37. Katske FA, Celis P (1991) Technique for removal of migrated double-J ureteral stent. Urology 37(6):579

38. Liang HL, Yang TL, Huang JS et al (2008) Antegrade retrieval of ureteral stents through an 8-French percutaneous nephrostomy route. AJR Am J Roentgenol 191(5):1530–1535

39. Ganatra AM, Loughlin KR (2005) The management of malignant ureteral obstruction treated with ureteral stents. J Urol 174(6):2125–2128

40. Alago W, Sofocleous CT, Covey AM et al (2008) Placement of transileal conduit retrograde nephro-ureteral stents in patients with ureteral obstruction after cystectomy: technique and outcome. AJR Am J Roentgenol 191(5):1536–1539

41. Tal R, Bachar GN, Baniel J, Belenky A (2004) External-internal nephro-uretero-ileal stents in patients with an ileal conduit: long-term results. Urology 63(3):438–441

42. Ingraham CR, Montenovo M (2016) Interventional and surgical techniques in solid organ transplantation. Radiol Clin N Am 54(2):267–280

43. Nikolic B, Rose SC, Ortiz J et al (2012) Standards of reporting for interventional radiology treatment of renal and pancreatic transplantation complications. J Vasc Interv Radiol 23(12):1547–1556

44. Kobayashi K, Censullo ML, Rossman LL, Kyriakides PN, Kahan BD, Cohen AM (2007) Interventional radiologic management of renal transplant dysfunction: indications, limitations, and technical considerations. Radiographics 27(4):1109–1130

45. Kolli KP, Laberge JM (2016) Interventional management of nonvascular renal transplant complications. Tech Vasc Interv Radiol 19(3):218–227

46. Dyer RB, Chen MY, Zagoria RJ, Regan JD, Hood CG, Kavanagh PV (2002) Complications of ureteral stent placement. Radiographics 22(5):1005–1022

Interventional Radiology in the Treatment of Abscess Collections

21

Anna Maria Ierardi, Salvatore Alessio Angileri,
Enrico Maria Fumarola, Filippo Piacentino,
Natalie Lucchina, Domenico Laganà,
and Gianpaolo Carrafiello

21.1 Introduction

An abscess is a localized collection of purulent fluid [1]. Perinephric and renal abscesses are uncommon but potentially lethal complications which may lead to sepsis from hematogenous spread of infection [2].

A renal abscess is confined to the renal parenchyma; a perinephric abscess is a pocket of pus in the perinephric space between the renal capsule and Gerota's fascia; perirenal abscesses may also develop from extension of inflammatory disease outside the Gerota's fascia [3].

The most common causes are either ascending infections of the lower urinary tract or hematogenous seeding from primary infectious sites [4].

Perinephric abscess may result from rupture of a renal abscess into the perirenal space but most often develops directly from hematogenous spread of infection. Alternative mechanisms include extension from extrarenal inflammatory processes such as diverticulitis and pyelosinus extravasation of infected urine [5].

Despite their rarity, also abscesses remain an important complication of renal transplantation [6].

Moreover, abscesses can develop secondary to spontaneous or iatrogenic infection after recent surgery [7]. They commonly manifest in the first postoperative month but can arise at any time.

Perinephric abscesses can result from infection of the surgical site, spontaneous or iatrogenic infection of a previously sterile fluid collection, or complicated pyelonephritis [8].

Common predisposing conditions are systemic diseases such as diabetes mellitus and renal or urologic diseases such as malignancy or renal stones [9].

Renal or perinephric hematoma, spontaneous, traumatic, or iatrogenic, can become infected [10].

Bacterial pyelonephritis is most common due to Gram-negative organisms such as *Escherichia coli* [11]. The following represents a description of indications, techniques, complications, and management of percutaneous drainage in patients with renal collections [12].

A.M. Ierardi (✉) • S.A. Angileri • E.M. Fumarola
G. Carrafiello
Diagnostic and Interventional Radiology Department,
ASST Santi Paolo e Carlo, Via A di Rudinì 8, Milan
20142, Italy
e-mail: amierardi@yahoo.it;
alessioangileri@gmail.com;
em.fumarola@gmail.com; gcarraf@gmail.com

F. Piacentino • N. Lucchina
Unit of Radiology, Uninsubria, Varese, Italy

D. Laganà
Unit of Radiology, Università Magna Graecia,
Catanzaro, Italy

© Springer International Publishing AG 2018
M. Tonolini (ed.), *Imaging and Intervention in Urinary Tract Infections and Urosepsis*,
https://doi.org/10.1007/978-3-319-68276-1_21

21.2 Indications

In most cases, small-sized renal abscesses <3 cm are successfully treated with intravenous antibiotics alone; small fluid collections can be sampled or aspirated for the assessment of optimal antibiotic coverage or for fluid characterization. If material appears infected, a drainage catheter may then be placed [13].

For instance, although fever, leukocytosis, malaise, anorexia, or other systemic symptoms point to an infection, these signs and symptoms may be absent in elderly, very ill, or immunocompromised patients [14].

Large (>5 cm) or rapidly enlarging collections and obstructing and infected collecting systems are readily amenable to percutaneous drainage [9].

21.3 Contraindications

Significant coagulopathy and severe compromised cardiopulmonary function or hemodynamic instability are common contraindications for all types of percutaneous procedures [15].

These contraindications should be addressed and corrected or controlled before the procedure whenever is possible. Percutaneous drainage is contraindicated in calcified masses. Septation and multiloculation are not absolute contraindications for percutaneous drainage because these conditions can be resolved by inserting several catheters or by septal perforation.

Pre-procedural planning may be the most important step of the procedure to avoid potential complications. Lack of a safe pathway to the abscess or fluid collection is a contraindication.

Inability of the patient to cooperate with, or to be positioned correctly for, the procedure may prevent the success of treatment [16].

21.4 Antibiotics Prophylaxis

The authors of the Society of Interventional Radiology (SIR) standards of practice guidelines for adult antibiotic prophylaxis consider percutaneous abscess drainage a dirty procedure, and, as such, routine pre-procedural prophylactic antibiotic administration is recommended [17].

21.5 Procedure

21.5.1 Approach

Pre-procedural planning represents the most important step in order to avoid complications, especially major vessel injuries and the formation of a pseudoaneurysm and/or bleeding.

First of all, aseptic technique is mandatory to prevent the spread of pathogens and the development of sepsis and septic shock.

Few recommendations can help to minimize the risk of complications: first of all, it is important to use the safest and most direct percutaneous route, as to minimize the length of the internal catheter; another concern is to avoid organs or vital anatomical structures—often that part can be achieved easier with an angled approach, which helps the needle to maintain a smooth coiling and an easier advancement of the wire. Finally, it can be helpful to place the drainage catheter in the most dependent portion of the cavity in order to facilitate the evacuation of the collection [2].

21.5.2 Imaging Diagnosis and Guidance

US, CT, and magnetic resonance imaging (MRI) are accurate modalities for diagnosis of renal and retroperitoneal abscess.

The US appearance of renal abscess is variable. It can appear as either a hyper- or hypoechoic focal mass or complex cystic structure. On CT renal or perirenal abscess appears as a low attenuation mass that may enhance after contrast administration, although not to the extent of a solid renal tumor.

CT and MRI reveal a heterogeneously enhancing, complex, cystic lesion with enhancing internal septa and a variable degree of infiltration of the perinephric space [12].

However, ultrasound is a useful real-time guidance for percutaneous catheter drainage (Fig. 21.1).

The combination of sonographic and fluoroscopic guidance is the most dynamic method because it provides multiplanar real-time visualization of needle advancement and direct visualization of dilator and catheter placement [11].

Conventional fluoroscopy fails to provide internal body detail, limiting its use to the drainage of large superficial fluid cavities or intraorgan cavities containing a sufficient amount of air that can be used for targeting and as an adjunctive modality to US and CT. A combination of initial US or CT guidance for the placement of the access needle and guidewire followed by fluoroscopic guidance for the wire and catheter manipulations and completion of the procedure can be useful for difficult drainages such as small or relatively deep cavities [2].

Intracavitary air may prevent optimal visualization of an abscess using US guidance.

CT may be used for air-containing cavities, for small or deep cavities, and for those with a potentially intervening hollow viscus or solid organ along the path of the access needle [18].

CT fluoroscopy using the "quick-check" technique has been shown to decrease total procedure time and patient radiation dose when compared to CT guidance without fluoroscopy [19].

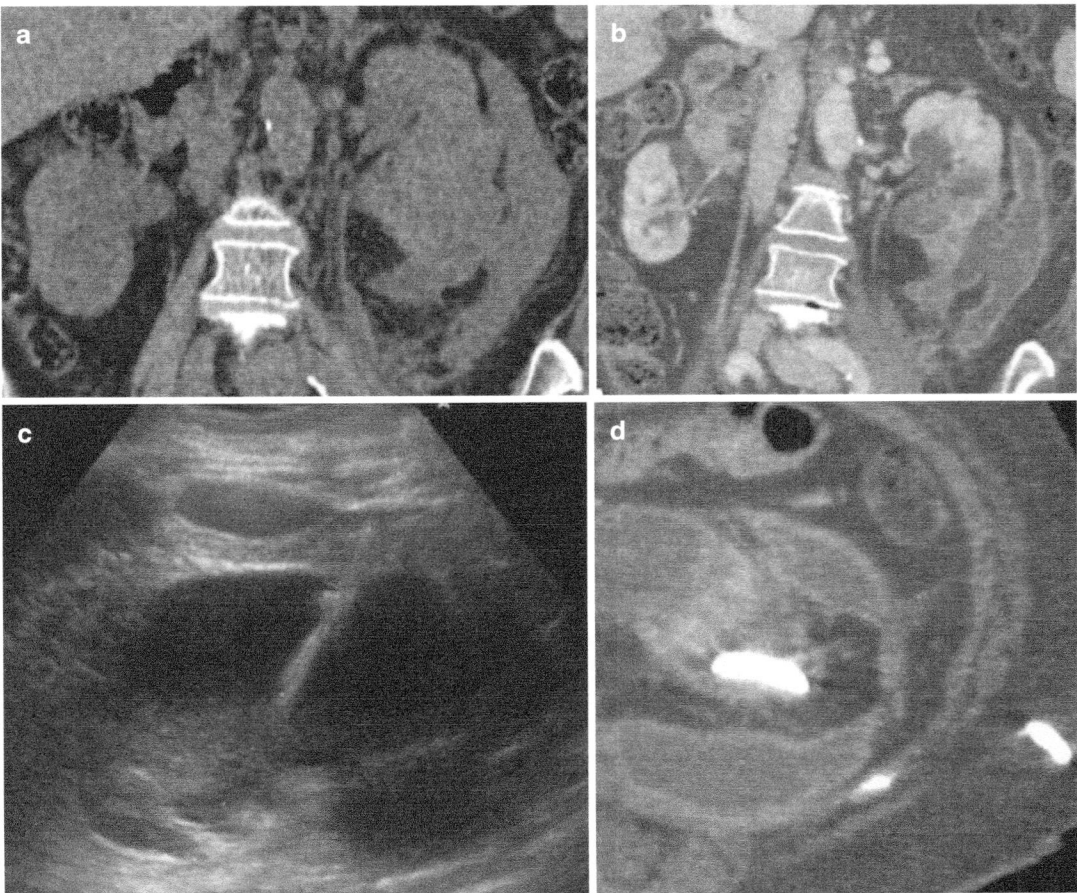

Fig. 21.1 (a) Unenhanced CT axial image shows a collection in the left perirenal space. (b) After administration of contrast media, an enhanced rim was shown, adjacent to renal parenchyma. (c) The drainage was deployed under US guidance. (d) One week later, contrast-enhanced CT showed partial resolution of the collection

21.5.3 Techniques

Two methods may be applied for the percutaneous approach to the collection and a safe deployment of a drainage catheter.

The Seldinger technique uses an 18-gauge sharp hollow needle (trocar) to puncture the rim of the fluid collection. Once punctured, the stylet is withdrawn, and the fluid is aspirated through the trocar needle to confirm intracavitary location. A 0.035-in. floppy-tipped guidewire is advanced through the lumen of the trocar, and the needle is then withdrawn, leaving the distal tip of the wire coiled in the collection. Imaging at this point in the procedure is useful to document appropriate placement of the wire prior to track dilation. Fascial dilators are then advanced over the wire with a stepwise increase in diameter to dilate the intended track of the catheter. Once the track is dilated, the drainage catheter, assembled with stiffener but without the trocar, is advanced along the wire to the previously marked depth of the collection. Once the track has been dilated, the drainage catheter, assembled with the stiffener but without the trocar, is advanced along the wire to the collection. Once in the exact point, the catheter is released from the metal cannula and the pigtail is formed. To secure the catheter in place, a string locking mechanism is used to fix the pigtail in the coiled position. The string is then cut and fixed to the stopcock. Catheters should be secured at the skin, preferably with an adhesive-backed locking device.

The trocar technique, the alternative to the Seldinger method, is performed using a direct puncture approach using the catheter with stylet in place. After access to the collection is obtained, the catheter is advanced and fed off the stiffener and stylet and is retained in place with the pigtail locking device. The trocar technique is faster than the Seldinger technique, obviates the need for an assistant, and is well suited for large or superficial fluid collections [20].

21.6   Success Rate

Curative drainage, defined as complete resolution of infection requiring no further operative intervention (Fig. 21.2), may be achieved in more than 80% of patients. Partial success is defined as either adequate drainage of the abscess with surgery subsequently performed to repair an underlying problem or as temporizing drainage performed to stabilize the patient's condition before surgery. Partial success occurs in 5–10% of patients. Failure occurs in 5–10% and recurrence in 5–10%. These results are similar for both abdominal and chest drainage procedures [16].

21.7   Complications

All complications are recorded and classified as minor and major.

Major complications were defined as complications that, if untreated, might threaten the patient's life, lead to substantial morbidity and disability, result in hospital admission, or substantially lengthen hospital stay.

Minor complications include conditions (like pain or mild hematuria) that do not lead to consequences, and require only symptomatic therapy and observation [16].

Complications after percutaneous drainage of renal and perirenal abscess are unusual: a transient febrile episode without sequelae in the first 12 h after placement of the catheter is the most common complication related to percutaneous abscess drainage [21], occurring in less than 10% of the patients [22].

The erosion or the inadvertent placement of the catheter into the gastrointestinal tract, the inadvertent dislodgment of the drainage catheter, and the renal vascular or ureteral injury [23] are less frequent, but they can also occur as complications after percutaneous drainage [24]. Hemorrhagic event represents a possible event, rarely requiring transfusion [16].

Another rare complication described in the literature is pyopneumothorax, resulted from an inappropriately placed drainage catheter that violated the pleural space [25].

21.8   Management

Daily catheter care with irrigation of the catheter, preferably every 8 h with at least 10 mL of sterile saline, is recommended. The decision to remove

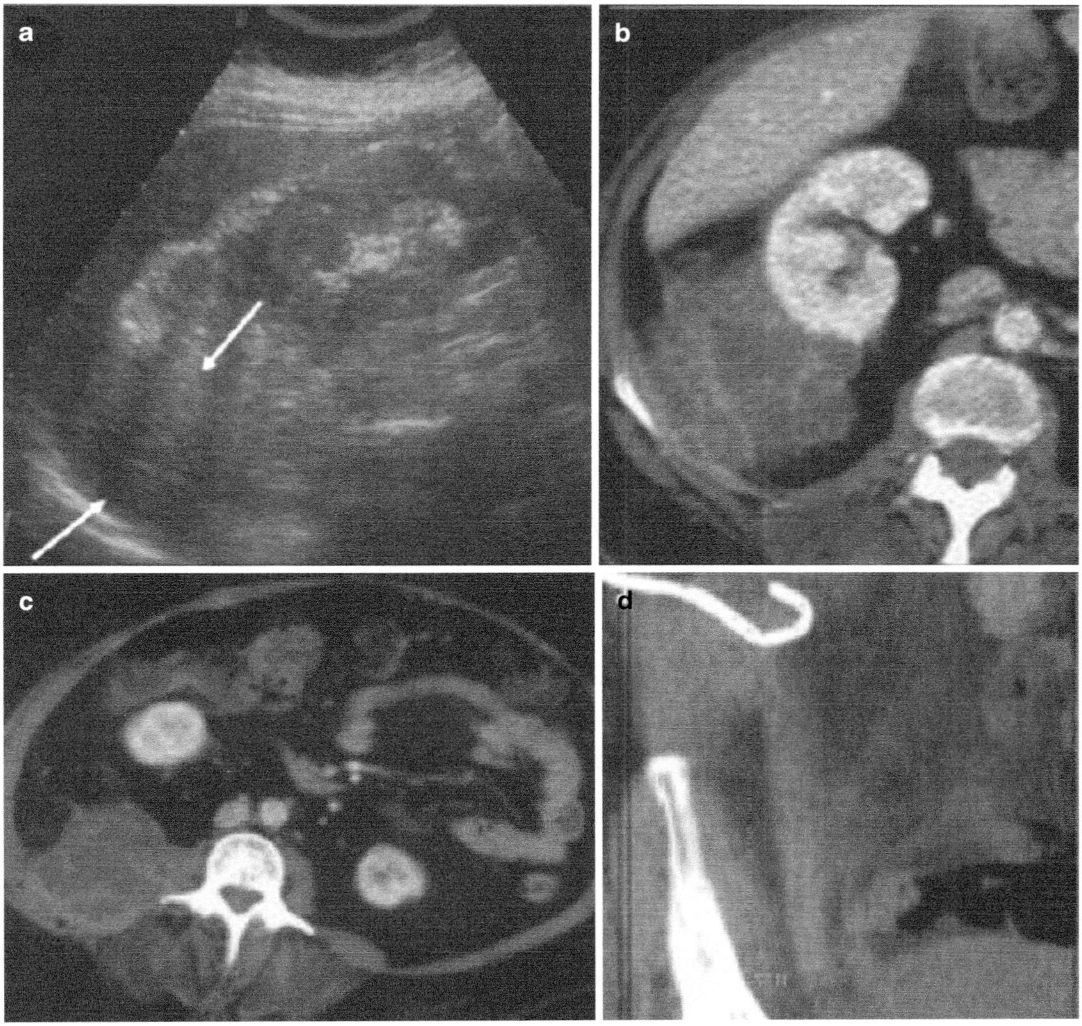

Fig. 21.2 (**a**) US showed a perirenal collection (*arrows*); (**b, c**) contrast-enhanced CT confirmed a multiloculated abscess; (**d**) unenhanced CT scan after 15 days showing almost complete resolution of the fluid collection and the pigtail drainage catheter

the catheter is multifactorial and includes normalization of temperature and white blood cell count as well as reduction of drainage volume to less than 10 mL/day [20].

21.9   Fluid Collections in the Transplanted Kidney

Perinephric fluid collections after renal transplantation are common and are associated with a number of serious complications, one of these is a perirenal abscess, which account for 2–30% of all aspirated fluid collections in the peritransplant period. Classically, these patients present with fever alone or with perigraft pain plus tenderness in a period ranging from the first 2–3 days to weeks after transplantation [6].

21.9.1 Lymphocele

Postoperative lymphoceles are caused by lymphatic leakage from the allograft bed or from the allograft itself and are the most common perirenal fluid collection, usually occurring weeks to months after transplantation [26].

Renal transplant patients are predisposed to prolonged lymphatic leakage as a result of graft rejection, the use of steroids or diuretics, or retransplantation [27].

Most lymphoceles are small and asymptomatic, and intervention is not necessary. However, some lymphoceles compress adjacent structures and may cause hydronephrosis, edema, or deep venous thrombosis in the ipsilateral lower extremity, and percutaneous aspiration of the fluid becomes indicated [28] (Fig. 21.3).

The most effective therapy is the combination of indwelling catheter drainage and sclerotherapy with a reported success rate of 68–100% [26].

Various sclerosing agents can be used with multiple treatments required in most cases, with the catheter left in place for anywhere from 4 to 35 days [29].

If an uninfected lymphocele recurs, it is usually treated by un-roofing into the peritoneal cavity by either open or laparoscopic technique [6].

21.9.2 Abscess

An abscess may arise from an infected wound or from a secondarily infected lymphocele, hematoma, or urinoma after attempts at aspiration or as a consequence of graft pyelonephritis [6] (Fig. 21.4).

Any perigraft fluid collection can become infected; usually, the affected patient presents with fever or local pain. US or CT findings usually are nonspecific, but air within the perirenal fluid collection strongly suggests a perirenal abscess. Also, in the clinical setting of fever and leukocytosis in a transplant patient, the detection of a perinephric fluid collection is presumptive evidence that the fluid is infected. In these situa-

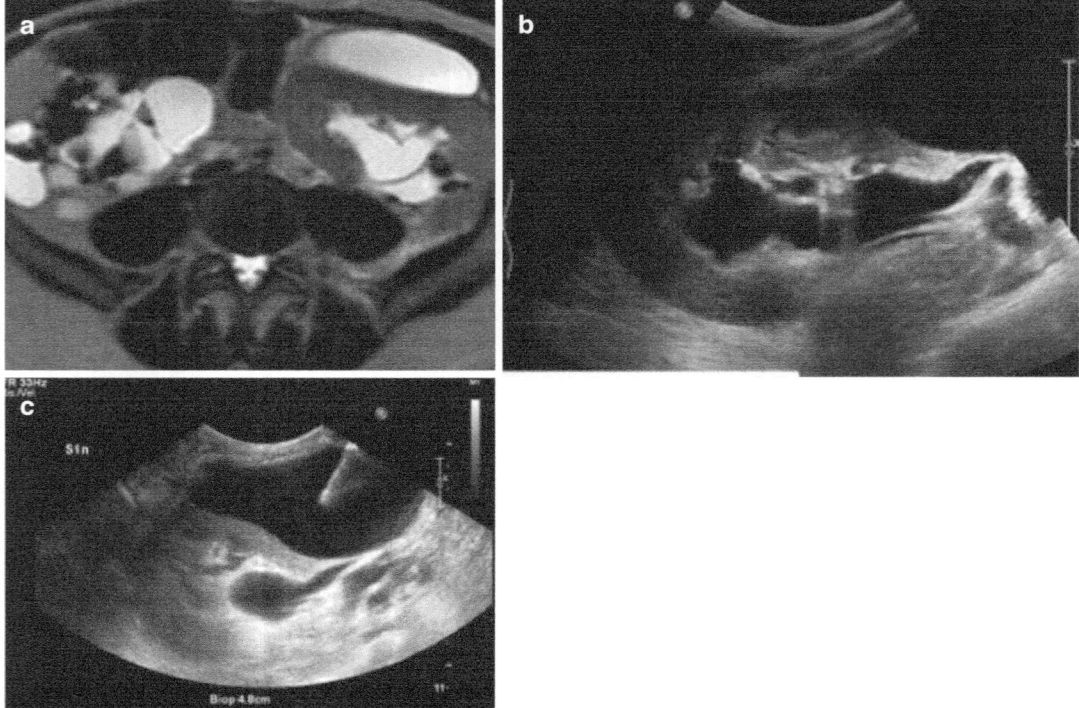

Fig. 21.3 (**a**) Axial RM T2 image showed a lymphocele. (**b**) US image confirmed the possibility to deploy the drainage. (**c**) Image performed during the deployment of the drainage

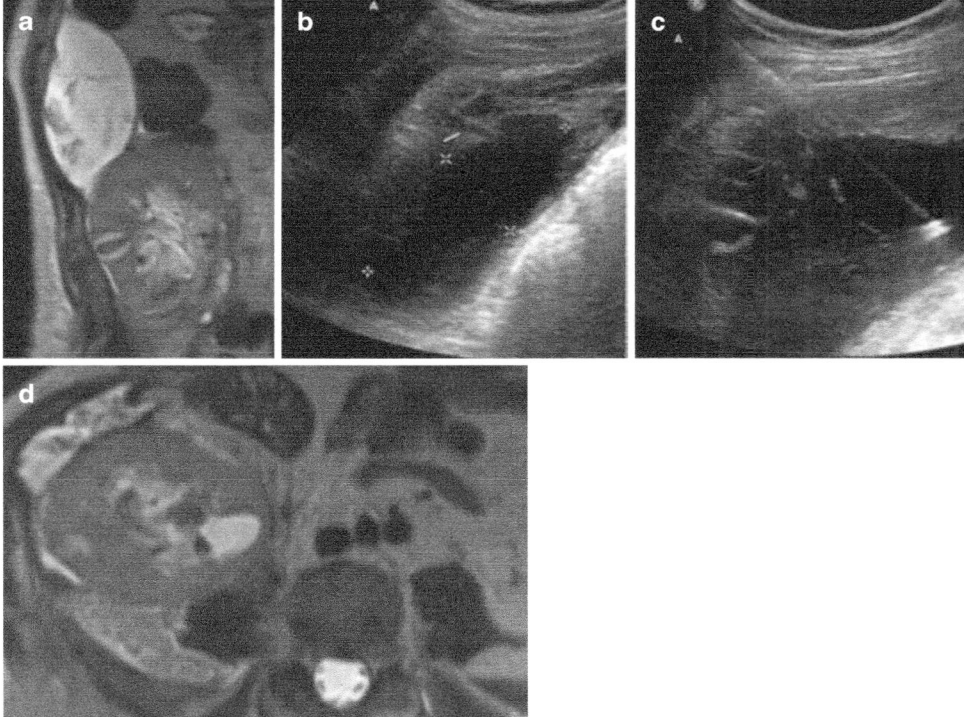

Fig. 21.4 (a) RM image showed an infected lymphocele. (b) US confirmed RM finding. (c) The same modality was used as guidance to deploy the drainage. (d) RM per-formed 10 days later demonstrated almost complete reso-lution cf the fluid collection

tions, ultrasound- or CT-guided needle aspiration may confirm the diagnosis and permit the planning of a percutaneous drainage [30].

Prompt surgical or percutaneous drainage combined with systemic antibiotics is mandatory because of the immunosuppressed state of transplant patients. Percutaneous drainage under US or CT guidance is associated with a high rate of success and a low complication rate [28], with the modalities previously described in this chapter [28].

If the fluid is purulent, microscopic examination of the fluid for pus cells and organisms is done, and antibiotic treatment is initiated. Open surgical drainage becomes necessary when the percutaneous drainage of the infected fluid collections is ineffective completely or partially [6].

Conclusions

Nowadays, the procedures described became the first choice in the treatment of abscess col-lections. They have resulted in reduced mor-bidity and mortality and have helped to reduce length of hospital stay and hospital costs. In conclusion, th-ee fundamental steps can be identified: pat ent selection, performing the prccedure, and correct management of the patient. In all three steps, interventional radi-ologist, suppoited by clinicians, has the most important role.

References

1. Hung CH, Liot JD, Yan MY, Chang CC (2007) Im mediate percutaneous drainage compared with sur-gical drainage of -enal abscess. Int Urol Nephrol 39:51–55. https://doi.org/10.1007/s11255-006-9033-5
2. Charles HW (2012) Abscess drainage. Semin Interv Radiol 29:325–336. https://doi.org/10.105 5/s-0032-1330068
3. Kr shna GS, Vijayalakshmidevi B, Lakshmi AY, Mutheswaraiah B, Sivakumar V (2012) Perinephric

abscess with extension into mediastinum and epidural space. Indian J Nephrol 22:224–225. https://doi.org/10.4103/0971-4065.98770

4. Dielubanza EJ, Mazur DJ, Schaeffer AJ (2014) Management of non-catheter-associated complicated urinary tract infection. Infect Dis Clin N Am 28:121–134. https://doi.org/10.1016/j.idc.2013.10.005

5. Coelho RF, Schneider-Monteiro ED, Mesquita JLB, Mazzucchi E, Marmo Lucon A, Srougi M (2007) Renal and perinephric abscesses: analysis of 65 consecutive cases. World J Surg 31:431–436. https://doi.org/10.1007/s00268-006-0162-x

6. Ahmadnia H, Yarmohamadi A (2003) Percutaneous drainage of perirenal abscess after kidney transplantation: a 4-year experience. Transplant Proc 35:2670–2671. https://doi.org/10.1016/j.transproceed.2003.08.074

7. Meng MV, Mario LA, McAninch JW (2002) Current treatment and outcomes of perinephric abscesses. J Urol 168:1337–1340. https://doi.org/10.1097/01.ju.0000027904.39606.32

8. Nixon JN, Biyyam DR, Stanescu L, Phillips GS, Finn LS, Parisi MT (2013) Imaging of pediatric renal transplants and their complications: a pictorial review. Radiographics 33:1227–1251. https://doi.org/10.1148/rg.335125150

9. Lee SH, Jung HJ, Mah SY, Chung BH (2010) Renal abscesses measuring 5 cm or less: outcome of medical treatment without therapeutic drainage. Yonsei Med J 51:569–573. https://doi.org/10.3349/ymj.2010.51.4.569

10. Dietrich CF, Lorentzen T, Appelbaum L, Buscarini E, Cantisani V, Correas JM, Cui XW, D'Onofrio M, Gilja OH, Hocke M, Ignee A, Jenssen C, Kabaalioğlu A, Leen E, Nicolau C, Nolsoe CP, Radzina M, Serra C, Sidhu PS, Sparchez Z, Piscaglia F (2016) EFSUMB guidelines on interventional ultrasound (INVUS), part III - abdominal treatment procedures (short version). Ultraschall Med 37:27–45. https://doi.org/10.1055/s-0035-1553965

11. Heller MT, Haarer KA, Thomas E, Thaete FL (2012) Neoplastic and proliferative disorders of the perinephric space. Clin Radiol 67:e31–e41

12. Demertzis J, Menias CO (2007) State of the art: imaging of renal infections. Emerg Radiol 14:13–22. https://doi.org/10.1007/s10140-007-0591-3

13. Lorenz JM, Al-Refaie WB, Cash BD, Gaba RC, Gervais DA, Gipson MG, Kolbeck KJ, Kouri BE, Marshalleck FE, Nair AV, Ray CE, Hohenwalter EJ (2015) ACR appropriateness criteria radiologic Management of Infected Fluid Collections. J Am Coll Radiol 12:791–799. https://doi.org/10.1016/j.jacr.2015.04.025

14. Siegel JF, Smith A, Moldwin R (1996) Minimally invasive treatment of renal abscess. J Urol 155:52–55

15. Patel IJ, Davidson JC, Nikolic B, Salazar GM, Schwartzberg MS, Walker TG, Saad WE, Standards of Practice Committee, with Cardiovascular and Interventional Radiological Society of Europe

(CIRSE) Endorsement, Standards of Practice Committee of the Society of Interventional Radiology (2013) Addendum of newer anticoagulants to the SIR consensus guideline. J Vasc Interv Radiol 24:641–645. https://doi.org/10.1016/j.jvir.2012.12.007

16. Wallace MJ, Chin KW, Fletcher TB, Bakal CW, Cardella JF, Grassi CJ, Grizzard JD, Kaye AD, Kushner DC, Larson PA, Liebscher LA, Luers PR, Mauro MA, Kundu S (2010) Quality improvement guidelines for percutaneous drainage/aspiration of abscess and fluid collections. J Vasc Interv Radiol 21:431–435. https://doi.org/10.1016/j.jvir.2009.12.398

17. Venkatesan AM, Kundu S, Sacks D, Wallace MJ, Wojak JC, Rose SC, Clark TWI, D'Othee BJ, Itkin M, Jones RS, Miller DL, Owens CA, Rajan DK, Stokes LS, Swan TL, Towbin RB, Cardella JF (2010) Practice guideline for adult antibiotic prophylaxis during vascular and interventional radiology procedures. J Vasc Interv Radiol 21:1611–1630. https://doi.org/10.1016/j.jvir.2010.07.018

18. Carlson SK, Bender CE, Classic KL, Zink FE, Quam JP, Ward EM, Oberg a L (2001) Benefits and safety of CT fluoroscopy in interventional radiologic procedures. Radiology 219:515–520. https://doi.org/10.1148/radiology.219.2.r01ma41515

19. Paulson EK, Sheafor DH, Enterline DS, McAdams HP, Yoshizumi TT (2001) CT fluoroscopy--guided interventional procedures: techniques and radiation dose to radiologists. Radiology 220:161–167. https://doi.org/10.1148/radiology.220.1.r01jl29161

20. Jaffe TA, Nelson RC (2016) Image-guided percutaneous drainage: a review. Abdom Radiol 41:629–636

21. Deyoe LA, Cronan JJ, Lambiase RE, Dorfman GS (1990) Percutaneous and perirenal drainage of renal abscesses: results in 30 patients. AJR Am. J. Roentgenol. 155:81–83

22. Rubilotta E, Balzarro M, Lacola V, Sarti A, Porcaro AB, Artibani W (2014) Current clinical management of renal and perinephric abscesses: a literature review. Urologia 81:144–147. https://doi.org/10.5301/urologia.5000044

23. Mueller PR, Ferrucci JT, Butch RJ, Simeone JF, Wittenberg J (1985) Inadvertent percutaneous catheter gastroenterostomy during abscess drainage: significance and management. Am J Roentgenol 145:387–391. https://doi.org/10.2214/ajr.145.2.387

24. vanSonnenberg E, Mueller PR, Ferrucci JT (1984) Percutaneous drainage of 250 abdominal abscesses and fluid collections. Part I: results, failures, and complications. Radiology 151:337–341. https://doi.org/10.1148/radiology.151.2.6709901

25. Lang EK (1990) Renal, perirenal, and pararenal abscesses: percutaneous drainage. Radiology 174:109–113. https://doi.org/10.1148/radiology.174.1.2294535

26. Johnson SP, Berry RS (2001) Interventional radiological Management of the Complications of renal transplantation. Semin Interv Radiol 18:047–058. https://doi.org/10.1055/s-2001-12838

27. Khauli RB, Stoff JS, Lovewell T, Ghavamian R, Baker S (1993) Post-transplant lymphoceles: a critical look into the risk factors, pathophysiology and management. J Urol 150:22–26

28. Kobayashi K, Censullo ML, Rossman LL, Kyriakides PN, Kahan BD, Cohen AM (2007) Interventional radiologic management of renal transplant dysfunction: indications, limitations, and technical considerations. Radiographics 27:1109–1130. https://doi.org/10.1148/rg.274065135

29. Pollak R, Veremis SA, Maddux MS, Mozes MF (1988) The natural history of and therapy for perirenal fluid collections following renal transplantation. J Urol 140:716–720

30. Bouali K, Magoteaux P, Jadot A, Saive C, Lombard R, Weerts J, Dallemagne B, Jehaes C, Delforge M, Fontaine F (1993) Percutaneous catheter drainage of abdominal abscess after abdominal surgery. Results in 121 cases. J Belg Radiol 76:11–14

Urinary Tract Infections in Infants and Children

22

Marcello Napolitano and Anna Ravelli

22.1 Introduction

Urinary tract is a common site of bacterial infection in children [1–5]. For many years urinary tract infections (UTIs) have been arousing the interest of scientific community; during the last decade, the UK National Institute for Clinical Excellence (NICE) and the American Academy of Pediatrics (AAP) published their guidelines to help the pediatricians in the diagnosis and management of this affection [2, 3]. Nevertheless, there is still uncertainty regarding *whether* or not and *what* examination is necessary to reach the correct diagnosis, identify the eventual complications, and continue the appropriate follow-up [3]. Clinical manifestation and laboratory analysis on blood sample are nonspecific for UTI and cannot make confidence about the diagnosis [3]. On the other hand, urine culture is useful, but it takes at least 24 h for the results [2]. Nowadays, thanks to the improvement of imaging techniques, several tools are available to study the urinary tract such as ultrasound (US), voiding cystourethrography (VCUG), dimercaptosuccinic acid (DMSA) scintigraphy, magnetic resonance urography

(MRU), computed tomography (CT), and videourodynamic study (VUDS) that can be combined in different way in top-down or bottom-up approach [6, 7]. Urinary tract infections can be distinguished in simple UTIs characterized by isolated bacteriuria and complicated UTIs characterized by the development of acute pyelonephritis (APN), acute focal bacterial nephritis also named acute lobar nephronia (AFBN or ALN), renal abscess, and/or pyonephrosis [4]. These entities may result in renal scar and lead to serious sequelae such as hypertension, proteinuria, and chronic kidney disease until renal failure [4, 5, 8, 9]. It is relevant to distinguish among the different forms of UTIs because their treatment is different [5, 9, 10]. UTIs are clearly a problem for affected children but represent also a distress for their parents and a challenge for the clinicians. In this context, the aim of this chapter is to clarify the role of the imaging in the management of infant and pediatric UTIs, focalizing on the complicated forms.

22.2 Definition, Incidence, and Risk Factors

Urinary tract infection is defined by the American Academy of Pediatrics as the presence of pyuria and at least 50,000 colony-forming units per mL of bacteria in a clean urine specimen [2].

In childhood, urinary tract infections are a frequent disease present in up to 6% of children

M. Napolitano (✉) • A. Ravelli
Dapartment of Radiology and Neuroradiology,
Children's Hospital Vittore Buzzi,
via Castelvetro 32, Milan 20154, Italy
e-mail: Marcello.napolitano@asst-fbf-sacco.it;
ellian@hotmail.it

© Springer International Publishing AG 2018
M. Tonolini (ed.), *Imaging and Intervention in Urinary Tract Infections and Urosepsis*,
https://doi.org/10.1007/978-3-319-68276-1_22

under the age of 7 years [11]; in particular, prevalence is about 5% in the subset of 2- to 24-month-old children according to AAP guidelines [2]. In young children from 0 to 6 months of age, UTIs are more diffuse among males and after 6 months among girls [11]. The exact incidence of complicated UTIs in children is not well established yet, but from some studies, it seems to be about 4% in children hospitalized for suspected acute focal bacterial nephritis, renal abscess, and/or pyonephrosis [4, 12–14]; in Taiwan the rate of ALN among children with febrile UTI results higher, about 8–10% [10, 15]. The microorganisms involved in the majority of UTIs are bacteria, first *Escherichia Coli*, followed by *Proteus* and *Pseudomonas* sp. [4, 14, 16, 17]. When infection is due to non-*E. Coli* organism, it is considered an atypical UTI [3].

Currently, some predisposing factors for UTIs have been identified: first, congenital malformations (megaureter, urethral valves, renal hypoplasia), vesicoureteral reflux (VUR), family history of renal disease, dysfunctional elimination syndrome (DES), poor urine flow, previous UTI, recurrent fever of uncertain origin, constipation, enlarged bladder, spinal lesion, abdominal mass, poor growth, high blood pressure, and for boys uncircumcision [2, 3, 11, 14].

The role of VUR is still controversial because in the past it was thought to be the main cause of UTI and renal damage, but now the association between VUR, reported in one-third of children with febrile UTIs, and renal injury does not appear so straightforward [6, 18–20]. Moreover, the pathogenesis of renal scar remains uncertain, even if VUR, delayed therapy, young age, and extension of renal injury seem to be risk factors [18]. The pathogenesis of AFBN is unclear; it is likely due to hematic or ascending infection from the lower urinary tract. At histological examination, acute focal bacterial nephritis shows hyperemia, interstitial edema, and leukocyte infiltration [14, 16]; area of acute pyelonephritis presents similar features but milder, while intraparenchymal abscess is a focal, purulent parenchymal cavity with peripheral wall and internal liquefaction and necrosis [5]. Pyonephrosis is another inflammatory condition included in the spectrum of complicated UTIs, usually when collecting systems are dilated or obstructed [4].

22.3 Clinical and Laboratory Features

Clinical and biochemical findings are not specific of a urinary tract infection, being common to other febrile infections not involving the bladder and/or kidneys [9, 21]. Children with UTI can be very asymptomatic, having only bacteriuria, or may manifest bladder symptoms and/or fever [3, 11]. The most common signs and symptoms of UTIs for infants younger than 3 months seem to be fever, vomiting, irritability, and lethargy and for older children also dysuria [3]; diarrhea, poor feeding, and dehydration have also been described in young infants [14]. According to AAP, there is fever if temperature is at least 38.0 °C [2]. Children with complicated UTIs generally present nonspecific symptoms similar to those of noncomplicated infections but more severe, with septic temperature, and rapid worsening of clinical condition [9, 14]; the differential diagnosis among different forms of febrile UTIs based only on clinical data is not simple [5].

Furthermore, urinary tract is commonly subdivided in upper and lower tract; usually, fever and bacteriuria in the presence or absence of lower back pain are considered linked to APN or upper urinary tract infection, while cystitis or lower urinary tract infection should be considered in the case of isolated bacteriuria, with no associated signs and symptoms. All other infants and children who have bacteriuria but no systemic symptoms or signs should be considered to have cystitis/lower urinary tract infection [3].

Urine collection is recommended in any case of febrile infant suspected to have an infectious involvement of urinary tract [2, 3]. The specimen for the culture of the pathogen and urinalysis, intended as the research of bacteria and leukocytes at microscope and leukocyte esterase and nitrite tests, has to be collected through the urethral catheterization or suprapubic aspiration to avoid any contamination. Positive microscopy, leukocyte esterase, and nitrite tests combined have a sensitivity of about 100% and specificity of 70% in detecting UTI [2]. Instead, blood analysis showing elevated inflammatory indices (white blood cell count (WBC), serum C-reactive protein (CRP), erythrocyte sedimentation rate (ESR)) is nonspecific [4].

22.4 Role of Imaging: *What and When?*

The management of children with febrile UTI is not univocally determined, and nowadays there is not a single accepted protocol to guide the practicing clinician among the several imaging modalities available. The goal of radiologic imaging is to prevent significant renal damage, avoid unnecessary examinations, and reduce subsequent stress for children and their families.

22.4.1 Ultrasound

US is considered the cornerstone of pediatric imaging in the evaluation of genitourinary district, due to its accessibility, noninvasiveness, and lack of exposure to radiation. It is the first-line modality to investigate renal and bladder involvement in course of acute febrile UTI; its role is to detect congenital urinary tract malformations predisposing to upper or lower urinary tract infection and to identify eventual complications such as pyonephrosis, acute lobar bacterial nephritis, and renal and perirenal abscesses, in order to guarantee a prompt treatment [2, 3, 6] (Fig. 22.1). Actually, routine use of prenatal ultrasonography has reduced the prevalence of unexpected urinary tract anomalies in infants, but absence of abnormalities in screening ultrasound does not completely exclude the presence of a structural abnormality of kidneys or bladder [2, 22].

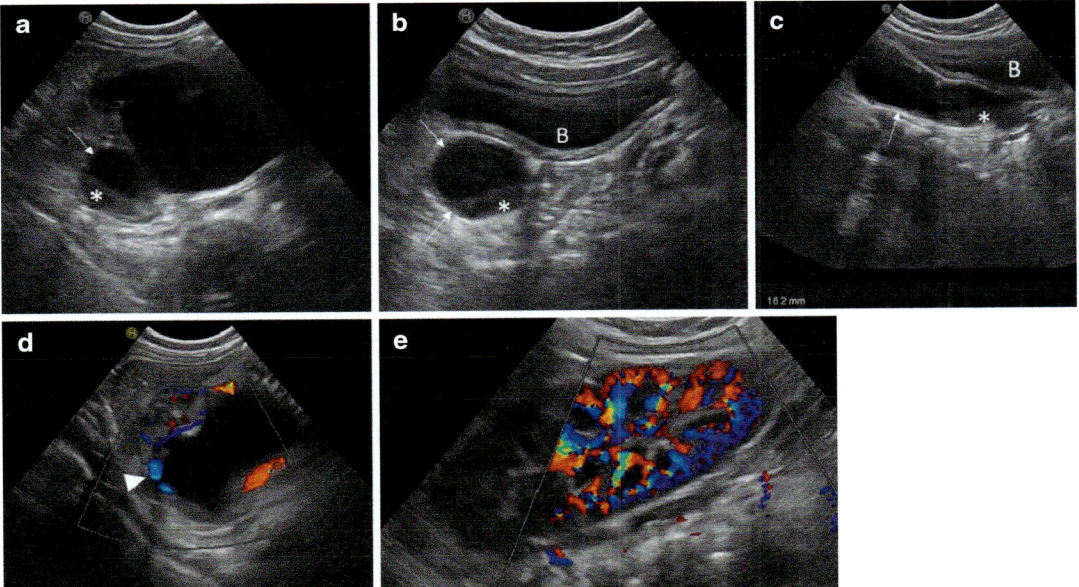

Fig. 22.1 A 5-month-old boy affected with megaureter and pyonephrosis. (**a**) US transverse image showing dilatation of pelvis and calyces of the right kidney with presence of debris (asterisk) in the calyces (arrow); (**b**) US transverse image showing dilatation of the distal tract of the right ureter (arrows) with hyperechoic debris in the dependent position (asterisk), B = bladder; (**c**) US longitudinal image showing the distal tract of the right ureter dilated (arrow) with declivous hyperechoic debris (asterisk), B = bladder; (**d**) US transverse image showing hydronephrosis of the right kidney with concomitant thinning of the renal parenchyma and decreased vascularization at color Doppler interrogation (arrowhead); (**e**) US longitudinal image with color Doppler analysis showing normal perfusion of the left kidney without signs of hydronephrosis

Several authors reported a poor accuracy of US in detecting urinary tract abnormality, with sensitivity ranging from 12 to 79% and specificity from 41 to 99%, [2, 19, 22–30], with a specific sensitivity for detecting VUR (evidence of urinary tract dilatation) of 10% and a positive predictive value of 40% [19]. According to recent guidelines from the American Academy of Pediatrics, 1–2% of US abnormalities lead to further investigations or surgery, while the rate of false positive is about 2–3%. However, for its advantages, US is commonly well accepted by parents, and benefits-harm balance is considered in favor of performing US in case of suspected acute febrile UTI [2].

According to NICE guidelines, it is possible to divide UTIs in three different categories: typical, atypical, and recurrent. Atypical UTI comprises *non-E. Coli* infections, presence of bladder or abdominal mass, high value of creatinine, sepsis, nonresponse to antibiotics within 48 h, and poor urine flow. Recurrent UTI can be defined as more than one episode of acute upper or lower urinary tract infection [3]. NICE guidelines give different recommendation regarding the use of ultrasound in case of febrile UTI either based on the type or on the age of the patient. Three different groups can be identified: (1) 0–6 months, (2) 6–36 months, and (3) >36 months.

Ultrasound is recommended during the acute infection in the presence of atypical or recurrent UTI for infants younger than 6 months, while for infants who has positive response to treatment within 48 h, US is recommended within 6 weeks from the acute episode. Ultrasound during the acute infection is recommended only in the presence of atypical UTI for patients with more than 6 months, while patients with recurrent UTI are recommended to undergo US within 6 weeks from the acute episode. Moreover, children who have positive response to antibiotics within 48 h should not undergo any imaging investigation.

Current practice guidelines of the American Academy of Pediatrics refer to infants and young children 2–24 months of age, recommending to perform US to detect complications if clinical situation is severe or there is no improvement of the clinical condition during the first

2 days of treatment. If the patient shows significant improvement of clinical situation, early US examination during the acute infection is not mandatory.

22.4.2 Voiding Cystourethrography

The goal of voiding cystourethrography (VCUG) is to identify genitourinary abnormalities which may favor urinary tract infection and lead to renal damage. Vesicoureteral reflux has been for long time the primary focus of imaging, because it was believed to be strongly associated with renal lesion. In healthy pediatric population, VUR prevalence has been estimated to range between 0.4 and 1.8%, while it is present in about one-third of children, who experienced febrile UTI [31, 32]. The real role of VUR, especially of high grade, in the development of APN, has not been clarified yet [2, 3, 11, 30, 33]. Association of VUR with UTI seems to have higher risk of renal damage, but it is also reported that pyelonephritis can develop in infants and children without any demonstrable VUR as well [31]. Currently, it does not exist any laboratory or clinical test to discover in advance infants and children with VUR, so VCUG remains the gold standard to detect and grade it. Moreover, this test allows to detect bladder dysfunction and also urethral abnormalities. It is clear that VCUG is an invasive procedure, uncomfortable for the little patients and not well accepted by their parents because of catheterization and use of ionizing radiation, so it should not be performed routinely. Regarding the average radiation dose derived from VCUG, it is not easy to estimate, because it depends on the fluoroscopy time and on the use of conventional or pulsed digital fluoroscopy. NICE and AAP give some indication about performing VCUG; NICE guidelines suggest to perform VCUG in infants younger than 6 months just in case of atypical or recurrent UTI, while in children aged 6–36 months, VCUG is recommended only in the presence of hydronephrosis on US, poor urine flow, and family history of vesicoureteral reflux and when *E. Coli* is not the pathogen responsible [3]. AAP is of the same opinion, suggesting not to perform VCUG always after the first episode of fever due to UTI, but just in case of complex clinical situation, US dilatation, renal scarring, suspected obstructive uropathy, or high-grade VUR, usually, the committee recommends to perform VCUG after the second episode of febrile UTI.

22.4.3 Dimercaptosuccinic Acid (DMSA) Scintigraphy

Technetium (Tc)-99m DMSA is considered the gold standard for detection and quantification of acute pyelonephritis and for identification of renal scarring in children [9, 34–36]; its sensitivity for renal cortical abnormalities has been reported to be higher than that of US or intravenous urography, ranging between 80 and 100% [37–39], while its sensitivity is still in discussion with respect to MRI [40–42]. Renal scar is one of the possible sequelae after a febrile UTI; generally, on DMSA it appears as photopenic area, due to focal ischemia and tubular dysfunction; it may appear as retraction of renal parenchyma with calices deformity. The affected kidney may become small and irregular in shape, in case of multifocal scars. Detection of scarring has a prognostic value, because it can lead to recurrent pyelonephritis in adulthood, renal hypertension, and renal insufficiency [40, 43, 44]. Although DMSA is very sensitive to detect focal renal defect, it does not allow to discriminate different underlying conditions [9, 18, 41]; in fact, acute pyelonephritis, permanent scar, cortical cysts, renal abscesses, hydronephrosis, and calculi appear in the similar way as focal tracer uptake defects [9, 41]. Then, it would be preferable to perform it no earlier than 6 months from the acute episode of febrile UTI so that acute temporary lesions have the time to heal [45]. This nuclear medicine technique has different disadvantages to take in consideration: first of all it is not radiation-free, even if the radiation dose is generally low (about 1 mSv) [46]; secondarily, it requires positioning of a cannula for intravenous administration of the radiotracer; it takes a long time because patients have to wait some hours after the injection before undergoing the scan; and finally the spatial resolution is poor [40, 42]. Current practice guidelines of the UK National Institute for Clinical Excellence recommend to perform DMSA 4–6 months after the acute infection in infants younger than 36 months in case of atypical or recurrent UTI and only in case of recurrent UTI for children 36 months old or older.

22.4.4 Magnetic Resonance Imaging

The use of magnetic resonance imaging in pediatric radiology is increasingly widespread, because it provides noninvasive evaluation, anatomical and functional information, high accuracy, and soft tissue contrast, without radiation exposure [4, 40–42]. In literature there are some studies which compare MRI with the gold standard DMSA for the identification of renal parenchymal defects in infants and children with febrile UTIs; different protocols were used, with or without dynamic contrast-enhancement technique, known as MR urography (MRU), which enables to study renal morphology and perfusion together with anatomical and functional status of the collecting system [40–42, 47]. Kavanagh et al. [42] reported a sensitivity of 77% and a specificity of 87% for detection of renal scarring and sensitivity of 75% and specificity of 98% for detection of focal parenchymal abnormality using a coronal fat-saturated T1-W sequence. The authors of the study reviewed the discordant DMSA/MRI cases and concluded that MRI seemed to be the more precise examination. Cerwinka et al. [40] reached a similar conclusion, even if in their study they used also T1-weighted post-contrast sequences. Kovanlikaya et al. [41] reported the sensitivity and the specificity of MRI in the detection of pyelonephritic lesions as about 91 and 89%, respectively. Vivier et al. [47] concluded that DWI sequences as well allow to detect a similar number of renal lesions with a sensitivity of 100% and specificity of 93.5%, compared to T1-weighted post-contrast images.

MRI is superior to DMSA in terms of contrast and spatial resolution; it can differentiate between acute pyelonephritis and renal scar, but it also allows to discriminate parenchymal defect among other renal lesions such as small cortical renal cyst, well identifiable on T2-weighted images, or nephrolithiasis [40, 41]. Moreover, MRI has the possibility to show the kidneys in multiple planes. Some authors have demonstrated that on post-gadolinium inversion recovery, MR images of acute pyelonephritis had hyperintense signal, while renal scar was seen as cortical thinning, parenchymal defect, or irregular contour without any signal change [39, 41]. However, MRI has some disadvantages such as the risks derived from sedation, necessary for infants and often for some young child, the limited accessibility and the elevated costs [40].

In our institution, the use of MRI in case of suspected urinary tract infection is accepted in case of complicated UTI, for instance when US reveals renal lesion suspected for abscess, pyelonephritis, or acute focal lobar nephritis; in such cases, we use a standard protocol, which consists of pre-contrast T2-weighted, DWI, and T1-weighted sequences followed by dynamic study with late urographic images, providing morphological evaluation of the collecting system; injection of furosemide just before dynamic acquisition is routinely performed. In our experience, MRI allows to identify and discriminate renal lesions and detect eventual underlying urinary tract anomalies, guiding the choice of subsequent management (Figs. 22.2, 22.3, 22.4, 22.5, and 22.6).

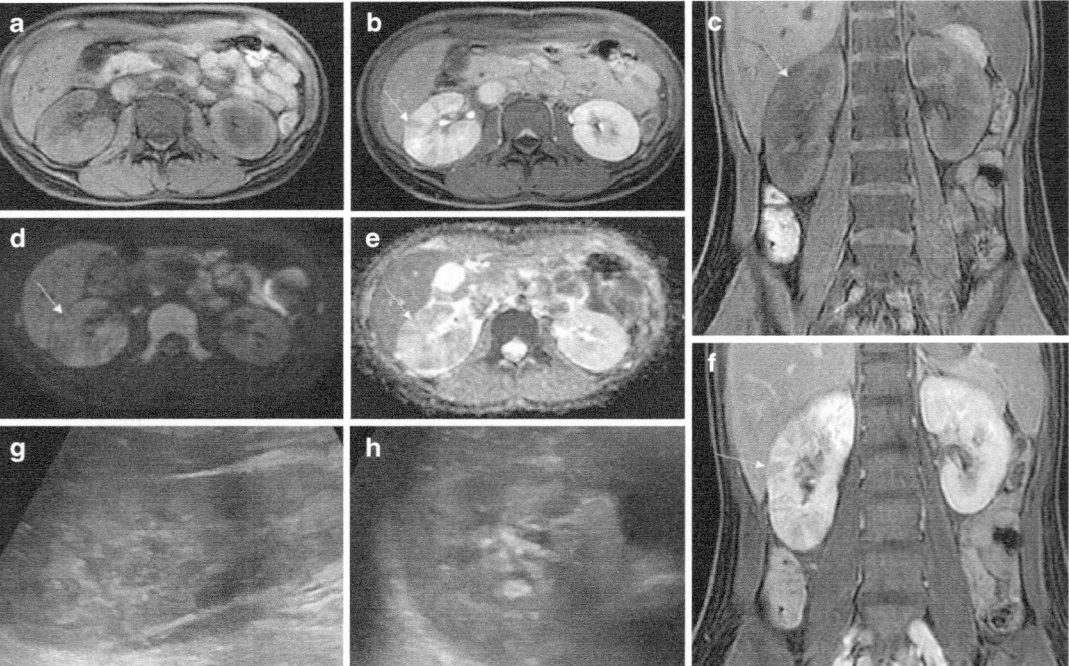

Fig. 22.2 A 16-year-old girl affected with acute pyelonephritis was admitted to hospital due to right lumbar pain, fever, and rise of white blood cell count. (**a**) Axial T1-weighted fat-suppressed MR image showing an enlarged right kidney with reduced corticomedullary differentiation; (**b**) axial T1-weighted fat-suppressed post-contrast image showing multiple wedge-shaped cortical hypovascular lesions in the right kidney (arrow) as for acute pyelonephritis; (**c**) coronal T1-weighted fat-suppressed image showing enlargement of the right kidney with some hypointense focal area in the cortex (arrow); (**d**) axial DWI b800 image showing striated appearance of renal parenchyma with areas of restricted signal (arrow); (**e**) ADC map confirming the parenchymal alterations seen in DWI image (arrow); (**f**) coronal T1-weighted fat-suppressed post-contrast image showing multiple wedge-shaped cortical hypovascular lesions in the right kidney (arrow). Ultrasonography ((**g**) longitudinal view, (**h**) transverse view) shows an enlarged right kidney with hyperechoic upper pole. There is no evidence of intraparenchymal abscess or mass

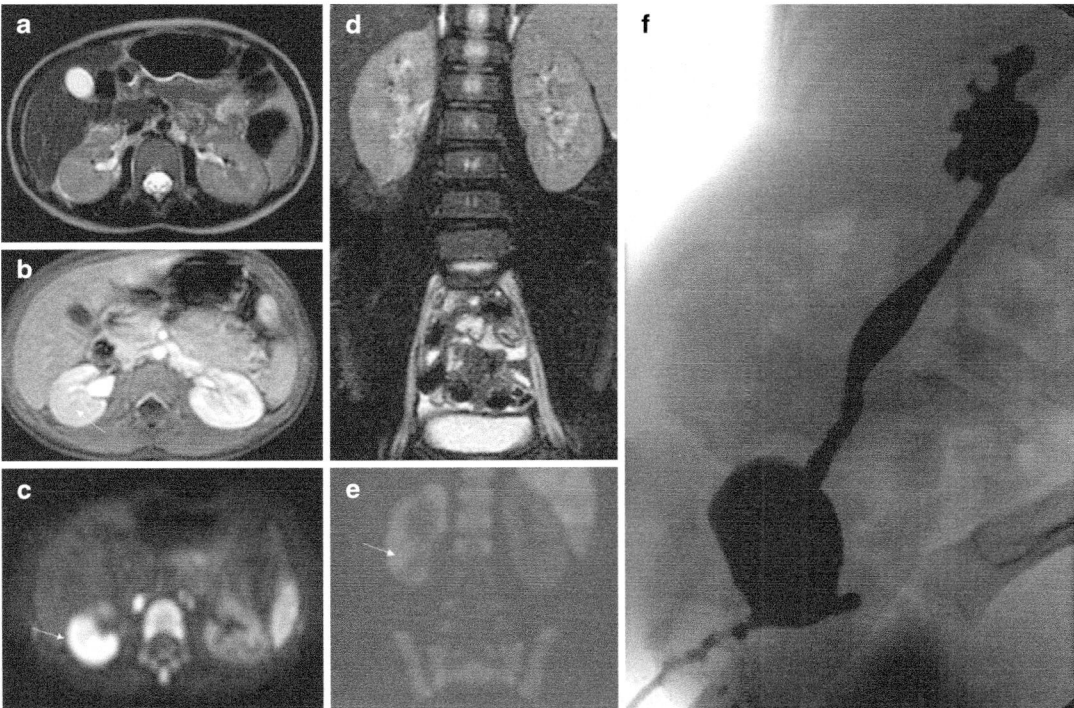

Fig. 22.3 A 6-year-old girl with history of recurrent pyelonephritis of the right kidney. (**a**) Axial T2-weighted image showing the right kidney smaller than left with an area of loss of corticomedullary differentiation; (**b**) axial T1-weighted fat-saturated post-contrast image showing hypoperfused-affected renal parenchyma (arrow); (**c**) axial DWI b = 800 image showing the pyelonephritic area characterized by hypersignal (arrow); (**d**) coronal T2-weighted image showing the right kidney smaller than left with loss of corticomedullary differentiation; (**e**) coronal DWIBS image showing hypersignal parenchyma as for pyelonephritis (arrow); (**f**) fluoroscopy image showing vesicoureteral reflux of III grade

22.4.5 Computed Tomography

Usually, computed tomography is not the favored imaging modality for pediatric patients, due to the use of ionizing radiation, need of iodinated contrast material, and sedation in infants and young children. However, CT is considered the gold standard in the diagnosis of acute focal bacterial nephritis, a form of localized, severe bacterial infection affecting single or multiple renal lobules, and associated with a very high risk of renal scarring [4, 9, 13, 16]. AFBN is a relatively recent entity, described for the first time in children in 1985 [48]. At histopathology, it is characterized by hyperemia, interstitial edema, and infiltration of white blood cells, without necrosis or liquefaction [16]. It is controversial if AFBN represents the midpoint between uncomplicated pyelonephritis and intrarenal abscess [4, 13, 49,

50]. In children with AFBN, vesicoureteral reflux has a similar incidence than in children with other type of UTI, ranging from 17% to 42% [18, 30]. So, it seems that VUR is not necessary for the development of AFBN [5]. It is important to differentiate AFBN from tumor or renal abscess, because therapy is different [4, 14]. Finally, CT maintains a role in detecting calculi, especially if wedged in the ureter and hidden to US.

22.4.6 Videourodynamic Study

The videourodynamic study (VUDS) has a role in the evaluation of children with pathologies involving the low urinary tract. VUDS, in fact, allows to assess the detrusor activity, detrusor sphincter dyssynergia, and intravesical pressure [51–53].

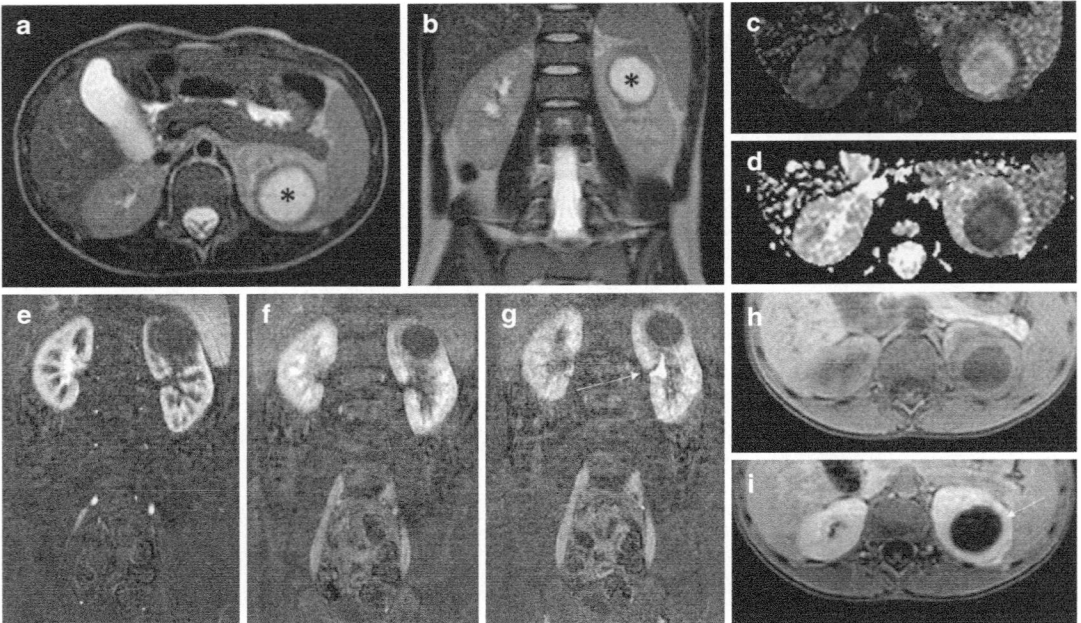

Fig. 22.4 A young boy with abscess in the left kidney. (**a**) Axial T2-weighted image showing round-shape intraparenchymal abscess with hypersignal core (asterisk) and hypointense border; (**b**) coronal T2-weighted image showing the abscess (asterisk) in the superior portion of the left kidney. Axial DWI b800 image (**c**) and ADC map (**d**) showing restriction of the signal of the abscess core. Coronal T1-weighted fat-suppressed post-contrast images in arterial (**e**), parenchymal (**f**), and excretory phase (**g**) showing the absence of vascularization inside the abscess and initial excretion of contrasted urine in left pelvis (arrow); (**h**) axial T1-weighted fat-suppressed image showing the hypointense core of the abscess; (**i**) axial T1-weighted fat-suppressed post-contrast image showing normal vascularization of the renal parenchyma around the abscess (arrow)

22.4.7 Voiding Urosonography

Contrast-enhanced voiding urosonography (VUS) has emerged in the last years as alternative imaging modality to assess VUR with a reported sensitivity and specificity of about 100% (95% CI 96.5–100%) compared with the gold standard VCUG [54, 55]. Moreover, Duran et al. demonstrated that VUS is a reliable technique also for evaluation of the neck of the bladder and the urethra in children [56].

22.5 Complicated UTIs: Imaging Findings

22.5.1 Acute Pyelonephritis (APN)

Typical US signs in case of APN include focal or diffuse increase of renal volume, reduction of corticomedullary differentiation, thickening of the walls of the upper urinary tract (pelvis and proximal ureter), hyperechogenicity of the renal sinus, and areas of altered parenchymal echogenicity [57]. Sensitivity of US in detecting APN is not very high (about 50–60%), and the examination can be totally normal, even in the presence of acute inflammation. Color and power Doppler analysis can increase sensitivity of conventional US until 80–85% compared to CT, depicting APN as hypovascular regions [58]. On contrast-enhanced CT scan, APN is characterized by striated appearance with hypovascular wedge-shaped areas of varying extension, parenchymal swelling, and reduction of corticomedullary differentiation [58, 59]. APN has similar appearance on gadolinium-enhanced MRI: on T1-weighted images, it has low signal, while on inversion recovery images, it has increased signal intensity compared to normal renal parenchyma [39, 41], while on diffusion-weighted images, APN appears bright [47].

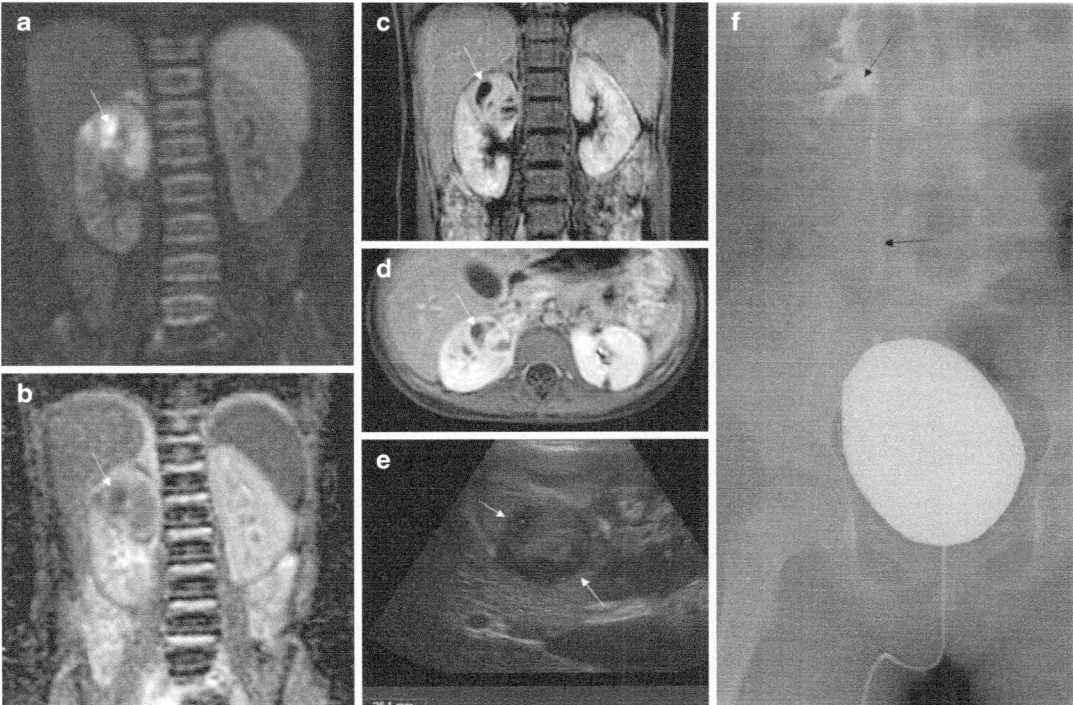

Fig. 22.5 A 5-year-old girl affected with complicated acute lobar nephronia. (**a**) Coronal DWI b800 image showing several hyperintense small foci of abscess located in the superior portion of the right kidney (arrow). (**b**) ADC map confirming multiple microabscesses with restricted signal in the superior portion of the right kidney (arrow). Coronal (**c**) and axial (**d**) T1-weighted fat-suppressed post-contrast images showing not enhanced foci of abscess (arrow); (**e**) US longitudinal image showing round-shape focal mass with inhomogeneous structure due to presence of fluid content (arrows); (**f**) cystourethrography showing vesicoureteral reflux of grade III (arrows)

22.5.2 Acute Focal Bacterial Nephritis (AFBN)

At ultrasonography, AFBN usually appears as circular, hypovascular lesion in the renal parenchyma, with ill-defined irregular margins and loss of corticomedullary differentiation. It can be hypo-, hyper- or isoechoic depending on the phase of the infection; in the early stage, it is more echoic and becomes hypoechoic later [9, 16, 60]. Among the imaging findings of AFBN, severe nephromegaly reflecting acute renal inflammation, and defined as renal length of greater than mean + 3 SD for age, demonstrated a diagnostic sensitivity of 90%, rising to 95% if associated with a focal renal mass, with specificity of about 86%, compared to the gold standard CT [61]. Non-enhanced CT images usually do not show any abnormality of the infected regions, becoming evident in post-contrast images as ill-defined, wedge-shaped hypoperfused areas of renal parenchyma [16, 62].

22.5.3 Renal Abscess

On US, typical signs of renal abscess consist of hypoechoic, usually round-shape area, with thick wall. Contrast-enhanced CT scan and post-contrast MR images typically show renal abscess as a rounded, well-defined lesion with avascular core and hypervascular, irregular peripheral walls, with restricted diffusion signal in DWI sequences and relative ADC map. Presence of intralesional air is suspected for abscess formation [63]. CT and MR scan allow precise

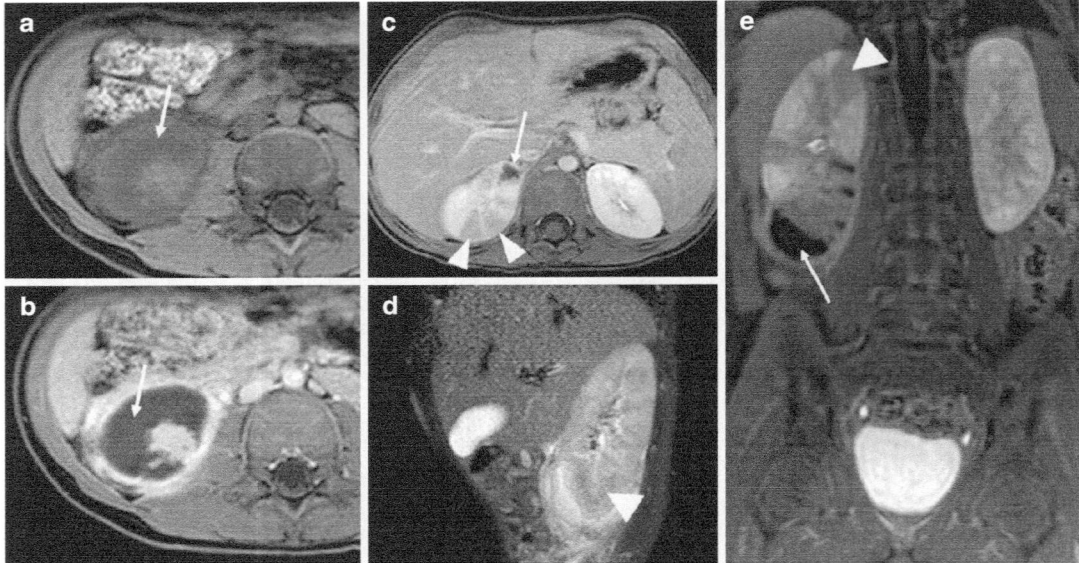

Fig. 22.6 A 3-year-old boy with complicated pyelone-phritis was admitted to hospital due to fever and vomit. He was treated with antibiotic therapy for pyelonephritis 1 month before, and parents referred recent mild abdominal trauma. At physical examination, he had positive right renal percussion. Axial T1-weighted pre-contrast (**a**) and post-contrast (**b**) MR images show a subcapsular hematic collection at the lower pole of the right kidney (arrow); (**c**) axial T1-weighted post-contrast image well depicts a small intraparenchymal abscess (arrow) and triangular-shape areas of pyelonephritis (arrowheads) in the upper pole of the right kidney; (**d**) sagittal T2-weighted fat-saturated image shows altered parenchymal signal in the lower pole of the right kidney (arrowhead) near the perirenal collection; (**e**) coronal T1-weighted post-contrast image shows a hypovascular triangular-shape area of pyelonephritis in the upper pole of the right kidney (arrowhead) and the subcapsular hematic collection at the lower pole (arrow)

evaluation of extrarenal extension of the purulent collection [64, 65]. (Fig. 22.4).

22.5.4 Pyonephrosis

Pyonephrosis refers to a collection of purulent material in the renal calices and pelvis, usually associated with congenital or acquired obstructions of the urinary tract [64]. It is infrequent in children and even rarer in neonates [66, 67]. US clearly shows dilatation of calices and renal pelvis, containing echoic debris in the dependent position (Fig. 22.7). Hydronephrosis without superinfection can be suspected on US in presence of dilated pelvocaliceal system without any evidence of internal echoes. Contrast-enhanced CT better shows dilatation of the collecting system with debris localized below the iodate urine and is useful to exclude associated parenchymal lesion and tumoral cause of obstruction, while in case of radiopaque calculi, non-enhanced CT can easily identify them [64].

22.5.5 Cystitis

Cystitis represents the infection of the lower urinary tract in absence of systemic symptoms. There are no specific signs of cystitis. US can demonstrate hyperechoic urine and increased bladder wall thickness, defined as detrusor muscle thickness greater than 3 mm for full bladder (Fig. 22.8) [68, 69]. However, these conditions are not pathognomonic for cystitis, being present also in other inflammatory or tumoral conditions, after

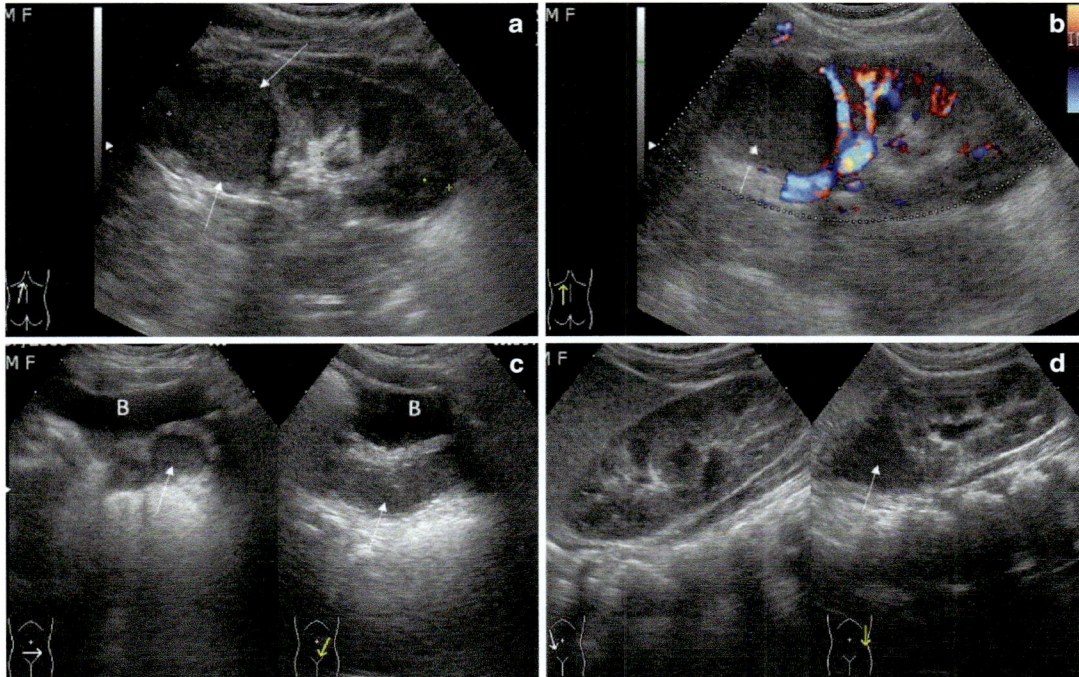

Fig. 22.7 A 2-year-old girl with left-sided infected ureterohydronephrosis of the upper pole collecting system in a patient with bilateral duplex collecting system. (**a**, **b**) Longitudinal US images showing dilatation of the superior district with hyperechoic debris without any internal vascularization (arrows) consistent with pyonephrosis; (**c**)

US images in transverse and longitudinal view showing debris within the dilated ureter (arrows) in proximity of the bladder (B); (**d**) US longitudinal images of the right and left kidneys showing pyonephrosis of the dilated left upper pole collecting system (arrow)

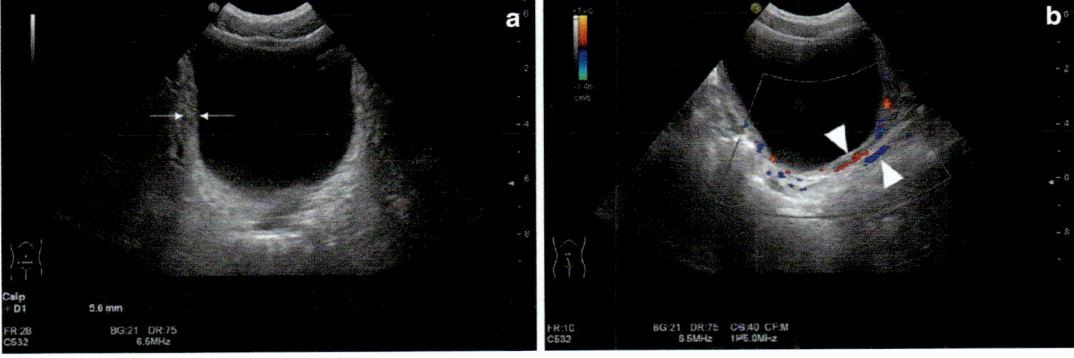

Fig. 22.8 A 7-year-old girl affected with cystitis. (**a**) US transverse image showing diffuse thickened bladder wall (arrows); (**b**) US longitudinal image showing increased vascularization of bladder wall (arrowheads)

specific chemotherapy (e.g., cyclophosphamide) and neurological disorders of the lower urinary tract [70–72].

22.6 Rare Urinary Tract Infections

22.6.1 Xanthogranulomatous Pyelonephritis (XGP)

XGP is believed to be a chronic obstructive pyelonephritis, more often superinfected by bacteria such as *Proteus mirabilis*, *E. coli*, and *Pseudomonas* species [73]. XGP is rare in children and commonly is sustained by a congenital or acquired obstruction of the urinary tract. Usually, XGP affects focally or extensively one kidney, inducing reactive hypertrophy of the contralateral. In 80% of the cases, the infection spreads to the perirenal space, sometimes forming fistulous tracts. When XGP manifests as palpable mass in the flank, Wilms' tumor has to be excluded by using fine-needle aspiration biopsy [74]. Microscopically, XGP is characterized by the presence of inflammatory cells, lipid-filled macrophages, necrosis, and fibrosis [73, 75]. At US examination, kidney with XGP appears enlarged and hyperechoic, and as the disease progress, areas of parenchymal necrosis and reduction of renal volume become evident [76]. CT scan and MR imaging are considered more sensitive than US, showing an enlarged kidney with loss of function; calcification is often present. Thanks to their panoramic field of view, CT and MRI allow to better identify extrarenal invasion of the nearby organs [77]. Partial or complete nephrectomy is actually the treatment of choice [73].

22.6.2 Fungal Infections

Fungal infections are rare in healthy children. The most affected are premature babies, and the most common responsible pathogen is *Candida albicans*. It is believed that pathogens reach kidneys primary by hematogenous diffusion [78]. US examination may show an enlarged kidney with hyperechoic cortex, which has to be differentiated from normal hyperechoic cortex of the newborn, with the presence of echoic fungus balls without acoustic shadowing into the collecting system, to thickening of the bladder walls with debris in the bladder lumen.

22.6.3 Tuberculosis (TB)

TB of urinary tract is a rare disease in children and represents less than 5% of cases of pediatric extrapulmonary disease [79, 80]. *Mycobacterium tuberculosis* affects kidneys by hematogenous dissemination. Imaging may be mute in acute phase, but if the disease progresses, it can cause parenchymal caseous necrosis with subsequent cavitation and formation of intraparenchymal calcifications, distortion, and stenosis of pelvocaliceal system, often present in end-stage renal TB. In rare case, TB infection can appear as hypoechoic/hypodense mass lesion, respectively, on US and CT [81–83].

22.6.4 Infected Urachus

Urachus is an embryological remnant of the allantois, not completely closed and transformed into the medial umbilical ligament. As the rest of the urinary tract, urachus remnant can become infected as well, showing thickening of the walls and increased vascularization on color Doppler investigation (Fig. 22.9).

22.7 Treatment, Prophylaxis, and Follow-Up

22.7.1 Treatment

Treatment of UTI is based on administration of antibiotic therapy. Early treatment, in absence of antibiogram response, is usually empiric and should be based on broad spectrum antibiotics. According to several authors, there is no significant difference in efficacy between oral and parenteral antibiotics [2, 84, 85]. The total duration of antibiotic therapy changes on the basis of

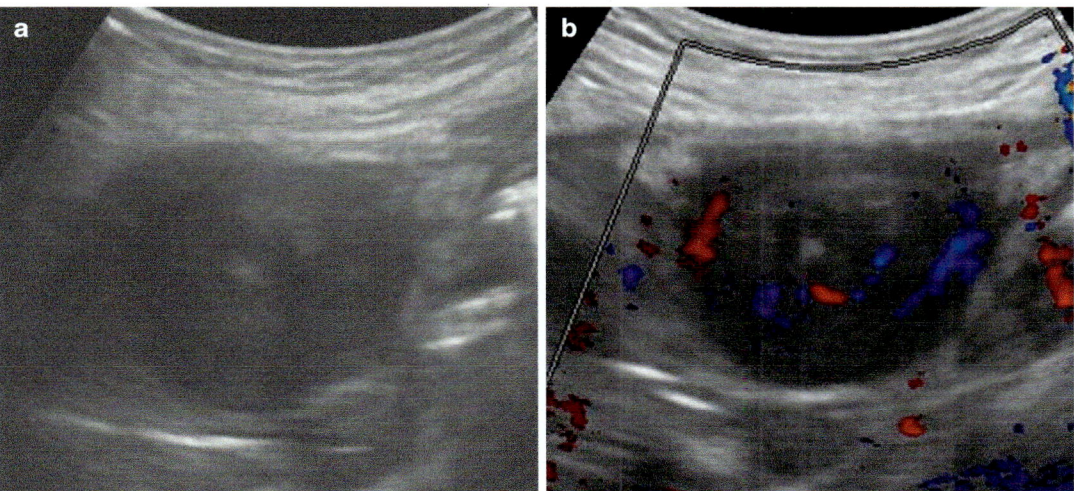

Fig. 22.9 A 1-year-old boy with infected urachus remnant. US transverse image showing hypoechoic markedly thickened urachus walls (**a**) with increased vascularization on color Doppler analysis (**b**)

the diagnosed renal lesion. Even if the optimal duration of antimicrobial treatment has not been determined yet, AAP recommends antibiotics for at least 7 days to treat UTI [2]. In case of AFBN, antibiotic therapy should be continued for at least 2–3 weeks, with intravenous administration at least until 2–3 days after defervescence [9, 16, 17]; however, it seems that the duration of therapy does not reduce the risk for renal scarring [18, 84]. Instead, in presence of renal abscess, the minimal duration of treatment should be 4 weeks, also when abscess requires surgical intervention (drainage) [49, 86]. Early drainage is recommended also in case of suspected pyonephrosis as diagnostic and therapeutic tool [59, 87]. Early diagnosis of first-time or recurrent UTI is relevant to promptly start the proper antibiotic therapy, in order to limit renal damage and risk of renal scarring [18, 88]. Instead, the value of treatment of the reflux, either medical or surgical, is still controversial, because the role of VUR in the pathogenesis of febrile UTI and renal scar remains unclear [2, 19, 84, 89].

22.7.2 Prophylaxis

The use of antimicrobial prophylaxis to prevent recurrence UTI in children with vesicoureteral reflux is still controversial. Several studies, conducted in the last decade, have suggested that prophylaxis does not manage to prevent recurrent febrile UTI as desired [90–94]; on the other hand, the most recent "Randomized Intervention for Children With Vesicoureteral Reflux study" reported that the risk of recurrence of febrile UTI was lower (about 50% less) in the group of children who received prophylaxis with respect to the children who had placebo [95]. Brandstrom as well reported a reduction of the infection rate in children who received antibiotic prophylaxis [11].

22.7.3 Follow-Up

Infants and children who become asymptomatic after the first episode of febrile UTI should not routinely undergo urinalysis but should be retested only in occasion of recurrent infections, in order to proceed as soon as possible with the most effective antibiotic therapy [2, 3].

References

1. Kass EH (1972) The search for asymptomatic pyelonephritis. N Engl J Med 287:563–564

2. American Academy of Pediatrics (2011) Steering committee on quality improvement, subcommittee on urinary tract infection: urinary tract infection: clinical practice guideline for the diagnosis and management of the initial UTI in febrile infants and children 2 to 24 months. Pediatrics 128:595–610
3. National Institute for Clinical Excellence (2007) Urinary tract infection in under 16s: diagnosis and management. Clinical guideline. . nice.org.uk/guidance/cg54
4. Bitsori M, Raissaki M, Maraki S, Galanakis E (2015) Acute focal bacterial nephritis, pyonephrosis and renal abscess in children. Pediatr Nephrol 30:1987
5. Sheu JN (2015) Acute lobar nephronia in children. Pediatr Neonatol 56(3):141–142
6. Ording-Müller LS (2011) Imaging in urinary tract infection: top-down or down-up? Pediatr Radiol 41(Suppl 1):96–98
7. Prasad MM, Cheng EY (2012) Radiographic evaluation of children with febrile urinary tract infection: bottom-up, top-down, or none of the above? Adv Urol 2012:716739
8. Alexander SE, Arlen AM, Storm DW et al (2015) Bladder volume at onset of vesicoureteral reflux is an independent risk factor for breakthrough febrile urinary tract infection. J Urol 193(4):1342–1346
9. Bibalo C, Apicella A, Guastalla V et al (2016) Acute lobar nephritis in children: not so easy to recognize and manage. World J Clin Pediatr 5(1):136–142
10. Cheng CH, Tsau YK, Chen SY et al (2009) Clinical courses of children with acute lobar nephronia correlated with computed tomographic patterns. Pediatr Infect Dis J 28(4):300–303
11. Brandström P, Esbjörner E, Herthelius M et al (2010) The Swedish reflux trial in children: I. Study design and study population characteristics. J Urol 184:274–279
12. Uehling DT, Hahnfeld LE, Scanlan KA (2000) Urinary tract abnormalities in children with focal bacterial nephritis. BJU Int 85(7):885–888
13. Klar A, Hurvitz H, Berkun Y et al (1996) Focal bacterial nephritis (lobar nephronia) in children. J Pediatr 128(6):850–853
14. Seidel T, Kuwertz-Bröking E, Kaczmarek S et al (2007) Acute focal bacterial nephritis in 25 children. Pediatr Nephrol 22:1897–1901
15. Huang HP, Lai YC, Tsai IJ et al (2008) Renal ultrasonography should be done routinely in children with first urinary tract infections. Urology 71(3):439–443
16. Rathore NH, Barton LL, Luisiri A (1991) Acute lobar nephronia: a review. Pediatrics 87:728–734
17. Cheng CH, Tsau YK, Lin TY (2006) Effective duration of antimicrobial therapy for the treatment of acute lobar nephronia. Pediatrics 117:84–89
18. Cheng CH, Tsau YK, Chang CJ et al (2010) Acute lobar nephronia is associated with a high incidence of renal scarring in childhood urinary tract infections. Pediatr Infect Dis J 29:624–628
19. Hoberman A, Charron M, Hickey RW et al (2003) Imaging studies after a first febrile urinary tract infection in young children. N Engl J Med 348:195–202
20. Arant BS Jr (1991) Vesicoureteric reflux and renal injury. Am J Kidney Dis 17:491–511
21. Garin EH, Olavarria F, Araya C et al (2007) Diagnostic significance of clinical and laboratory findings to localize site of UTI. Pediatr Nephrol 22:1002–1006
22. Juliano TM, Stephany HA, Clayton DB et al (2013) Incidence of abnormal imaging and recurrent pyelonephritis after first febrile urinary tract infection in children 2 to 24 months old. J Urol 190(4 Suppl):1505–1510
23. Rickwood AM, Carty HM, McKendrick T et al (1992) Current imaging of childhood urinary infections: prospective survey. BMJ 304(6828):663–665
24. Zamir G, Sakran W, Horowitz Y et al (2004) Urinary tract infection: is there a need for routine renal ultrasonography? Arch Dis Child 89(5):466–468
25. Mahant S, Friedman J, MacArthur C (2002) Renal ultrasound findings and vesicoureteral reflux in children hospitalised with urinary tract infection. Arch Dis Child 86(6):419–420
26. Lee JH, Kim MK, Park SE (2012) Is a routine voiding cystourethrogram necessary in children after the first febrile urinary tract infection? Acta Paediatr 101(3):e105–e109
27. Preda I, Jodal U, Sixt R et al (2007) Normal dimercaptosuccinic acid scintigraphy makes voiding cystourethrography unnecessary after urinary tract infection. J Pediatr 151(6):581–584
28. Tsai JD, Huang CT, Lin PY et al (2012) Screening high-grade vesicoureteral reflux in young infants with a febrile urinary tract infection. Pediatr Nephrol 27(6):955–963
29. Preda I, Jodal U, Sixt R et al (2010) Value of ultrasound in evaluation of infants with first urinary tract infection. J Urol 183:1984–1988
30. Logvinenko T, Chow JS, Nelson CP (2015) Predictive value of specific ultrasound findings when used as a screening test for abnormalities on VCUG. J Pediatr Urol 11(4):176.e1–176.e7
31. Sargent MA (2000) What is the normal prevalence of vesicoureteral reflux? Pediatr Radiol 30(9):587–593
32. Skoog SJ, Peters CA, Arant BS Jr et al (2010) Pediatric vesicoureteral reflux guidelines panel summary report: clinical practice guidelines for screening siblings of children with vesicoureteral reflux and neonates/infants with prenatal hydronephrosis. J Urol 184(3):1145–1151
33. Lin KY, Chiu NT, Chen MJ et al (2003) Acute pyelonephritis and sequelae of renal scar in pediatric first febrile urinary tract infection. Pediatr Nephrol 18(4):362–365
34. Jakobsson B, Nolsted L, Svennson L et al (1992) 99m Technetium-dimercaptosuccinic acid scan in the diagnosis of acute pyelonephritis in children: relation to clinical and radiological findings. Pediatr Nephrol 6(2):328–334

35. Rushton HG (1997) The evaluation of acute pyelo-nephritis and renal scarring with technetium 99m-dimercaptosuccinic acid renal scintigraphy: evolving concepts and future directions. Pediatr Nephrol 11:108–120

36. MacKenzie JR (1996) A review of renal scarring in children. Nucl Med Commun 17:176–190

37. Elison BS, Taylor D, Van der Wall H et al (1992) Comparison of DMSA scintigraphy with intravenous urography for the detection of renal scarring and its correlation with vesicoureteric reflux. Br J Urol 69(3):294–302

38. Björgvinsson E, Majd M, Eggli KD (1991) Diagnosis of acute pyelonephritis in children: comparison of sonography and 99mTc-DMSA scintigraphy. AJR Am J Roentgenol 157(3):539–543

39. Lonergan GJ, Pennington DJ, Morrison JC et al (1998) Childhood pyelonephritis: comparison of gadolinium-enhanced MR imaging and renal cortical scintigraphy for diagnosis. Radiology 207(2):377–384

40. Cerwinka WH, Grattan-Smith JD, Jones RA et al (2014) Comparison of magnetic resonance urography to dimercaptosuccinic acid scan for the identification of renal parenchyma defects in children with vesico-ureteral reflux. J Pediatr Urol 10(2):344–351

41. Kovanlikaya A, Okkay N, Cakmakci H et al (2004) Comparison of MRI and renal cortical scintigraphy findingsin childhood acute pyelonephrit: preliminary experience. Eur J Radiol 49(1):76–80

42. Kavanagh EC, Ryan S, Awan A et al (2005) Can MRI replace DMSA in the detection of renal parenchy-mal defects in children with urinary tract infections? Pediatr Radiol 35(3):275–281

43. Jacobson SH, Eklof O, Goran Eriksson C et al (1989) Development of hypertension and uraemia after pyelonephritis in childhood: 27 year follow-up. BMJ 299(6701):703–706

44. Berg UB (1992) Long term follow-up of renal mor-phology and function in children with recurrent pyelonephritis. J Urol 148:1715–1720

45. Stokland E, Hellstrom M, Jakobsson B et al (1999) Imaging of renal scarring. Acta Paediatr Suppl 88:13–21

46. Smith T, Evans K, Lythgoe MF et al (1996) Radiation dosimetry of technetium-99m-DMSA in children. J Nucl Med 37(8):1336–1342

47. Vivier PH, Sallem A, Beurdeley M et al (2014) MRI and suspected acute pyelonephritis in children: com-parison of diffusion-weighted imaging with gado-linium-enhanced T1-weighted imaging. Eur Radiol 24(1):19–25

48. Lawson GR, White FE, Alexander FW (1985) Acute focal bacterial nephritis. Arch Dis Child 60:475–477

49. Cheng CH, Tsai MH, Su LH et al (2008) Renal abscess in children: a 10-year clinical and radiologic experience in a tertiary medical center. Pediatr Infect Dis J 27:1025–1027

50. Cheng CH, Tsau YK, Lin TY (2010) Is acute lobar nephronia the midpoint in the spectrum of upper uri-nary tract infections between acute pyelonephritis and renal abscess? J Pediatr 156:82–86

51. Concodora CW, Reddy PP, VanderBrink BA (2017) The role of video urodynamics in the management of the valve bladder. Curr Urol Rep 18(3):24

52. Podesta ML, Castera R, Ruarte AC (2004) Videourodynamic findings in young infants with severe primary reflux. J Urol 171(2 Pt 1):829–823

53. Lee NG, Gana R, Borer JG et al (2012) Urodynamic findings in patients with Currarino syndrome. J Urol 187(6):2195–22C0

54. Darge K (2008) Voiding urosonography with ultra-sound contrast agents for the diagnosis of vesicoure-teric reflux in children. II comparison with radiological examinations. Pediatr Radiol 38(1):54–63

55. Berrocal T, Gayá F, Arjonilla A et al (2001) Vesicoureteral reflux: diagnosis and grading with echo-enhanced cystourethrography versus voiding cystourethrography. Radiology 221:359–365

56. Duran C, Valera A, Alguersuari A et al (2009) Voiding urosonography: the study of the urethra is no longer a limitation of the technique. Pediatr Radiol 39(2):124–131

57. Dacher JN, Avni F, François A et al (1999) Renal sinus hyperechogenicity in acute pyelonephritis: description and pathological correlation. Pediatr Radiol 29(3):179–182

58. Dacher JN, Pfister C, Monroc M et al (1996) Power Doppler sonographic pattern of acute pyelonephri-tis in children: comparison with CT. AJR Am J Roentgenol 166(5):1451–1455

59. Demertzis J, Menias CO (2007) State of the art: imaging of renal infections. Emerg Radiol 14(1): 13–22

60. Boam WD, Miser WF (1995) Acute focal bacterial pyelonephritis. Am Fam Physician 52:919–924

61. Cheng CH, Tsau YK, Hsu SY et al (2004) Effective ultrasonographic predictor for the diagnosis of acute lobar nephronia. Pediatr Infect Dis J 23:11–14

62. Rauschkolb EN, Sandler CM, Patel S et al (1982) Computed tomography of renal inflammatory disease. J Comput Assist Tomogr 6:502–506

63. Joseph RC, Amendola MA, Artze ME et al (1996) Genitourinary tract gas: imaging evaluation. Radiographics 16(2):295–308

64. Yu M, Robinson K, Siegel C et al (2017) Complicated genitourinary tract infections and mimics. Curr Probl Diagn Radiol 46(1):74–83

65. Soulen MC, Fishman EK, Goldman SM et al (1989) Bacterial renal infection: role of CT. Radiology 171(3):703–707

66. Sharma S, Mohta A, Sharma P (2004) Neonatal pyo-nephrosisDOUBLEHYPHENa case report. Int Urol Nephrol 36(3):313–315

67. Patel R, Nwokoma N, Ninan GK (2013) Primary neonatal MRSA pyonephrosis. Int Urol Nephrol 45:939–942

68. Kuzmić AC, Brkljacić B, Ivanković D (2001) Sonographic measurement of detrusor muscle

thickness in healthy children. Pediatr Nephrol 16(12):1122–1125

69. Cvitković-Kuzmić A, Brkljacić B, Ivanković D et al (2002) Ultrasound assessment of detrusor muscle thickness in children with non-neuropathic bladder/sphincter dysfunction. Eur Urol 41(2):214–218

70. Abilov A, Ozcan R, Polat E et al (2013) Rare cause of dysuria: eosinophilic cystitis. J Pediatr Urol 9(1):e6–e8

71. Sauvage P, Bientz J, Boilletot A et al (1982) Cyclophosphamide haemorragic cystitis in a child. Radiological and endoscopic aspects. Chir Pediatr 23(2):125–127

72. Netto JM, Pérez LM, Kelly DR et al (1999) Pediatric inflammatory bladder tumors: myofibroblastic and eosinophilic subtypes. J Urol 162(4):1424–1429

73. Iumanne S, Shoo A, Akoko L et al (2016) Case report: Xanthogranulomutous pyelonephritis presenting as "Wilms' tumor". BMC Urol 16(1):36

74. Rao AG, Eberts PT (2011) Xanthogranulomatous pyelonephritis: an uncommon pediatric renal mass. Pediatr Radiol 41(5):671–672

75. Li L, Parwani AV (2011) Xanthogranulomatous pyelonephritis. Arch Pathol Lab Med 135(5):671–674

76. Cousins C, Somers J, Broderick N et al (1994) Xanthogranulomatous pyelonephritis in childhood: ultrasound and CT diagnosis. Pediatr Radiol 24(3):210–212

77. Verswijvel G, Oyen R, Van Poppel H et al (2000) Xanthogranulomatous pyelonephritis: MRI findings in the diffuse and the focal type. Eur Radiol 10(4):586–589

78. Mesini A, Bandettini R, Caviglia I et al (2017) Candida infections in paediatrics: results from a prospective single-centre study in a tertiary care children's hospital. Mycoses 60(2):118–123

79. Hageman J, Shulman S, Schreiber M et al (1980) Congenital tuberculosis: critical reappraisal of clinical findings and diagnostic procedures. Paediatrics 66:980–984

80. Starke JR, Smith KC (2003) Textbook of pediatric infectious diseases. In: Feigin R, Cherry J (eds) Tuberculosis. Lipincott Williams and Wilkins, Philadelphia, pp 1337–1379

81. Cremin BJ (1987) Radiological imaging of urogenital tuberculosis in children with emphasis on ultrasound. Pediatr Radiol 17(1):34–38

82. Santra A, Mandi F, Bandyopadhyay A (2016) Renal tuberculosis presenting as a mass lesion in a two-year-old girl: report of a rare case. Sultan Qaboos Univ Med J 16(1):e105–e108

83. Merchant S, Bharati A, Merchant N (2013) Tuberculosis of the genitourinary system: urinary tract tuberculosis - renal tuberculosis: part I. Indian J Radiol Imaging 23:46–63

84. Hoberman A, Wald ER, Hickey RW et al (1999) Oral versus initial intravenous therapy for urinary tract infection in young febrile children. Pediatrics 104:79–86

85. Hodson EM, Willis NS, Craig JC (2007) Antibiotics for acute pyelonephritis in children. Cochrane Database Syst Rev 4:CD003772

86. Angel C, Shu T, Green J et al (2003) Renal and peri-renal abscess in children: proposed physiopathologic mechanisms and treatment algorithm. Pediatr Surg Int 19:35–39

87. Schneider K, Helmig FJ, Eife R et al (1989) Pyonephrosis in childhood-is ultrasound sufficient for diagnosis? Pediatr Radiol 19(5):302–307

88. American Academy of Pediatrics (1999) Practice parameter: the diagnosis, treatment, and evaluation of the initial urinary tract infection in febrile infants and young children. Pediatrics 103:843–852

89. Gordon I, Barkovics M, Pindoria S et al (2003) Primary vesicoureteric reflux as a predictor of renal damage in children hospitalized with urinary tract infection: a systematic review and meta-analysis. J Am Soc Nephrol 14:739–744

90. Pennesi M, Travan L, Peratoner L et al (2008) Is antibiotic prophylaxis in children with vesicoureteral reflux effective in preventing pyelonephritis and renal scars? A randomized, controlled trial. Pediatrics 121(6):e1489–e1494

91. Garin EH, Olavarria F, Garcia Nieto V et al (2006) Clinical significance of primary vesicoureteral reflux and urinary antibiotic prophylaxis after acute pyelonephritis: a multicenter, randomized, controlled study. Pediatrics 117(3):626–632

92. Montini G, Rigon L, Zucchetta P et al (2008) Prophylaxis after first febrile urinary tract infection in children? A multicenter, randomized, controlled, noninferiority trial. Pediatrics 122(5):1064–1071

93. Roussey-Kesler G, Gadjos V, Idres N et al (2008) Antibiotic prophylaxis for the prevention of recurrent urinary tract infection in children with low grade vesicoureteral reflux: results from a prospective randomized study. J Urol 179(2):674–679

94. Craig J, Simpson J, Williams G (2009) Antibiotic prophylaxis and recurrent urinary tract infection in children. N Engl J Med 361(18):1748–1759

95. RIVUR Trial Investigators, Hoberman A, Greenfield SP, Mattoo TK et al (2014) Antimicrobial prophylaxis for children with vesicoureteral reflux. N Engl J Med 370(25):2367–2376

Printed by Printforce, the Netherlands